Attention Deficit Hyperactivity Disorder

Medical Psychiatry

1. Handbook of Depression and Anxiety: A Biological Approach, *edited by Johan A. den Boer and J. M. Ad Sitsen*
2. Anticonvulsants in Mood Disorders, *edited by Russell T. Joffe and Joseph R. Calabrese*
3. Serotonin in Antipsychotic Treatment: Mechanisms and Clinical Practice, *edited by John M. Kane, H.-J. Möller, and Frans Awouters*
4. Handbook of Functional Gastrointestinal Disorders, *edited by Kevin W. Olden*
5. Clinical Management of Anxiety, *edited by Johan A. den Boer*
6. Obsessive-Compulsive Disorders: Diagnosis • Etiology • Treatment, *edited by Eric Hollander and Dan J. Stein*
7. Bipolar Disorder: Biological Models and Their Clinical Application, *edited by L. Trevor Young and Russell T. Joffe*
8. Dual Diagnosis and Treatment: Substance Abuse and Comorbid Medical and Psychiatric Disorders, *edited by Henry R. Kranzler and Bruce J. Rounsaville*
9. Geriatric Psychopharmacology, *edited by J. Craig Nelson*
10. Panic Disorder and Its Treatment, *edited by Jerrold F. Rosenbaum and Mark H. Pollack*
11. Comorbidity in Affective Disorders, *edited by Mauricio Tohen*
12. Practical Management of the Side Effects of Psychotropic Drugs, *edited by Richard Baton*
13. Psychiatric Treatment of the Medically Ill, *edited by Robert G. Robinson and William R. Yates*
14. Medical Management of the Violent Patient: Clinical Assessment and Therapy, *edited by Kenneth Tardiff*

15. Bipolar Disorders: Basic Mechanisms and Therapeutic Implications, *edited by Jair C. Scares and Samuel Gershon*
16. Schizophrenia: A New Guide for Clinicians, *edited by John G. Csernansky*
17. Polypharmacy in Psychiatry, *edited by S. Nassir Ghaemi*
18. Pharmacotherapy for Child and Adolescent Psychiatric Disorders: Second Edition, Revised and Expanded, David R. Rosenberg, Pablo A. Davanzo, and Samuel Gershon
19. Brain Imaging In Affective Disorders, *edited by Jair C. Scares*
20. Handbook of Medical Psychiatry, *edited by Jair C. Scares and Samuel Gershon*
21. Handbook of Depression and Anxiety: A Biological Approach, Second Edition, *edited by Siegfried Kasper, Johan A. den Boer, and J. M. Ad Sitsen*
22. Aggression: Psychiatric Assessment and Treatment, *edited by Emitl Coccaro*
23. Depression in Later Life: A Multidisciplinary Psychiatric Approach,*edited by James Ellison and Sumer Verma*
24. Autism Spectrum Disorders, *edited by Eric Hollander*
25. Handbook of Chronic Depression: Diagnosis and Therapeutic Management, *edited by Jonathan E. Alpert and Maurizio Fava*
26. Clinical Handbook of Eating Disorders: An Integrated Approach, *edited by Timothy D. Brewerton*
27. Dual Diagnosis and Psychiatric Treatment: Substance Abuse and Comorbid Disorders: Second Edition, *edited by Henry R. Kranzler and Joyce A. Tinsley*
28. Atypical Antipsychotics: From Bench to Bedside, *edited by John G. Csernansky and John Lauriello*
29. Social Anxiety Disorder, *edited by Borwin Bandelow and Dan J. Stein*
30. Handbook of Sexual Dysfunction, *edited by Richard Balon and R. Taylor Segraves*
31. Borderline Personality Disorder, *edited by Mary C. Zanarini*
32. Handbook of Bipolar Disorder: Diagnosis and Therapeutic Approaches, *edited by Siegfried Kasper and Robert M. A. Hirschfeld*
33. Obesity and Mental Disorders, *edited by Susan L. McElroy, David B. Allison, and George A. Bray*
34. Depression: Treatment Strategies and Management, *edited by Thomas L. Schwartz and Timothy J. Petersen*
35. Bipolar Disorders: Basic Mechanisms and Therapeutic Implications, Second Edition, *edited by Jair C. Soares and Allan H. Young*
36. Neurogenetics of Psychiatric Disorders, *edited by Akira Sawa and Melvin G. McInnis*
37. Attention Deficit Hyperactivity Disorder: Concepts, Controversies, New Directions, *edited by Keith McBurnett and Linda Pfiffner*

Attention Deficit Hyperactivity Disorder

Concepts, Controversies, New Directions

Edited by
Keith McBurnett
University of California, San Francisco, USA
Linda Pfiffner
University of California, San Francisco, USA

CRC Press
Taylor & Francis Group
Boca Raton London New York

CRC Press is an imprint of the
Taylor & Francis Group, an **informa** business

CRC Press
Taylor & Francis Group
6000 Broken Sound Parkway NW, Suite 300
Boca Raton, FL 33487-2742

Printed on acid-free paper
Version Date: 20130125

International Standard Book Number-13: 978-0-8247-2927-1 (Hardback)

Visit the Taylor & Francis Web site at
http://www.taylorandfrancis.com

and the CRC Press Web site at
http://www.crcpress.com

Preface

This book bridges the gap between the several existing introductory works on attention deficit hyperactivity disorder and those more advanced texts that focus on a narrow issue or subpopulation. It targets readers in training (medical and nursing students, residents, graduate students, etc.) rather than a lay audience, and thus it is a natural companion to the attention deficit hyperactivity disorder section in the *Diagnostic and Statistical Manual of Mental Disorders* -IV-TR. Although it can be used as an introductory text, it also covers specialized topics that will be of interest to seasoned clinicians and to anyone affected by attention deficit hyperactivity disorder who wishes to broaden their understanding of the disorder.

We asked experts around the world to contribute chapters, with the guideline that they be brief and concise. We granted significant "wiggle room" when contributors needed more length. Some topics received extra emphasis, in order to present readers with more of what they might need to know rather than what they already know about attention deficit hyperactivity disorder. For example, because most of what is known about the disorder comes from research with school-age boys, we thought it essential to include chapters spanning ages and genders. We also overweighted psychosocial approaches to treatment, because the sub-modalities of evidence-based psychosocial treatment are rarely presented. Coverage of medication was limited to the essentials, because pharmacotherapy of attention deficit hyperactivity disorder is already widely disseminated online and in book form and because continuing medical education and pharmaceutical-medical liaisons are sources of continual updates for the prescribing community.

This book also asks readers to challenge their assumptions about attention deficit hyperactivity disorder. The chapter by Pelham is an iconoclastic manifesto on the primary importance of psychosocial treatment. It stems from the fact that the first reported result of the Multimodal Treatment of ADHD Study—that well-managed pharmacotherapy is more effective than psychosocial treatment, and that little is gained from adding psychosocial treatment to pharmacotherapy alone—is often over-interpreted. By considering a broader context, Pelham's chapter stimulates the reader into becoming more sophisticated about medication versus psychosocial issues. Diller's chapter reminds the reader that, even with the amount of research currently available on the disorder, much work remains to be done before some fundamental questions can be put to rest. Regardless of the reader's viewpoint, the chapters in the "Controversies" section will leave the reader better able to defend their views.

Our choice of emphases should not be misconstrued. Our personal views are that attention deficit hyperactivity disorder is a valid and under-treated disorder, that multimodal treatment (medication *and* psychosocial) is often the best treatment, that federal funding of research on this and related disorders should be quadrupled, and that major revisions are needed to how treatment is provided and reimbursed. Everyone is affected by attention deficit hyperactivity disorder, whether they have it or not. Given the worldwide estimated prevalence of 5.29%, chances are that one out of every 20 people one encounters (including drivers of other cars) has the disorder. Untreated and under-treated, it closes off many paths to better education, better jobs, better health, and better social relationships. It is a costly disorder for everyone. We know a great deal about identifying and helping individuals with attention deficit hyperactivity disorder, but we mustn't allow ourselves to smugly think we know enough. If our book stimulates readers to consider new views on it and to develop their own insights, it will have done its job.

We owe a debt of gratitude for the scholarly efforts of the contributors to this book. Special thanks are due to Russell Schachar, Joel Nigg, and Glen Elliott, who helped in the conceptualization and early planning.

Keith McBurnett
Linda Pfiffner

Contents

SECTION V: SPECIAL POPULATIONS

SECTION VI: CONTROVERSIES

SECTION VII: CONSENSUS

SECTION VIII: NEW DIRECTIONS

Contributors

Howard Abikoff Department of Child and Adolescent Psychiatry, New York University School of Medicine, New York, New York, U.S.A.

Ann Abramowitz Department of Psychology, Emory University, Atlanta, Georgia, U.S.A.

Eleanor Ainslie Institute for Pediatric Neuroscience, NYU Child Study Center, New York University School of Medicine, New York, New York, U.S.A.

T. Banaschewski Department of Child and Adolescent Psychiatry, Central Institute of Mental Health, Mannheim, Germany

Joseph Biederman Clinical Research Program in Pediatric Psychopharmacology, Massachusetts General Hospital, Harvard Medical School, Boston, Massachusetts, U.S.A.

Thomas A. Blondis University of Chicago School of Medicine, Chicago, Illinois, U.S.A.

Juliana Sanchez Bloom The Children's Hospital of Philadelphia, Philadelphia, Pennsylvania, U.S.A.

Laurie Miller Brotman NYU Child Study Center, New York University School of Medicine, New York, New York, U.S.A.

Kerry A. Brown La Rabida Children's Hospital, Chicago, Illinois, U.S.A.

Ruth C. Brown Alvin V. Baird Attention and Learning Disabilities Center, James Madison University, Harrisonburg, Virginia, U.S.A.

F. Xavier Castellanos Institute for Pediatric Neuroscience, NYU Child Study Center, New York University School of Medicine, New York, New York, U.S.A.

Jennifer Crosbie Department of Psychiatry, Hospital for Sick Children, University of Toronto, Toronto, Ontario, Canada

Laurent Demanez Department of Otorhinolaryngology, University of Liege, Liege, Belgium

Douglas Derryberry Department of Psychology, Oregon State University, Corvallis, Oregon, U.S.A.

Lawrence Diller Private Practice, Walnut Creek, and University of California San Francisco, San Francisco, California, U.S.A.

Carey B. Dowling Alvin V. Baird Attention and Learning Disabilities Center, James Madison University, Harrisonburg, Virginia, U.S.A.

George J. DuPaul College of Education, Lehigh University, Bethlehem, Pennsylvania, U.S.A.

Leah Ellenberg University of Southern California School of Medicine, Los Angeles, California, U.S.A.

Glen R. Elliott The Children's Health Council, Palo Alto, and University of California San Francisco, San Francisco, California, U.S.A.

Steven W. Evans Alvin V. Baird Attention and Learning Disabilities Center, James Madison University, Harrisonburg, Virginia, U.S.A.

Greg A. Fabiano Center for Children and Families, State University of New York at Buffalo, Buffalo, New York, U.S.A.

Richard Gallagher Department of Child and Adolescent Psychiatry, NYU School of Medicine, New York, New York, U.S.A.

Elizabeth M. Gnagy Center for Children and Families, State University of New York at Buffalo, Buffalo, New York, U.S.A.

Kathleen Kiely Gouley NYU Child Study Center, New York University School of Medicine, New York, New York, U.S.A.

Andrew R. Greiner Center for Children and Families, State University of New York at Buffalo, Buffalo, New York, U.S.A.

H. Heinrich Department of Child and Adolescent Psychiatry, University of Göttingen, Göttingen and Department of Child and Adolescent Psychiatry, University of Erlangen, Erlangen, Germany

Lisa Hilley Department of Psychiatry, University of California San Francisco, San Francisco, California, U.S.A.

Stephen P. Hinshaw Department of Psychology, University of California Berkeley, Berkeley, California, U.S.A.

Betsy Hoza Department of Psychology, University of Vermont, Burlington, Vermont, U.S.A.

Cynthia L. Huang-Pollock Department of Psychology, Pennsylvania State University, University Park, Pennsylvania, U.S.A.

George W. Hynd Purdue University, West Lafayette, Indiana, U.S.A.

Charlotte Johnston Department of Psychology, University of British Columbia, Vancouver, British Columbia, Canada

Nichole Jurbergs Department of Psychology, Louisiana State University, Baton Rouge, Louisiana, U.S.A.

Nina M. Kaiser Department of Psychiatry, University of California San Francisco, San Francisco, California, U.S.A.

Mary Lou Kelley Department of Psychology, Louisiana State University, Baton Rouge, Louisiana, U.S.A.

Joel Kramer Departments of Neurology and Psychiatry, University of California San Francisco Medical Center, San Francisco, California, U.S.A.

Angela Liang Child Development Center, University of California Irvine, Irvine, California, U.S.A.

Keith McBurnett Department of Psychiatry, University of California San Francisco, San Francisco, California, U.S.A.

Bruce D. McCandliss Sackler Institute for Development Psychology, Weill Medical College of Cornell University, New York, New York, U.S.A.

James J. McGough Division of Child and Adolescent Psychiatry, UCLA Semel Institute for Neuroscience and Human Behavior and UCLA Child and Adolescent Psychopharmacology Program and ADHD Clinic, Los Angeles, California, U.S.A.

Amori Yee Mikami Department of Psychology, University of Virginia, Charlottesville, Virginia, U.S.A.

G.H. Moll Department of Child and Adolescent Psychiatry, University of Göttingen, Göttingen and Department of Child and Adolescent Psychiatry, University of Erlangen, Erlangen, Germany

William E. Pelham Jr. Center for Children and Families, State University of New York at Buffalo, Buffalo, New York, U.S.A.

Linda J. Pfiffner Department of Psychiatry, University of California San Francisco, San Francisco, California, U.S.A.

Steven R. Pliszka Division of Child and Adolescent Psychiatry, University of Texas Health Science Center at San Antonio, San Antonio, Texas, U.S.A.

Michael I. Posner Department of Psychology, University of Oregon, Eugene, Oregon, U.S.A.

Jefferson Prince Clinical Research Program in Pediatric Psychopharmacology, Massachusetts General Hospital, Harvard Medical School, Boston, Massachusetts, U.S.A.

Marjorie A. Reed Department of Psychology, Oregon State University, Corvallis, Oregon, U.S.A.

Abram Rosenblatt Department of Psychiatry, University of California San Francisco, San Francisco, California, U.S.A.

A. Rothenberger Department of Child and Adolescent Psychiatry, University of Göttingen, Göttingen, Germany

Russell Schachar Department of Psychiatry, Hospital for Sick Children, University of Toronto, Toronto, Ontario, Canada

Douglas Scoular Department of Psychology, University of British Columbia, Vancouver, British Columbia, Canada

J. Sergeant Department of Clinical Neuropsychology, Vrije Universiteit Amsterdam, Amsterdam, The Netherlands

Edmund J. S. Sonuga-Barke Institute for Disorders of Impulse and Attention, University of Southampton, Southampton, U.K.

Mark A. Stein Department of Psychiatry and HALP Clinic and ADHD Research Center, University of Illinois at Chicago, Chicago, Illinois, U.S.A.

James M. Swanson Child Development Center, University of California Irvine, Irvine, California, U.S.A.

Leanne Tamm Center for Advanced ADHD Research, Treatment, and Education, University of Texas Southwestern Medical Center, Dallas, Texas, U.S.A.

Daniel A. Waschbusch Center for Children and Families, State University of New York at Buffalo, Buffalo, New York, U.S.A.

Karen C. Wells Department of Psychiatry, Duke University Medical Center, Durham, North Carolina, U.S.A.

Tim L. Wigal Child Development Center, University of California Irvine, Irvine, California, U.S.A.

Timothy E. Wilens Clinical Research Program in Pediatric Psychopharmacology, Massachusetts General Hospital, Harvard Medical School, Boston, Massachusetts, U.S.A.

Perry A. Zirkel College of Education, Lehigh University, Bethlehem, Pennsylvania, U.S.A.

Section I: Assessment

1

The Diagnosis and How We Got There

Keith McBurnett
Department of Psychiatry, University of California San Francisco, San Francisco, California, U.S.A.

The standard for diagnosing attention deficit hyperactivity disorder (ADHD) is to apply diagnostic criteria from DSM-IV (1). These criteria were derived using the most empirically sound methods ever used to formulate criteria for a psychiatric disorder. They have been adopted almost universally, and yet somehow they manage to foster both consensus and controversy about what ADHD is and how it should be identified. This chapter outlines the historical and scientific underpinnings of DSM-IV ADHD, and implications for ADHD in DSM-V.

The history of psychiatric diagnosis can be divided into two eras: before DSM-III and after DSM-III. There are several good accounts of the early history of psychiatric diagnosis, so only a brief synopsis need be covered here. One interesting historical fact is that the reason that we have a *Diagnostic and Statistical Manual of Mental Disorders* instead of simply a *Diagnostic Manual of Mental Disorders* is because the DSM was developed from national statistical records. The U.S. Constitution mandates the collection of census data for purposes of representation and taxation. Over time, questions were added to the census to gather additional informational. The first tallies of mental disorders (intended to learn about the institutionalized population) were obtained in the 1840 census, although categories at that time were only idiocy/insanity. In 1918, the Census Bureau published *The Statistical Manual for the Use of Hospitals for Mental Diseases* (2), which was updated in 10 editions through 1942. There were several other important influences leading to the first DSM, but the Census Bureau's *Statistical Manual* can fairly be described as the key precursor (hence the retention of the term *Statistical Manual* despite the smaller role now played by statistics).

Other milestones were the *Standard Nomenclature of Diseases* (3) and the addition of mental disorders to the international classification of diseases, ICD-6 (4). The mental disorders section in ICD-6 was influenced by the attention given to mental disorders by the military, which came to the realization during World War II that recruitment, fitness for duty, and rehabilitation of psychological injury would be enhanced if mental disorders could be better tracked. This was one reason why, when the American Psychiatric Association adopted the first DSM (5), it did not address disorders of children, even though preliminary nomenclature for child disorders had appeared as early as 1886 (6) and was included in the *Standard Nomenclature*.

DSM-II (7) listed a new broad category, "Behavior Disorders of Childhood and Adolescence" and a subordinate subcategory of "Hyper-kinetic Reaction of Childhood." The diagnostic methodology of the era was to obtain insightful descriptions so that a trained clinician could recognize a disorder when presented in the clinic. This is an intuitively appealing process, deeply rooted in Platonic and rational traditions. It is, essentially, a match to prototype method. There is nothing inherently wrong about this method—we use it everyday to identify all manner of things. Problems arise when it is applied to conceptual entities like disease states, especially abnormal behavioral syndromes. Differences in training, experience, cultural background, and theoretical orientation cause clinicians to gather information selectively and to weigh data differently. These difficulties might be surmounted by standardizing diagnostic training, but the more mercurial problem is that nature does not present mental disorders in discrete categories. Individual cases display different patterns of prototypical features, and it is the exceptional case that closely approximates one prototype and has few features of others. We can easily recognize those cases that clearly fit or do not fit a category. Those cases that only moderately fit are the ones that cause disagreement.

How good are we at matching to a prototypical description? Most of us would trust our own skill, but we might be more skeptical of the skills of others. Such skepticism appears warranted for the descriptive approach. When pairs of clinicians were asked to diagnose the same case independently using DSM-II, they often failed to agree on the results. Such unreliability threatens the validity of the diagnosis. After all, if diagnosticians disagree, at least one of them has given the wrong diagnosis and there is not an easy way to know which. An unreliable diagnosis cannot possibly be valid, or to use more precise psychometric terms, reliability places a ceiling on validity.

One cost of diagnostic unreliability is its hindrance of research. Feighner and colleagues at Washington University addressed this problem by developing specific criteria for several mental disorders (8). As these research diagnostic criteria (RDC) were further developed (9), they were shown to increase the reliability of psychiatric diagnosis. This benefit partly derived from the efforts to make the criteria clear and specific, and to generally focus on behavior rather than inferred states or traits. Improved reliability also derived from the use of multiple criteria. Thus, RDC nudged the diagnostic process from its total reliance on clinical judgment toward incorporating aspects of measurement theory.

The RDC approach was adopted for DSM-III (10), resulting in generally good diagnostic reliability. Hyperkinetic reaction was dropped in favor of attention deficit disorder (ADD), largely in response to reports of inattentive behavior and impaired performance on laboratory measures of attention in children with the disorder (11,12). DSM-III distinguished between ADD with hyperactivity and ADD without hyperactivity. Both types were considered to have significant attention problems and impulsiveness and were distinguished only by the severity of hyperactivity. An important result of this distinction was the emergence of a small research literature on ADD without hyperactivity. However, when the DSM was revised only 7 years later, the DSM-III-R (13) committee was not convinced that the then available research on ADD without hyperactivity was sufficient to validate the subtype. ADD without hyperactivity was not killed off, but it was relegated to a fate close to death: it was stripped of its diagnostic criteria and relegated to a catchall category of undifferentiated attention deficit hyperactivity disorder (UADHD). This had a chilling effect on research into an inattentive type. Not only did UADHD have no DSM-III-like RDC, it had no DSM-II-like clinical description. The real diagnosis (ADHD) could be met by having any 8 from a list of 13 symptoms of hyperactivity, impulsivity, and inattention.

The application of measurement theory to psychiatric diagnosis made a quantum leap in the development of behavior disorder diagnoses in DSM-IV (14). The DSM-IV committee explicitly sought to substitute the reliance on expert clinical opinion wherever possible in favor of generating questions to be addressed with empirical data. Proposals for changes to the DSM were widely solicited. Proposed changes were evaluated with literature reviews, secondary analyses of existing data, and newly designed field trials of proposed diagnostic criteria. For ADHD, three reviews were commissioned (15–17), and a nationwide field trial of all of the symptoms from the attention and disruptive behavior disorders was funded.

The DSM-IV committee gave the job of executing the field trial for attention and disruptive behavior disorders to Ben Lahey. Lahey, working closely with the rest of the committee, was methodical in using psychological measurement to address proposed changes. A large set of proposed symptoms of ADHD and disruptive behaviors was collected from 440 subjects in 11 different sites, including items proposed as sluggish cognitive tempo (SCT) identified from DSM-III era research. Impairment was captured as overall impairment and as domain-specific (e.g., academic, sociobehavioral) impairment. The latent structure (how well symptoms tend to aggregate and appear related to a single dimension) of ADHD symptoms was investigated using factor analysis. At one level, factor analysis identifies latent (meaning not observable, but detectable with statistics) groups of items. At the level of the item, it measures how closely each item is associated with each of the latent dimensions. The results confirmed prior hypotheses that ADHD symptoms appear grouped into only two dimensions: inattention and hyperactivity-plus-impulsivity. After these two sets of symptoms were demarcated, each item was tested for its symptom utility (18). Symptom utility means how well a symptom predicts the presence of the rest of its symptom group, combined with how well its absence (finding that it is not present) predicts the absence of the rest of its symptom group. The symptom utility analyses found that most symptoms functioned well, with the notable exception of the SCT symptoms. There was no problem with the positive predictive power of SCT symptoms: their presence was strongly associated with the presence of the group of inattentive symptoms. However, when SCT symptoms were not present, other inattentive symptoms were sometimes present and sometimes not. Thus, the SCT symptoms failed to meet the negative predictive power requirement. They were dropped from further investigation.

Lahey now had his final symptom lists. The final task was to use statistical measurement to empirically find the best cutpoints. A cutpoint, or diagnostic threshold, is the number of symptoms from a symptom group that are required to be present in order to determine that an individual has or exhibits that symptom group. (In other words, should we require four inattention symptoms, or five, or six or seven, in order to conclude that an individual case has inattention?) The committee took the innovative approach of selecting cutpoints based on how well different cutpoints predicted impairment, and by looking at how reliable were the categorical decisions made by using different cutpoints in test-retest and cross-diagnostician analyses. The final cutpoints could then be used in a two-by-two contingency table for subtyping ADHD: exceeding the inattention cutpoint but not that for hyperactivity-impulsivity would place a case in the box for predominantly inattentive type; if vice-versa, the box for predominantly hyperactive-impulsive type; if both, the combined type; and if neither, no ADHD diagnosis. (The reader is encouraged to retrieve the original report of these analyses to see the clear relationships between numbers of symptoms and impairment) (19). In toto, the data indicated that the best cutpoints were at six of the nine inattention symptoms, and five of the nine hyperactivity-impulsivity symptoms. However, for the hyperactivity-impulsivity symptoms, a cutpoint of five symptoms was supported by some of the data, but other data showed little difference between five or six symptoms. Given this ambiguity, the committee found favor in the symmetry of requiring six of nine symptoms for both categories. The committee also favored the use of a more stringent cutpoint in order to protect against overdiagnosis. After the criteria were finalized, a cross-validation study applied the new criteria to existing real-world clinical cases. The study confirmed the association of cutpoints with domain-specific criteria, and concluded that DSM-IV was superior to DSM-III-R in subcategorical homogeneity (the similarity of cases within a type) and in exhaustiveness (ability to classify all apparent cases) (20).

It is often overlooked that DSM-IV ADHD diagnosis is based on the "or rule." This procedure identifies a symptom as present if either the teacher or the parent reports the symptom as being present. So a cutpoint of six symptoms using the or rule is considerably less stringent than using the same cutpoint with a single informant. Using a single informant (generally this would be the primary caretaker), particularly when relying on a symptom checklist, will bias the results toward underdiagnosing ADHD. This bias might be mitigated when using a clinical interview with a parent who is keenly aware of school-based impairment, but this is an inference. Single-informant diagnoses will almost certainly be confirmable cases of DSM-IV ADHD, but they will not represent the population defined by DSM-IV criteria because they will tend to be more severe. There may also be a bias against identifying the inattentive type when relying on parent report only, because teachers appear to be more sensitive to inattention symptoms than are parents. The ice becomes much thinner when we try to apply DSM-IV criteria beyond the age range from which they were derived, due in part to the fact that the classic "or rule" cannot be implemented.

As well-derived as DSM-IV ADHD was, imperfections slowly began to appear. By requiring six symptoms of hyperactivity-impulsivity instead of five, cases that might otherwise be classified as combined type were instead assigned to predominantly inattentive. This meant that the inattentive type was made less homogenous simply by being contaminated with a few extra cases of combined type. One result was that correlates such as anxiety that were previously associated with DSM-III ADD without hyperactivity were not clearly associated with DSM-IV predominantly inattentive type, and the higher prevalence of girls in DSM-III ADD without hyperactivity (vs. with hyperactivity) was lessened in DSM-IV inattentive versus combined type (21). The elimination of SCT symptoms was questioned, and it was found that if SCT items were evaluated only in a subset of cases with predominantly inattentive type (the only type that would be expected to exhibit SCT), their symptom utility was perfectly adequate. Even the grouping of inattentive type in the same general category with other types of ADHD was assailed by airing a laundry list of reasons why the inattentive type might actually be a separate disorder altogether (22).

As we approach DSM-V, we face more questions than before about how to conceptualize and diagnose ADHD. If we continue to apply statistical methods to diagnoses, using methods such as latent class analysis, we must grapple with a proliferation of empirically derived categories that do not clearly map onto clinical observations and that rely on the severity of symptoms as one boundary between categories. If we appeal to genotypes, or to neuropsychological endophenotypes, we must reconcile that those variables do not fall into well-demarcated categories any better than behavioral symptoms do. The prospects that we might reverse engineer or reverse translate from genotypes or endophenotypes to refined behavioral diagnoses (phenotypes), and then discover a wealth of validity in the new diagnoses, are not likely. This is not to say that the holy grail of a laboratory test for ADHD is entirely futile. It may be possible at some stage to incorporate nonbehavioral laboratory tests into the diagnostic criteria. At this juncture, however, we seem destined to rely on behavior to diagnose ADHD when DSM-V arrives.

Some changes to the diagnostic system can be predicted. The requirement that the disorder must be present by the age of seven will almost surely be modified. Not only does this requirement ignore the normal development of attention problems, it also has been shown to lack validity (23,24). There may be proposals to adjust the content of some items to make them more applicable to older adolescents and adults. Another question is whether to adjust symptom cutpoints. It has been argued that, because the base rate of ADHD symptoms is lower in the population of girls compared to boys, the cutpoints should be lower for girls. This can be readily determined using DSM-IV field trial methods by testing the relationship of symptoms to impairment within gender. It has also been suggested that cutpoints be lowered for older age ranges, particularly for hyperactivity-impulsivity, because of the observed declines in symptoms as age increases. Because so many children with combined type drop a few symptoms of hyperactivity-impulsivity as they mature, the predominantly inattentive type in adulthood consists of both lifelong inattentives and what we might call residual combined type.

It also seems clear that SCT will be reconsidered as symptoms of ADD. Because this would mean that an inattentive category would no longer share the same cognitive symptoms as a hyperactive category, the idea of separating these types into entirely different categories may gain traction. Looking back, perhaps the successive approximations of ADHD across DSM editions might inform DSM-V. DSM-III and IV were correct in separating types. But DSM-III-R might have been right in lumping together cases that exhibit some combination of hyperactivity-impulsivity and attention problems, and it might have erred only in not specifying a separate category of predominantly inattention/SCT. One thing is certain; DSM-V will not be the final resolution of the ADHD nosology. There is far more research that is needed than can be done before its publication.

REFERENCES

1. American Psychiatric Association. Diagnostic and Statistical Manual of Mental Disorders. 4th ed., text revision. Washington, D.C.: American Psychiatric Press, 2000.
2. Bureau USC ed. The Statistical Manual for the Use of Hospitals for Mental Diseases. 10th ed. Washington, D.C.: U.S. Government Printing Office, 1918–1942.
3. National Conference on Nomenclature of Disease. In: Logie HB. A Standard Classified Nomenclature of Disease New York: Commonwealth Fund, 1933.
4. WHO. Manual of the International Statistical Classification of Diseases, Injuries, and Causes of Death. 6th ed. Geneva: World Health Organization, 1948.
5. American Psychiatric Association. Diagnostic and Statistical Manual for Mental Disorders. Washington, D.C.: American Psychiatric Press, 1952.
6. New York Medico-Legal Society. International Committee on the International Statistics of the Insane and Classification of Mental Diseases. New York: New York Medico-Legal Society, 1886.
7. American Psychiatric Association. Diagnostic and Statistical Manual of Mental Disorders. 2nd ed. Washington, D.C.: APA, 1968.
8. Feighner J, Robins E, Guze S, Woodruff R, Winokur G, Munoz R. Diagnostic criteria for use in psychiatric research. Arch Gen Psychiatry 1972; 26:57–63.
9. Spitzer RL, Endicott J, Robins E. Research diagnostic criteria: rationale and reliability. Arch Gen Psychiatry 1978; 35:773–82.
10. American Psychiatric Association. Diagnostic and Statistical Manual of Mental Disorders. 3rd ed. Washington, D.C.: APA, 1980.
11. Douglas VI, Peters KG. Toward a clearer definition of the attentional deficit of hyperactive children. In: Hale GA, Lewis M, eds. Attention and Cognitive Development. New York: Plenum Press, 1979:173–247.
12. Dykman RA, Ackerman PT, Oglesby DM. Selective and sustained attention in hyperactive, learning-disabled, and normal boys. J Nerv Ment Dis 1979; 167: 288–97.
13. American Psychiatric Association. Diagnostic and Statistical Manual of Mental Disorders. 3rd edition-Revised. Washington, D.C.: APA, 1987.
14. American Psychiatric Association. Diagnostic and Statistical Manual for Mental Disorders. 4th ed. Washington, D.C.: APA, 1994.
15. Biederman J, Newcorn JH, Sprich S. Comorbidity of attention-deficit/hyperactivity disorder. In: Widiger TA, Frances AJ, Pincus HA, Ross R, First M, Davis W, eds. DSM-IV Sourcebook. Washington, D.C.: American Psychiatric Press, 1997.
16. Lahey BB, Carlson CL, Frick PJ. Attention-deficit disorder without hyperactivity. In: Widiger TA, Frances AJ, Pincus HA, Ross R, First MB, Davis W, eds. DSM-IV Sourcebook, Vol. 3. Washington, D.C.: American Psychiatric Association, 1997.
17. McBurnett K. Attention-deficit/hyperactivity disorder: review of diagnostic issues. In: Widiger TA, Frances AJ, Pincus HA, Ross R, First M, Davis W, eds. DSM-IV Sourcebook, Vol. 3. Washington, D.C.: American Psychiatric Association, 1997:111–44.

18. Frick PJ, Lahey BB, Applegate B, et al. DSM-IV field trials for the disruptive behavior disorders: symptom utility estimates. J Am Acad Child Adolesc Psychiatry 1994; 33:529–39.
19. Lahey BB, Applegate B, McBurnett K, et al. DSM-IV field trials for attention deficit/hyperactivity disorder in children and adolescents. Am J Psychiatry 1994; 151:1673–85.
20. McBurnett K, Pfiffner LJ, Willcutt E, et al. Experimental cross-validation of DSM-IV types of attention-deficit/hyperactivity disorder. J Am Acad Child Adolesc Psychiatry, 1998; 38:17–24.
21. McBurnett K, Pfiffner LJ, Ottolini YL. Types of ADHD in DSM-IV. In: Accardo P, Blondis T, Stein MA, eds. The Attention Deficit Disorders. New York: Marcel Dekker, 2000:229–40.
22. Milich R, Balentine AC, Lynam DR. ADHD combined type and ADHD predominantly inattentive type are distinct and unrelated disorders. Clin Psychol: Sci Pract 2001; 8:463–88.
23. Applegate B, Lahey BB, Hart EL, et al. Validity of the age-of-onset criterion for ADHD: a report from the DSM-IV field trials. J Am Acad Child Adolesc Psychiatry 1997; 36:1211–21.
24. Barkley RA, Biederman J. Toward a broader definition of the age-of-onset criterion for attention-deficit hyperactivity disorder. J Am Acad Child Adolesc Psychiatry 1997; 36:1204–10.

2

Differential Diagnosis of Attention and Auditory Processing Disorders

Laurent Demanez
Department of Otorhinolaryngology, University of Liege, Liege, Belgium

INTRODUCTION

Children with central auditory processing disorders (CAPD) and those with attention deficit hyperactivity disorders (ADHD) may have difficulty in following directions, behave as though they have a hearing loss, frequently ask for repeated directions, and often display difficulty listening selectively in background noise, despite normal hearing (1,2).

CAPD have been observed in various clinical populations such those where morphological or functional disorders of the CNS are suspected: language disorders, dyslexia, learning disabilities, prematurity, attention deficit disorders (3–13). Does these pathologies are independent developmental disorders or simply comorbid?

DEFINITION OF CENTRAL AUDITORY PROCESSING DISORDERS

Central auditory processing disorders (CAPD) can be defined as syndromes in which hearing impairment is not due to a loss of peripheral auditory function. Since 19th century, only a few classical clinical presentations have been described mostly after large bitemporal lesions. In cortical deafness, the patient does not hear any sound stimulus and behaves like a profoundly deaf person (14,15). Auditory agnosie is defined as an incapacity to recognize any sound or noise although they are detected. In verbal deafness (16), the disability is limited to spoken language. Verbal expression as well as lecture and writing are preserved. Amusia is the incapacity to recognize or appreciate music (17). Depending on the extent and the importance of the lesion, there is a continuum between these various forms of central deafness which are sometimes associated to others cognitive or sensory disorders.

In addition to these major disorders, many other minor central auditory deficits can be frequently identified. The most common one is probably the impairment of intelligibility with low redundant messages which, of course, can also be associated with a peripheral deficit. In children delayed learning, with normal intelligence and normal peripheral auditory function, can be due to CAPD (18,19). Obscure auditory dysfunction or King-Kopetzky syndrome (20) occurs in patients presenting hearing disabilities despite a normal peripheral auditory function. Hemianacusia (14) is for the auditory modality the equivalent of hemianopsia for the visual modality. It signals a damage of unilateral, temporal, or callosal lesion. Hemianacusia is suggested by a severe or, more often, complete extinction of the contralateral ear, exclusively observed on verbal dichotic tests. In adults over 60 years old, the involution of the central auditory pathways, in particular the demyelinization of the transcallosal connexions, increase the hearing disabilities created by an inner ear lesion (21).

Because these disabilities can be due to other dysfunctions such as language processing disorders or attention deficits, the American Speech-Language-Hearing Association (ASHA) convened a task force in 1996 to develop a consensus statement. The task force defined the Central Auditory Processes (CAP) as the auditory system mechanisms and functions responsible for the following behavioral phenomena: sound localization and lateralization, auditory discrimination, auditory pattern recognition, temporal aspects of audition including temporal resolution (i.e., detection of changes in frequency, amplitude and duration of auditory stimuli, and detection of time intervals between auditory stimuli), temporal masking (i.e., obscuring of probe by pre- or poststimulatory presentation of masker), temporal integration (i.e., summation of power over durations less than 200–400 msec), and temporal ordering (i.e., detection of sequence of sounds over time), auditory performance with competing acoustic signals, and auditory performance with degraded acoustic signals (22).

Beside the above definition which concerns processes specifically dedicated to audition, attention, memory, long-term language representations, and other nondedicated neurocognitive mechanisms are involved in the processing of acoustic signals.

The current model of CAP, whereby a listener actively controls processing, requires reciprocity between bottom-up and top-down processes. This model and the association of both CAPD and metacognitive deficit, necessitate comprehensive intervention programming targeting development of both basic auditory and metalinguistic skills and metacognitive strategies.

CAPD is an observed deficiency in one or more of the above-listed behaviors. For some individuals, CAPD is presumed to result from the dysfunction of processes and mechanisms specifically dedicated to the auditory system. For others, CAPD may originate from a more general dysfunction, such as an attention deficit or neural timing deficit, which affects performance across modalities (i.e., visual, sensitive...). It is also possible for CAPD to reflect coexisting dysfunction of both types (22). Thus, besides pure auditory mechanisms, learning, long-term phonological representation, and other higher level neurocognitive processes, memory and attention are considered in the definition of CAPD. The deployment of these nondedicated global mechanisms and processes in the service of central auditory processing underlies the frequently observed clinical association between CAPD and speech and language disorders, learning disabilities, attention deficit disorders with or without hyperactivity, psychological, emotional, and social problems (21).

Recently, APD has been more widely defined as a deficit in the processing of information that is specific to the auditory modality. The problem may be exacerbated in unfavorable acoustic environments. It may be associated with difficulties in listening, speech understanding, language development, and learning. In its pure form, however, it is conceptualized as a deficit in the processing of auditory input (23). This definition tends toward the view of the potential for interaction between disorders originating at both nondedicated processes and mechanisms in the processing of acoustic information.

Prevalence of CAPD

There is a lack of well-designed epidemiological studies on the prevalence of CAPD. Based on the prevalence of comorbid associations (e.g., serous otitis media, language impairment and learning disabilities, attention deficit disorders), the prevalence of CAPD in children has been estimated to be between 2% and 3% (18). In the aging population, this prevalence ranges from a low of 17% to a high of 90% (18,24) according to the central tests administered and the inclusion or exclusion of subjects with peripheral hearing loss or cognitive deficits (21).

Appeal Signs of CAPD

In children, many appeal signs, although not specific, raise the likelihood of CAPD. Particularly in noisy or low-redundancy listening situations, the child can behave as if he or she has peripheral hearing loss, which is within normal limits. They have difficulty following long or complicated verbal instructions, request they be repeated, or are unable to remember them. They have verbal IQ scores often lower than performance scores or significant scatter across subtests, e.g. math- and language-based subtests, or subtests that tap auditory perceptual skills. Many of these children have significant reading problems, are poor spellers, and have poor handwriting. To minimize over referrals, CAP questionnaires have been designed to assess the teacher's and parent's perception of a child's auditory processing (25,26).

In adults, by far the most frequent symptom of CAPD is the inability to understand speech in low redundant conditions. The most commonly reported symptoms include: poor utilization of prosodic information, difficulty localizing sound sources or following complex auditory directions, subjective tinnitus, typically localized to the midline of the head, or unusual auditory sensations, e.g. marked decrease in the appreciation of music.

Beside children with learning disabilities and adults with poor in noise intelligibility, a large population can take benefit of central auditory testing. Many reports indicate that patients who have degenerative neurological diseases, multiple sclerosis among others, can have auditory deficits (27). A CAP deficit should be the first sign of senile demence or Alzheimer's disease (28). Occasionally patients with mass lesion of the brain may consult an ENT specialist before a diagnosis is made. Sometimes the auditory complains of patients who have received head trauma can be objectively acknowledged as central processing disorder.

Central Auditory Processing Tests

Tests of central auditory function can be categorized in a variety of ways, e.g., monotic, diotic, dichotic, speech, or nonspeech tests. In the author's commitment, we will follow the lead of Baran and Musiek (29) and categorize central tests in the following manner: low-redundancy speech tests, dichotic speech tests, temporal processing tasks, and binaural interaction tests.

Low-redundancy Speech Tests

Filtered, compressed, expanded, interrupted, and reverberated speech signals have all been used as central low-redundancy tests.

Since from the reports of Bocca et al. (30), low-pass filtering is by far the best known low-redundancy test. In the time compression or expansion technique, the temporal characteristics of the signal are electronically altered without affecting the frequency spectrum (31). Increasing the reverberation time of the speech signal provides an additional method of reducing the extrinsic redundancy (32).

A final method of reducing the redundancy of the speech signal is to imbed the signal in a background of noise (33–36). In spite of specific spectrum noise, cocktail babble has been used as competing signal (37).

Dichotic Speech Tests

Dichotic speech tests involve tests in which a different speech material is presented to both ears in a simultaneous or overlapping manner (38). Based on her observations, Kimura developed a model to describe dichotic speech perception (39,40). When the central auditory nervous system is stimulated with dichotic speech materials, the weaker ipsilateral ascending pathways tend to be suppressed, and the neural impulses travel up the predominant contralateral pathways to reach the auditory temporal areas. Because the language processing region resides in the left hemisphere for most individuals, stimuli presented to the left ear must ultimately cross over from the right hemisphere to the left-dominant hemisphere, via the corpus callosum. This longer route for left ear presented stimuli induces a Right Ear Advantage (REA) apparent only upon dichotic stimulation. Dichotic speech tests are particularly sensitive to lesions of the auditory cortices and corpus callosum and to a lesser degree to brainstem lesions.

One of the most common dichotic tests in use today in English speaking countries is the Dichotic Digits Test (DDT) (41). For each stimulus presentation four digits are presented to the patient with two digits presented to each ear in a dichotic fashion.

The Competing Sentences Test (CST) developed by Willford (42) is easier and more convenient for child testing and uses a target sentence presented to one ear at 35 db re: spondee threshold and a competing sentence at 50 db re: spondee threshold. Perhaps the most widely used dichotic speech test is the Staggered Spondaic Word (SSW) Test, first described by Katz in 1962 (43). In this procedure, two spondees (compound words with equal stress) are presented in an overlapped fashion so that the second syllable of the first spondee occurs at the same time as the first syllable of the second spondee.

Temporal Processing Tests

Temporal processing is critical to a wide variety of everyday listening tasks, such as environmental signals, melodies, and speech. Many speech sounds are characterized by rapid frequency and intensity transitions that provide information for their identification. The temporal aspects of audition include many processes among which only few are well-codified clinically and widely used.

Temporal resolution refers to the ability of the ear to follow relatively slower transitions (infra 500 Hz) in the amplitude envelope of a stimulus. It has most often been investigated using either the Gap Detection method (44) or the Temporal Modulation Transfer Function (TMTF) method (45).

Temporal masking may be forward or backward type. Forward type refers to masking that occurs when the masking sound comes before the signal, while backward masking means the reverse.

Temporal integrations or summation describe the function relating signal detection threshold to its duration. Stable above 200 msec, the threshold increases as the signal duration decreases (approximately 3 db for every division of duration by two) (46).

Due to equipment sophistication involved in administering these tasks combined with the lack of standardized test protocols, these temporal processing functions are not explored in widespread clinical practice not withstanding their good clinical potential (18,19).

A fourth temporal processing concerns an ordering or sequencing task, i.e., to make discrimination based on the temporal order of auditory stimuli.

Pinheiro and Musiek (47) introduced a test of temporal processing involving triads of tone bursts, the Pitch Pattern Sequence Test (PPST). The subject has to report the pattern perceived from a sequence of three tone bursts: two of one frequency and one of another.

A related test of temporal ordering is the Duration Pattern Test (DPT) described by Pinheiro and Musiek (48). The test is similar to the PPST, but has as its elements 1000 Hz tones which vary only in duration (either 250 or 500 msec with a 300 msec interstimulus interval).

Binaural Interaction Tests

Binaural interaction tests encompass those tests that require the interaction of both ears in order to effect integration of information that is separated by time, intensity, or frequency factors to the two ears. Functions that rely on binaural interaction include binaural fusion, localization (determining direction of the source) and lateralization (place perception in the head) of auditory stimuli, binaural release from masking, and detection of signals in noise.

The task of integrating a portion of one signal presented to one ear and a complementary portion presented to the other ear is referred to as binaural fusion in literature. This task assesses the ability of the CANS to take disparate information presented to the two ears and to unify this information into one perceptual event. The two most used tests in this category of task include the Rapidly Alternating Speech Perception (RASP) and the Band-Pass Binaural Fusion test.

RASP is a procedure in which sentence material is switched rapidly between ears at selected periodic intervals causing unintelligibility when monauraly presented (49). It seems this test should be sensitive only to grossly abnormal brainstem pathology (42).

The test of binaural fusion uses stimuli (mono- or bisyllables) which are band passed so that a low-pass band (500–800 Hz) segment is presented to one ear and a high-pass band (1815–2500 Hz) segment to the other (50). The poor sensibility and acoustic technical problems preclude the wide use of these two last tests.

Interaural difference timer tasks involve the use of pairs of tonal or click stimuli that are presented to both ears simultaneously. Either the onset time or the intensity of the stimulus to one ear is manipulated relative to the other ear. The listener is required to indicate when he or she perceives the signal as lateralizing to one side or the other (27,50,51).

The binaural release from masking refers to the improvement in intelligibility under noise in phase conditions when a speech signal is presented out of phase rather than in phase condition (52,53). Any acoustical stimulus presented in phase to the two ears results in a perception located in the midline of the head, whereas presented 180° out of phase, it will be perceived at the ears. When both speech and noise were in phase (homophasic condition) and perceived both at midline, the speech intelligibility is lower than when the speech is 180° out of phase and noise is in phase (antiphasic) and respectively perceived at the ears and at the midline. The difference in binaural threshold between homophasic and antiphasic condition constitutes the Masking Level Difference (MLD). Variation of the size of the MLD depends on the type of stimuli and masker and of the specific protocol used. It may be as high as 10 to 15 dB when pure tones are used instead of approximately 5 db with speech material (54). Experimental results have shown that the MLD is highly sensitive to brainstem dysfunction while largely unaffected by rostral brainstem and cortical lesions (55,56).

RELATIONS OF APD WITH ADHD

The characteristics of ADHD are defined in the *Diagnostic and Statistical Manual of Mental Disorders* (DSM-IV) (57). As said before, comparison of the definition of APD and ADHD reveals much overlap in behavior which could reflect a single developmental disorder (58). It has even been suggested that this difficult differential diagnosis may depend upon whether it is the audiologist or the psychologist who first evaluated the child (1). Nevertheless, some observations illustrating the differences between APD and ADHD support the clinical utility of these diagnosis (18).

The attention deficits of ADHD are typically restricted to sustained attention (59). They are supramodal, i.e., affecting more than one sensory modality (1). In contrast, subjects with APD experience selective and divided attention deficits restricted to the auditory modality. According to a recent study of Seikel et al. (60), inattention and distractibility seem to be the predominant overlapping symptomatology in APD and ADHD. APD should be characterized by a selective attention deficit associated with language processing and academic difficulties. On the other hand, ADHD should be characterized by a behavioral deregulation with inappropriate motor activity, restlessness, and socially inappropriate interaction profiles.

About this relation between APD and ADHD, some authors have suggested that auditory processing assessment could be useful in the evaluation of the methylphenidate (Ritalin®) treatment efficacy in ADHD. Another point is to know if a child with ADHD should be tested with or without treatment since this one could mask a true APD. An elegant way to answer to these questions is to statistically evaluate the effect of Ritalin upon APD. If APD are improved it can be assumed that there is a common neurodevelopmental disorder with ADHD. On the contrary, no modification of APD would lead to the conclusion of their comorbidity.

To date, only four studies have investigated the effects on Ritalin on auditory process of children with ADHD and/or APD. Three of them have demonstrated a significant improvement of APD in small group of children with ADHD (58,61,62) and in the last one no differences were found in a group of 66 children (63). Methodology, small group, and variation in the inclusion criteria may have influenced the significant medication effect found on the three first studies. Two of them (61,62) evaluated a population of children diagnosed with ADHD for two successive conditions: first without the treatment and then with it, so the improvement observed may be due to a learning effect. In the third one (58), a placebo was used in a double-blind session but the sample population was small ($N = 15$).

The Tillery study was made on a larger sample ($N = 32$). All the children were diagnosed with ADHD and APD. They were submitted to three CAP tests (the SSW, PS, and speech-in-noise tests) and to the Auditory Continuous Performance Test (ACPT), a measure of attention/impulsivity. The study was double-blind and placebo-controlled in a split-unit design. No effect of the Ritalin on the three CAP measures used was observed. However, improvement of ACPT performance was show in the Ritalin group. This underlies the probability that APD and ADHD are independent problems and that, although the treatment improved attention and lessened impulsivity, it was not sufficient to alleviate the auditory dysfunction (63).

CONCLUSIONS

APD refer to an observed deficit in one or more of the central auditory processes responsible for the following behaviors: sound localization and lateralization, auditory discrimination, auditory pattern recognition, temporal aspects of audition including temporal resolution, temporal masking, temporal integration and temporal ordering, auditory performance with competing acoustic signals, and auditory performance with degraded acoustic signals (22).

APD have been frequently observed in association with many other neuromorphological disorders including ADHD, the most common neurobehavioral disorder of childhood affecting 3% to 5% of children aged 2 to 8 years.

Many studies have been made on the co-occurrence of APD and ADHD. A few of them tried to evaluate the efficacy or the effectiveness of the ADHD pharmacological treatment on APD. Some of them seem to show a direct association between ADHD and APD but some methodological mistakes may have been made. On the contrary, a more recent study has demonstrated that these pathologies are two independent problems even if they frequently occurred together.

REFERENCES

1. Keller W. Auditory processing disorder or attention deficit disorder? In: Katz J, Stecker N, Henderson D, eds. Central Auditory Processing: A Transdisciplinary View. St. Louis, MO: Mosby, 1992:107–14.
2. Keller W. The relationship between attention deficit hyperactivity disorder, central auditory processing disorders, and specific learning disorders. In: Masters G, Stecker N, Katz J, eds. Central Auditory Processing Disorders: Mostly Management. Boston, MA: Allyn & Bacon, 1998:33–48.
3. Demanez L, Boniver V, Dony-Closon B, et al. Central auditory processing disorders: some cohorts studies. Acta Otorhinolaryngol Belg 2003; 57:291–9.
4. Persinger MA, Chellew-Belanger G, Tiller SG. Bilingual men but not women display less left ear but not right ear accuracy during dichotic listening compared to monolinguals. Int J Neurosci 2002; 112:55–63.
5. Stephens D, Zhao F. The role of a family history in King Kopetzky syndrome (obscure auditory dysfunction). Acta Otolaryngol 2000; 120:197–200.
6. Zhao F, Stephens D. Subcategories of patients with King-Kopetzky syndrome. Br J Audiol 2000; 34:241–56.
7. Saunders GH, Haggard MP. The clinical assessment of obscure auditory dysfunction. 1. Auditory and psychological factors. Ear Hear 1989; 10:200–8.
8. Saunders GH, Haggard MP. The clinical assessment of "Obscure Auditory Dysfunction" (OAD). 2. Case control analysis of determining factors. Ear Hear 1992; 13:241–54.
9. Bench J, Maule R. The use of internal speech by children with auditory processing problems. Audiology 1997; 36:312–24.
10. Jansson-Verkasalo E, Ceponiene R, Valkama M, et al. Deficient speech-sound processing, as shown by the electrophysiologic brain mismatch negativity response, and naming ability in prematurely born children. Neurosci Lett 2003; 348:5–8.
11. McFarland DJ, Cacace AT. Potential problems in the differential diagnosis of (central) auditory processing disorder (CAPD or APD) and attention-deficit hyperactivity disorder (ADHD). J Am Acad Audiol 2003; 14:278–80.
12. Chermak GD, Hall JW III, Musiek FE. Differential diagnosis and management of central auditory processing disorder and attention deficit hyperactivity disorder. J Am Acad Audiol 1999; 10:289–303.
13. Shriberg LD, Flipsen P Jr, Kwiatkowski J, et al. A diagnostic marker for speech delay associated with otitis media with effusion: the intelligibility-speech gap. J Clin Ling Phon 2003; 17:507–28.
14. Michel F, Peronnet F, Schott B. A case of cortical deafness: clinical and electrophysiological data. Brain Lang 1980; 10:367–77.
15. Freud S. Zur auffassung des aphasien. Eine kritische studie. Leipzig 1891.
16. Lichteim L. On aphasia. Brain 1885; 7:433–84.
17. Lechevalier B, Lamber J, Eustache F, Platel H. Agnosies auditives et syndromes voisins. Etude clinique, cognitive et psychopathologique. Encyclopedie Médico-chirurgicale, Neurologie. Paris: Elsevier SAS, 1999:1–9.
18. Chermak GD, Musiek FE. Central Auditory Processing Disorders. New Perspectives. San Diego, CA: Singular Publishing Group, 1997.

19. Bellis TJ. Central Auditory Processing Disorders. From Science to Practice. San Diego, CA: Singular Publishing Group, 1996.
20. Saunders GH, Haggard MP. The clinical assessment of obscure auditory dysfunction. 1. Auditory and psychological factors. Ear Hear 1989; 10:200–8.
21. Baran JA, Musiek FE. Central auditory disorders. In: Luxon LM, ed. Textbook of Audiological Medicine. London: Martin Dunitz, 2003:495–511.
22. American Speech-Language-Hearing Association Task Force on Central Auditory Processing Consensus Development. Central auditory processing current status of research and implications for clinical practice. Am J Audiol 1996; 5:41–54.
23. Jerger J, Musiek F. Report of the Consensus Conference on the Diagnosis of Auditory Processing Disorders in School-Aged Children. J Am Acad Audiol 2000; 11:467–74.
24. Cooper JC Jr, Gates GA. Hearing in the elderly–the Framingham cohort, 1983–1985: Part II. Prevalence of central auditory processing disorders. Ear Hear 1991; 12:304–11.
25. Fisher LI. Learning disabilities and auditory processing. In: Van Hattam RJ, ed. Administration of Speech Language Services in Schools: A Manual. San Diego, CA: College-Hill Press, 1985:231–91.
26. Anderson KL. Screening instruments for targeting educational risk. In: Johnson CD, Benson PV, Seaton JB, eds. Educational Audiology Handbook. San Diego, CA: Singular Publishing Group, 1997.
27. Levine RA, Gardner JC, Fullerton BC, et al. Effects of multiple sclerosis brainstem lesions on sound lateralization and brainstem auditory evoked potentials. Hear Res 1993; 68:73–88.
28. Gates GA, Cobb JL, Linn RT, et al. Central auditory dysfunction, cognitive dysfunction, and dementia in older people. Arch Otolaryngol Head Neck Surg 1996; 122:161–7.
29. Baran JA, Musiek FE. Behavioral assessment of the central auditory nervous system. In: Rintelmann W, ed. Hearing Assessment. Austin, TX: Pro-Ed Publishers, 1991:549–602.
30. Bocca E, Calearo C, Cassinari V. A new method for testing hearing in temporal lobe tumours: preliminary report. Acta Otolaryngol 1954; 44:219–21.
31. Fairbanks G, Everitt W, Jaeger R. Methods for time or frequency compression–expansion of speech. Trans IRE-PGA 1954; 2:7–12.
32. Helfer KS, Wilber LA. Hearing loss, aging, and speech perception in reverberation and noise. J Speech Hear Res 1990; 33:149–55.
33. Lafon JC. Le Test Phonétique et la Mesure de l'Audition. Editions Centrex, Eindhoven, 1964.
34. Keith RW. SCAN: A Screening Test for Auditory Processing Disorders. San Antonio, TX: The Psychological Corporation, 1986.
35. Keith RW. SCAN-A: A Screening Test for Auditory Processing Disorders in Adolescents and Adults. San Antonio, TX: The Psychological Corporation, 1994.
36. Cherry R. The selective auditory attention test (SAAT). St. Louis, MO: Auditec of St. Louis, 1980.

37. Jerger J, Jerger S. Auditory findings in brain stem disorders. Arch Otolaryngol 1974; 99:342–50.
38. Broadbent DE. The role of auditory localization in attention and memory span. J Exp Psychol 1954; 47:191–6.
39. Kimura D. Some effects of temporal-lobe damage on auditory perception. Can J Psychol 1961; 15:156–65.
40. Kimura D. Cerebral dominance and the perception of verbal stimuli. Can J Psychol 1961; 15:166–71.
41. Musiek FE. Assessment of central auditory dysfunction: the Dichotic Digit Test revisited. Ear Hear 1983; 4:79–83.
42. Willford J A, Burleigh JM. Sentence procedures in central testing. In: Katz J, ed. Handbook of Clinical Audiology. Baltimore, MD: Williams & Wilkins, 1994:256–68.
43. Katz J. The use of staggered spondaic words for assessing the integrity of the central auditory system. J Auditory Res 1962; 2:327–37.
44. Grose JH. Gap detection in multiple narrow bands of noise as a function of spectral configuration. J Acoust Soc Am 1991; 90:3061–8.
45. Viemeister NF. Temporal modulation transfer functions based upon modulation thresholds. J Acoust Soc Am 1979; 66:1364–80.
46. Cranford JL, Stream RW, Rye CV, et al. Detection v discrimination of brief-duration tones. Findings in patients with temporal lobe damage. Arch Otolaryngol 1982; 108:350–6.
47. Pinheiro ML, Musiek FE. Assessment of Central Auditory Dysfunction: Foundations and Clinical Correlates. Baltimore, MD: Williams & Wilkins, 1985.
48. Musiek FE, Baran JA, Pinheiro ML. Duration pattern recognition in normal subjects and patients with cerebral and cochlear lesions. Audiology 1990; 29: 304–13.
49. Hennebert D. Intégration de la perception auditive et l'audition alternante. Acta Otorhinolaryngol Belg 1955; 9:344–6.
50. Matzker J. Two new methods for the assessment of central auditory functions in case of brain diseases. Ann of Otol Rhinol Laryngol 1959; 68:1155–97.
51. Pinheiro ML, Tobin H. The interaural intensity difference as a diagnostic indicator. Acta Otolaryngol 1971; 71:326–8.
52. Licklider JCR. The influence of interaural phase relation upon the masking of speech by white noise. J Acoust Soc Am 1948; 20:150–9.
53. Hirsh IJ. The infuence of interaural phase on interaural summation and inhibition. J Acoust Soc Am 1948; 20:536–44.
54. Noffsinger D, Schaefer AB, Martinez CD. Behavioral and objective estimates of auditory brainstem integrity. Semin Hear 1984; 5:337–49.
55. Levine RA, Gardner JC, Fullerton BC, et al. Multiple sclerosis lesions of the auditory pons are not silent. Brain 1994; 117 (Pt. 5):1127–41.
56. Lynn GE, Gilroy J, Taylor PC, et al. Binaural masking-level differences in neurological disorders. Arch Otolaryngol 1981; 107:357–62.
57. American Psychiatric Association. DSM IV. Critères Diagnostiques (Washington, D.C. 1994) Traduction française. Paris: Masson, 1996.

58. Cook JR, Mausbach T, Burd L, et al. A preliminary study of the relationship between central auditory processing disorder and attention deficit disorder. J Psychiatry Neurosci 1993; 18:130–7.
59. Hooks K, Milich R, Lorch EP. Sustained and selective attention in boys with attention deficit hyperactivity disorder. J Clin Child Psychol 1994; 23:69–77.
60. Chermak GD, Somers EK, Seikel JA. Behavioral signs of central auditory processing disorder and attention deficit hyperactivity disorder. J Am Acad Audiol 1998; 9:78–84.
61. Gascon GG, Johnson R, Burd L. Central auditory processing and attention deficit disorders. J Child Neurol 1986; 1:27–33.
62. Keith RW, Engineer P. Effects of methylphenidate on the auditory processing abilities of children with attention deficit-hyperactivity disorder. J Learn Disabil 1991; 24:630–6.
63. Tillery KL, Katz J, Keller WD. Effects of methylphenidate (Ritalin) on auditory performance in children with attention and auditory processing disorders. J Speech Lang Hear Res 2000; 43:893–901.

Section II: Clinical Conceptualizations

3

Clinical Testing of Intelligence, Achievement, and Neuropsychological Performance in ADHD

Leah Ellenberg

University of Southern California School of Medicine, Los Angeles, California, U.S.A.

Joel Kramer

Departments of Neurology and Psychiatry, University of California San Francisco Medical Center, San Francisco, California, U.S.A.

According to the DSM-IV, diagnosis of attention deficit hyperactivity disorder (ADHD) is primarily based on behavioral criteria. If an individual manifests six of nine symptoms of ADHD, inattentive type or ADHD, impulsive hyperactive type in two or more settings with a history of onset before age seven, ADHD may be diagnosed. However, a more complete assessment of an individual who meets behavioral criteria for ADHD is often necessary for several reasons. To firmly establish the diagnosis of ADHD, it is important to rule out other disorders that may have similar behavioral manifestations. After confirmation of the diagnosis of ADHD, the possibility of comorbid disorders must be evaluated since they may effect treatment. Finally, an assessment of an individual's patterns of strengths and weaknesses in various neurocognitive and emotional realms is critical in designing a treatment program in areas such as academic accommodations, career planning, and therapeutic modalities. To that end, a comprehensive neuropsychological evaluation including assessment of intelligence, neuropsychological functioning, academic achievement and psychological functioning is often clinically indicated for individuals with ADHD.

USE OF INTELLIGENCE TESTING IN ADHD

In order to establish a differential diagnosis of ADHD, several conditions that include problems in attention most be ruled out. According to the DSM-IV, individuals with mental retardation and pervasive developmental disorders may meet behavioral criteria for ADHD and need to be differentiated from individuals with true ADHD. In addition, individuals with low average or borderline IQs may be misclassified as having ADHD when they fail to perform adequately in the school setting. Therefore, an accurate assessment of IQ is crucial in evaluating individuals who are underperforming in school and seem to be inattentive or excessively active to see if they are capable of meeting the demands placed upon them. Conversely, an individual who is gifted and placed in an unstimulating or restricted school environment may exhibit symptoms of ADHD due to lack of challenge.

Studies have generally shown that mixed groups of individuals with ADHD have slightly lower IQs than control samples. However, these studies generally do not differentiate between subtypes of ADHD or individuals with ADHD who have a comorbid learning disorder.

By far, the most commonly used IQ measure in assessing individuals with ADHD is the Wechsler Intelligence Scale for Children-IV (WISC-IV). Other tests that have been used are the Kaufman Assessment Battery and the Cognitive Skills Index (CSI).

The WISC-IV has been separated by means of factor analysis into four indexes: verbal comprehension, perceptual organization, working memory, and processing speed. Research has shown that the Working Memory Index score cannot be used to diagnose ADHD as it is not routinely lower in samples of children with the disorder. One of the two subtests that comprise the index, digit span, involves repeating digits forward and backward. However, in the total score there is no differentiation between digits forward, a fairly simple task and digits backwards, which places a larger load on sustained attention and working memory (the ability to hold information in mind to manipulate it). Letter-number sequencing, new on the WISC-IV, is difficult for some younger children to understand. Deficits on these tests may be related to factors other than distractibility, such as slow mental processing, language comprehension difficulties, auditory processing problems, or poor hearing.

Other indicators on the WISC-IV are important in ascertaining the particular neuropsychological profile of the individual being assessed. A discrepancy between the verbal comprehension and perceptual organization composites can delineate strengths and weaknesses important in educational planning. The processing speed index, which assesses the ability to quickly perform straightforward perceptual motor tasks, is an important determinant of functioning in individuals with ADHD. An individual with ADHD, impulsive hyperactive type may show rapid processing but make errors because of performing impulsively without adequate oversight. Other individuals, particularly those diagnosed with ADHD, inattentive type, may show significantly lowered processing speed. This may result in slow reading and difficulty rapidly performing academic tasks.

ACHIEVEMENT TESTING IN ADHD

Due to the high comorbidity rate between ADHD and learning disabilities, an assessment of an individual's academic strengths and weaknesses is an important part of the evaluation of ADHD. The core symptoms of ADHD often result in problems attending to classroom instructions and directions as well as difficulty carrying out independent assignments and complex or multimodal tasks. In addition, an individual with ADHD may have school problems because of a modality-specific comorbid learning disorder such as dyslexia (a language-based reading disorder), dysgraphia (a writing disorder), or a math learning disability. The most widely used tests in the neuropsychological arena to assess academic achievement are the Woodcock-Johnson Tests of Achievement-III, the Wechsler Individual Achievement Test (WIAT), and the Wide Range Achievement Test-IV (WRAT-IV). The WRAT-IV, which screens word reading, spelling, and math calculation takes the shortest amount of time to administer but has limited subtests. The WIAT includes reading, comprehension, and writing subtests and was standardized with the WISC-IV, providing comparable norms. The Woodcock-Johnson Achievement Test has a large number of subtests and was standardized with the Woodcock-Johnson Test of Cognitive Ability. It has the widest use among educators.

In the past, many achievement tests had a common disadvantage in that they did not have a timed component. For this reason, many individuals showed better performance on the screening measures than was evident by monitoring classroom performance. The Woodcock-Johnson III includes measures of reading, math, and writing fluency that help assess an individual's ability to perform tasks rapidly, often necessary in the classroom. Supplementing these achievement strategies with other times tests such as the Gray Oral Reading Test-4 or the Nelson Denny Reading Test is important to assess an individual with ADD in terms of understanding actual classroom functioning.

Accurate assessment of cognitive and achievement functioning is necessary to assess the desirability of instituting classroom modifications or accommodations for students with ADHD. Individuals with ADHD may qualify for accommodations based on the Individuals with Disabilities Education Act (IDEA) or under a 504 plan. In order to render students eligible, an academic as well as psychoeducational or neuropsychological evaluation is necessary.

NEUROPSYCHOLOGICAL TESTING IN AD/HD

ADHD has been conceptualized as a disorder of executive functioning, including attention difficulties with sustained and behavioral inhibition (1–8).

There is a great deal of evidence suggesting that individuals with ADHD show neuropsychological deficits on tests of executive functioning. However, there are significant differences between tests in terms of the effect size and specificity of an ADHD diagnosis based on test performance. It is apparent that the use of neuropsychological tests alone cannot provide reliable clinical diagnosis of ADHD. However, neuropsychological test performance may be very important in determining the severity and extent of life disturbances in an individual with ADHD, as well as being crucial for educational and treatment planning.

Specific tests of executive functioning that have differentiated groups with and without ADHD are the Stroop Color-Word Interference Test, Trails B, Design Fluency, Wisconsin Card Sort Test, Rey-Osterrieth Complex Figure, Continuous Performance Test, and the Controlled Oral Word Association Test.

In addition to assessment of executive functioning, several other neuropsychological domains are important to evaluate in individuals with ADHD. Short-term memory and working memory are often affected. The degree and nature of an individual's memory impairment may have important implications for treatment strategies. In addition, individuals with a comorbid learning disability are at risk for even greater short-term memory problems (9).

In the school setting, children with dyslexia are sometimes misclassified as having ADHD because of difficulty comprehending written directions as well as inattentiveness and distractibility during reading tasks. There may also be behavior problems related to self-esteem issues around the reading disability. It is important to do a thorough neuropsychological assessment of the underpinnings of reading, particularly phonemic awareness and rapid naming, to differentiate between the two disorders. Individuals with attentional problems sometimes show difficulty with rapid linguistic retrieval and verbal fluency (10). However, most studies indicate that children with reading disability only, without ADHD, show deficits in phonological processing, which are not generally shown in children with ADHD (11).

Clinical evaluation of the speed of mental processing of an individual with ADHD is important for treatment planning. Some individuals with ADHD show very high psychomotor speed, often combined with many attentional errors as material becomes more complex. On the other hand, some individuals with ADHD, primarily ADHD, inattentive type, show very slow mental processing. Individuals with the first pattern may need to be taught strategies for slowing down and checking work.

Individuals with the latter pattern may need extended time for completion of tests and to be taught strategies for organizing their approach to complex or multifaceted tasks.

Assessment of Psychological Functioning in ADHD

Assessment of psychological and emotional functioning is important in ADHD for several reasons. To begin with, there is a high comorbidity with anxiety and mood disorders in ADHD. In addition, an individual's motivation, anxiety level, frustration tolerance, and self-esteem are important in determining prognosis and designing an efficacious treatment plan.

Many symptoms consistent with ADHD, inattentive type are also found in depression and it is important to rule out depression as underlying difficulties in attention, concentration, and executive function. In children, the Childhood Depression Inventory may be useful. For teenagers, the Achenbach Youth Self-Report includes a number of emotional symptoms. For adults, a Minnesota Multiphase of Personality Inventory-2 (MMPI-2) and the Beck Depression Inventory may help to evaluate the presence and degree of depression. The presence of concomitant anxiety or mood disorders may have implications for medication management as well as treatment modalities.

IMPLICATIONS FOR TREATMENT

In addition to self-report forms, it is important to query individuals familiar with the patient as to daily functioning. Parents may be asked to complete such behavior rating scales as the Achenbach Child Behavior Checklist or the Behavior Inventory of Executive Functions (BRIEF). Teachers can complete an Achenbach Teacher Report or school version of the BRIEF.

CONCLUSIONS AND TREATMENT IMPLICATIONS

Complete neuropsychological assessment can aid in diagnosis and treatment planning for ADHD. To begin with, conditions which may meet behavioral criteria for ADHD such as low IQ or depression must be ruled out. When ADHD has been confirmed, evaluation of comorbid learning or emotional disorders is important in designing a comprehensive treatment plan. Academic accommodations will differ if a student has learning problems because of ADHD alone or whether there are concomitant learning disabilities. If ADHD alone is affecting learning, accommodations involving more individual attention and repetition of procedures and instructions may be helpful. In addition, the extent to which executive functioning is disrupted will be important to determine the strategy that will be most effective. Individuals with ADHD often have trouble with multistep or complicated projects. Writing assignments may be particularly difficult and the nature and extent of these difficulties need to be determined so that remediation can be specific.

Individuals with ADHD and a concomitant learning disability appear to be more impaired than those with ADHD alone on tasks of executive functioning as well as having further specific needs such as work on phonological processing for individuals who are dyslexic (12).

The presence or absence of deficits in processing speed affects academic accommodations. Individuals with ADHD and processing speed deficits require extra time for tests, and this accommodation is increasingly being provided by schools and outside testing agencies. In addition, individuals with ADHD who have working memory deficits may need additional time to reread passages to ensure comprehension and may also require extra time for adequate performance.

Individuals with comorbid emotional or self-esteem issues may benefit from psychotherapy in addition to other treatment modalities. When executive functioning deficits are significant, which may occur even when medication management is effective, resource specialist help or educational therapy in school may be indicated. For adults who continue to have executive function deficits after medication management, the use of educational therapists or "life coaches" may be indicated. Neuropsychological evaluation can provide a detailed neurocognitive, psychological, and behavioral profile that will help guide therapy by delineating the nature and extent of specific problem areas and areas of compensating strengths in an individual with ADHD (13).

REFERENCES

1. Barkley RO. Behavioral inhibition, sustained attention and executive functions: constructing a unifying theory of ADHD. Psychol Bull 1994; 121:65–94.
2. Schriber HE, Jarorsky DJ, Robinson JE, Stern RA. Rey-Osterrieth complex figure performance in adults with attention deficit hyperactivity disorder: a validation study of the Boston Qualitative Scoring System. Clin Neuropsychol. 1999; 13:509–20.
3. Doyle AE, Biederman J, Seidman LJ, Weber W, Faraone SV. Diagnostic efficiency of neuropsychological test scores for discriminating boys with and without attention deficit-hyperactivity disorder. J Consult Clin Psychol 2000; 58:477–88.
4. Grodzinsky GM, Barkley RA. Predictive power of frontal lobe tests in the diagnosis of attention deficit hyperactivity disorder. Clin Neuropsychologist 1999; 13:12–21.
5. Perugini EM, Harvey EA, Lovejoy DW, Sandstrom K, Webb AH. The predictive power of combined neuropsychological measures for attention-deficit/hyperactivity disorder in children. Child Neuropsychol 2000; 5:101–14.

6. Shallice Q, Marzocchi GM, Cosser S, Del Savio M, Neuter RF, Rumiatiri. Executive function profile of children with attention deficit hyperactivity disorder. Develop Neuropsychol 2002; 21:43–71.
7. Seidman LJ, Beiderman J, Faraone SV, Weber W, Ouellette C. Toward defining a neuropsychology of attention deficit-hyperactivity disorder: performance of children and adolescents from a large clinically referred sample. J Consult Clin Psychol 1997; 65:150–60.
8. Rapport LJ, VanVoorhis A, Tzelepisa A, Friedman SR. Executive functioning in adult attention-deficit hyperactivity disorder. Clin Neuropsychologist 2001; 4:479–91.
9. Johnson BD, Altmaier EM, Richman LC. Attention deficits and reading disabilities: are immediate memory defects additive? Develop Neuropsychol 1999; 15:213–26.
10. Grodzinsky GM, Diamond R. Frontal lobe functioning in boys with attention deficit/hyperactivity disorder. Develop Neuropsychol 1992; 8:427–45.
11. Pennington BF, Groiffer D, Welsh MC. Contracting cognitive deficits in attention deficit/hyperactivity disorder versus reading disability. Develop Psychol 1993; 29:511–23.
12. Kibby M, Marcotte A, Stern C, Wilson J, Kiessling L. Influence of co-morbid reading disorders on cognitive functioning in children diagnosed with attentional problems. 1999, Boston, International Neuropsychological Society.
13. Aro T, Ahonen T, Tolvanen A, Lyytinen H. Contribution of ADHD characteristics to the academic treatment outcome of children with learning difficulties. Develop Neuropsychol 1999; 15:291–305.

4

Self-Esteem and Self-Perceptions in ADHD

Nina M. Kaiser
Department of Psychiatry, University of California San Francisco, San Francisco, California, U.S.A.

Betsy Hoza
Department of Psychology, University of Vermont, Burlington, Vermont, U.S.A.

Attention deficit hyperactivity disorder (ADHD) is characterized by problems with hyperactivity/impulsivity and/or inattention (1). Children with ADHD also often experience severe functional impairments in the form of behavior problems, peer rejection, and/or academic and family-related dysfunction (2–4). In nondisordered populations, incompetencies such as these generally are associated with low self-esteem and/or depression (5–8). Research on the self-esteem and self-perceptions of children with ADHD is much more controversial, however, and at this time, there exist two opposing points of view. Some researchers have discovered children with ADHD to have lowered self-views as compared to controls (9–11). In contrast, there exists an increasingly larger body of research demonstrating overly positive self-views in children with ADHD (12–16). The topic of self-perceptions in children with ADHD thus is a matter of some contention, and the somewhat speculatory nature of this chapter is merely a reflection of the current state of research in this area.

As Hoza and colleagues (13) noted, dividing research on self-concept in children with ADHD into the categories of research on global self-esteem, research on domain-specific self-perceptions, and research on task-specific self-perceptions somewhat clarifies a picture that appears at first glance to be rather hazy. In the current chapter, we therefore consider each of these constructs in turn, and review both the literature indicative of lowered self-views in children with ADHD as well as that indicating unrealistically positive self-views in these children. As our particular interest lies in overly positive self-perceptions, termed "positive illusions" in our recent research (13), we also will discuss the specificity of self-enhancement findings to ADHD populations, as well as potential mechanisms that may explain this phenomenon. Finally, we will reflect upon the relevance of self-esteem and self-perception research to clinical interventions for children with ADHD.

GLOBAL SELF-ESTEEM

Research focusing on the global self-esteem of children with ADHD as compared to controls has generally shown that the estimates of self-esteem provided by children with ADHD are either lower or approximately equivalent to those provided by comparison children (9,11). For example, Treuting and Hinshaw (11) compared the self-esteem of aggressive boys with ADHD, nonaggressive boys with ADHD, and comparison boys. They discovered that the aggressive subgroup of boys with ADHD reported lower levels of self-esteem than did either nonaggressive boys with ADHD or comparison boys, but failed to discover any significant differences between the nonaggressive ADHD group and the comparison group.

Similarly, Hoza and colleagues (14) compared the estimates of global self-worth provided by children with ADHD to those provided by comparison children. Results indicated that the reports of self-esteem provided by children with ADHD did not differ significantly from the appraisals provided by comparison children, despite the numerous functional impairments typically associated with the diagnosis of ADHD. This finding was replicated by Hoza et al. (13) with a substantially larger sample. The self-esteem of boys with ADHD, therefore, may be unjustifiably positive.

DOMAIN-SPECIFIC SELF-PERCEPTIONS OF COMPETENCE

As with research on self-esteem, a great deal of past research has examined absolute levels of self-perceptions of competence (i.e., examining subjective self-perceptions without comparing them to an external criterion). The results of this research are similar to those reviewed for self-esteem. Again, some research suggests that children with ADHD exhibit lower absolute perceptions of domain-specific competence (10), while other research indicates that children with ADHD provide estimates of their competence that are similar to those provided by comparison children (14). For example, Hoza and colleagues (14) investigated self-perceptions of scholastic competence, social acceptance, athletic competence, physical appearance, and behavioral conduct in boys with ADHD and comparison boys. They discovered that the self-reports of children with ADHD differed from those of control children only in the domain of behavioral conduct, boys with ADHD reported lower levels of competence (i.e., poorer behavioral conduct) than control boys. Hoza et al. (13) utilized a larger sample in order to perform a between-groups comparison (ADHD vs. control) of absolute levels of self-perceived competence in the above domains, although the researchers chose not to examine the domain of physical appearance. Results indicated that the absolute self-perceptions of boys with ADHD did not differ significantly from those of comparison boys in any of the four domains. These findings indicate that the self-perceptions of children with ADHD may be overly positive.

Several researchers have commented that it is necessary to compare self-views to objective criteria in order to determine their value or accuracy (13,17). Some children's positive self-views may be realistic reflections of actual competence, while other children may be overly positive reporters of their own competencies. As Hoza and colleagues (13) note, it is likely that these two groups of children differ on dimensions that are relevant to adjustment and response to clinical intervention.

Recent research comparing the domain-specific self-perceptions of children with ADHD to control children therefore has compared the perceptions of each child to ratings provided by external raters in order to obtain an index of over- and underestimation (13,18). For example, Hoza and colleagues (13) examined the self-perceptions of children with ADHD and comparison children relative to competence ratings completed by the boys' teachers. These researchers discovered that the reports of children with ADHD regarding their own competence were more inflated relative to teacher reports than the reports provided by comparison children. Further, the researchers found that children with ADHD provided the most positive self-reports in domains in which the teachers had rated them as being most impaired.

Hoza et al. (18) replicated these results with a separate sample of children with ADHD. This study further extended previous work by examining the self-perceptions of children with ADHD and control children in comparison to competence ratings provided by the children's mothers and fathers as well as to ratings supplied by the children's teachers. Regardless of which comparison rater was utilized as the criterion (i.e., mother, father, or teacher), results indicated that children with ADHD overestimated their competence to a greater degree relative to the criterion than the comparison children. These results lend additional support to the hypothesis that children with ADHD provide overly positive reports of their own abilities.

TASK-SPECIFIC SELF-PERCEPTIONS OF COMPETENCE

In addition to examinations of the domain-specific self-perceptions of children with ADHD versus comparison children, both on an absolute level and in comparison to criteria, children's task-specific evaluations of competence have been examined on laboratory tasks where actual performance on the task is known. For example, Hoza and colleagues (15) administered a find-a-word puzzle task to both boys with ADHD and comparison boys. The researchers found that in comparison to the group of control boys, the group of boys with ADHD solved fewer puzzles, stopped early more frequently, and were able to find fewer words on a subsequent generalization task. Further, research assistants rated the boys with ADHD as trying less hard and less cooperating than control boys. Despite the poorer performance of the ADHD group on the behavioral measures and the lower ratings of effort and cooperation that this group of boys received, the pretask performance expectations and posttask evaluations of performance provided by boys with ADHD were not significantly different from those of control boys. These findings further support the idea that children with ADHD provide evaluations of their own competence that are positively biased.

Hoza et al. (16) further investigated the construct of positive illusions through an examination of the self-ratings of boys with ADHD on a social laboratory task. Specifically, both boys with ADHD and control boys were asked to convince a child confederate to attend a camp under either a success or a failure manipulation. In addition, following the manipulation, an adult research assistant also provided each boy with either positive or negative feedback regarding his performance on the task. Consistent with similar research in the academic domain, the boys with ADHD provided more positive ratings of the child confederate and of their own performance on the task than did the comparison boys. For a subset of the dependent variables, these differences between boys with ADHD and comparison boys were even more marked after the boys had experienced the failure manipulation. Evidence that self-reports of the boys with ADHD were overly positive, came from objective raters, who evaluated the boys with ADHD as being less socially effective than the control boys. These findings are further evidence toward the conclusion that children with ADHD are overly positive reporters of their own performance. In addition, they indicate that these children may be most unrealistic about their performance when they have failed at a task.

This finding is consistent with research demonstrating that children with ADHD manifest positive illusions to the greatest degree in their domains of greatest deficit (13,18). In other words, the discrepancies between positive illusory estimates of their own competence provided by children with ADHD and the competence ratings provided by adults familiar with the children are greatest in the domains where children are evaluated as being least competent by the adult raters. Thus, aggressive children with ADHD provide the most inflated evaluations of their own competence in the behavioral domain, while low-achieving children with

ADHD provide the most inflated estimates of competence in the academic domain (13).

Comorbid depressive symptoms, on the other hand, appear to exert a different effect upon the self-views of children with ADHD than do the comorbidities described above. In fact, comorbid depression appears to alleviate the positive bias to a certain extent (13,14,18). For example, although Hoza and colleagues (13) discovered that the absolute self-perceptions of children with ADHD and control children did not differ significantly, subgrouping the children with ADHD into those with and without comorbid depressive symptoms produced an interesting pattern of results. The self-perceptions of boys with ADHD and comorbid depressive symptoms were significantly lower than the self-perceptions of both, the boys with ADHD but without comorbid depression and the comparison boys. These two latter groups did not differ significantly from one another. Further, when the researchers examined the boys' self-perceptions relative to ratings provided by the boys' teachers, they discovered that the boys with ADHD and comorbid depressive symptoms provided estimations in key domains (e.g., social) that were similarly realistic to those provided by comparison boys. Boys with ADHD but without depressive symptoms, on the other hand, overestimated their competence in multiple domains as compared to both of the other groups. In the behavioral conduct domain, however, both groups of boys with ADHD overestimated their competence relative to control boys, although the effect size was smaller for boys with ADHD and co-occurring depression than for nondepressed boys with ADHD. Consistent with research demonstrating a link between depression and diminished self-esteem in nondisordered populations (19), therefore, it appears as if comorbid depressive symptoms may lessen positive illusory tendencies in children with ADHD.

ARE POSITIVE ILLUSIONS SPECIFIC TO ADHD?

Specific ADHD-related behaviors appear to be associated with positive illusory beliefs of self-competence, although there is currently a paucity of research addressing this issue. However, Owens and Hoza (20) studied the presence and extent of overly positive views of academic self-competence in children with symptoms characteristic of ADHD, and discovered that hyperactive/impulsive symptoms were more closely related to positive illusions of academic competence than were inattentive symptoms. In other words, the self-reports of children exhibiting hyperactive/impulsive symptoms were found to be overly positive when compared both to the children's own achievement test scores and to their teachers' reports. Both control children and children with primarily inattentive symptoms provided more accurate self-reports of their academic competence.

Despite this tie to hyperactive/impulsive symptoms, a core component of ADHD, it seems likely that positive illusions also are associated with other disruptive behavior disorders. In the past, overly positive self-esteem and self-perceptions have been linked to problems such as peer rejection (21–23) and aggression (17,24–29). Further, comparisons performed between children diagnosed with conduct problems or oppositional-defiant disorder (ODD) and comparison children indicate that children with these externalizing disorders provide estimates of their own social competence that do not differ significantly from those provided by control children, despite parents' and teachers' reports to the contrary (30). It therefore appears at this time that the positive illusory bias is a construct that is indeed correlated with specific dimensions of psychopathology, namely those associated with the disruptive behavior disorders and specifically with ADHD. The common comorbidity among ADHD and other disruptive behavior disorders (31) may at least partially account for the presence of positive illusions in both ADHD and other behavior-disordered populations.

POTENTIAL MECHANISMS

There are several potential explanations for the existence of positive illusory self-perceptions. First, it seems possible that these inflated self-perceptions reflect other impairments associated with ADHD. For example, Barkley (32) has proposed that the primary dysfunction in ADHD is a deficit in executive functioning, specifically a lack of behavioral inhibition that can account for all of the impairments that are commonly associated with ADHD. Barkley hypothesized that tasks such as the inhibition of task-irrelevant responses, execution of goal-directed responses, sensitivity to response feedback, and persistence toward a specific goal all can be subsumed under the general category of behavioral inhibition. A deficit in behavioral inhibition therefore would cause impairments in self-control and self-regulation much like those demonstrated in ADHD. It seems likely that accurate self-perception requires the ability to self-regulate in response to external feedback, and an impairment in executive functioning thus may prevent children with ADHD from being aware of their deficits. Indeed, past research has demonstrated a connection between impaired executive functioning and diminished self-awareness (33).

Research on clinical assessment (3) and cognitive interventions (34) also emphasizes the idea that children with ADHD may lack certain cognitive skills relevant to self-perception. For instance, clinicians are encouraged to discount the self-reports of externalizing children in the assessment and diagnostic process (3). In addition, cognitive treatment strategies such as self-instructing, problem solving, self-reinforcement, and self-redirection appear ineffective when used as primary interventions to ameliorate the problems of children with ADHD (3,34). In fact, current empirically supported treatments for ADHD are all treatments that emphasize altering the environment of the child rather than fostering changes within the child (35). Current clinical wisdom therefore accentuates the possibility that these children lack the self-regulatory abilities necessary to effectively process and apply external criticism in order to regulate their own behavior.

Alternatively, another group of researchers has proposed a self-protective interpretation of the positive illusory bias (12,36). This explanation posits that overly positive views of self-competence are a façade for actual insecurities on the part of children with ADHD, serving the function of preventing these children from feeling inadequate as a result of their deficits. There is some evidence to support this hypothesis, most notably in the social domain. For example, Ohan and Johnston (36) presented children with ADHD with a social task, and then asked the children to evaluate their own performance. The researchers found that children with ADHD who initially provided overly positive estimates of their performance on the task were able to provide more realistic evaluations of their performance after an adult research assistant gave them positive, task-specific feedback. Similarly, Diener and Milich (12) discovered that providing boys with ADHD with positive feedback that was supposedly from a peer partner in a laboratory interaction task served the function of reducing overly positive performance evaluations on the part of the boys with ADHD to a more realistic level.

However, evidence regarding the validity of the self-protective hypothesis has been inconsistent across domains. Ohan and Johnston (36) also presented their ADHD and control sample with an academic task. As expected, the boys with ADHD provided pretask estimates of their performance that were similarly high to those of comparison boys, even though the boys with ADHD subsequently performed at a significantly lower level than the comparison boys. Contrary to findings in the social domain, however, providing the boys with positive feedback resulted in increased performance evaluations from both boys with ADHD and control boys in this condition, as compared to boys who received either average or no feedback regarding their performance. These results are inconsistent with the self-protective hypothesis. Ohan and Johnston posited that academic tasks may be less salient than social tasks for children with ADHD. If children with ADHD view academic competence as being less important, they may be able to discount their failure in the academic domain. If this is the case, then these children would have no reason to self-protect. Alternatively, Ohan and Johnston suggested that the explanation for positive illusory estimates of competence may vary from domain to domain. They proposed the possibility that although positive biases in the social domain may be best explained by the self-protective hypothesis, overly positive estimates of academic competence may reflect children's actual judgments of their academic performance.

This suggestion is consistent with research from the adult social psychology literature that points toward another potential explanation for inability to acknowledge incompetence. Kruger and Dunning (37) claim that individuals who are incompetent are, by definition, less able to recognize competence (and thus incompetence) in themselves or in others. If this is the case, the skills deficits demonstrated by children with ADHD ironically may prevent them from realizing their own incompetence. If these children do not understand what it means to be competent, they are free to consider themselves as being competent. This explanation should be considered in future research.

CLINICAL RELEVANCE

Research on the self-perceptions of children with ADHD is relevant in shaping clinical interventions. Although many clinicians, parents, and researchers cite increased levels of self-esteem as a key treatment goal (38), there exist several studies demonstrating poorer treatment response in subsets of externalizing children with either elevated self-esteem (39) or self-confidence (40). This research highlights the possibility that current clinical practice may promote inaccurate and overly positive self-perceptions in these children, therefore making them more resistant to therapeutic change. It seems likely that the failure of these children to recognize their own incompetence in essential domains of functioning means that they see no need for improvement and thus have no motivation for treatment. In fact, Gresham et al. (21) suggest that this population of children may best be served by interventions targeting self-control and "humility training" (p. 405), the goal of which would be to decrease these children's self-views to a more realistic level. However, this is a radical departure from common clinical intuition, and we feel that outcomes associated with a positive illusory style of self-perception over time should be examined before definite recommendations are made.

The competing explanations for the existence of positive illusions imply different effective treatments for children with positive illusory biases, and it consequently is impossible for us to make specific recommendations at this time. If the positive illusions of children with ADHD stem from cognitive skill deficits, then this bias may not be easily altered by feedback of any kind. Current behavioral treatments that operate by modifying the child's environment through the use of incentives may therefore remain the best strategy. The self-protective hypothesis, however, implies that clinicians and parents may need to praise the successes of children with ADHD and downplay their failures. Taking this tactic may permit positive illusory children with ADHD to relax their defenses, evaluate their competence more realistically, and therefore perhaps understand the necessity of change. Finally, accepting Kruger and Dunning's (37) explanation of positive illusions as the inevitable consequence of incompetence implies that teaching positive illusory children to become competent in their domains of greatest deficit may ameliorate positive illusory self-perceptions. All of these recommendations, however, are purely speculatory at this time; at present, it seems most prudent to recommend that clinicians continue to employ existing interventions in order to increase the competence of children with ADHD (consequently making these children's competence more congruent with their self-views). Future researchers must determine the true cause of positive illusions and the function that these illusions serve prior to amending existing interventions.

REFERENCES

1. American Psychiatric Association. Diagnostic and Statistical Manual of Mental Disorders. 4th ed., text revision. Washington, D.C.: Author, 2000.
2. Anastopoulos AD, Barkley RA. Attention deficit-hyperactivity disorder. In: Walker DE, Roberts MC, eds. Handbook of Clinical Child Psychology. 2nd ed. New York: John Wiley & Sons, 1992:413–30.
3. Hinshaw SP. Attention-deficit/hyperactivity disorder: the search for viable treatments. In: Kendall PC, ed. Child and Adolescent Therapy: Cognitive Behavioral Procedures. 2nd ed. New York: Guilford, 2000:88–128.
4. Hoza B, Owens JS, Pelham WE. Attention-deficit/hyperactivity disorder. In: Ammerman RT, Hersen M, Last CG, eds. Handbook of Prescriptive Treatments for Children and Adolescents. Boston: Allyn & Bacon, 1999:63–83.
5. Cole DA. Relation of social and academic competence to depressive symptoms in childhood. J Abnorm Psychol 1990; 99:422–9.
6. Cole DA. Preliminary support for a competency-based model of depression in children. J Abnorm Psychol 1991; 2:181–90.
7. Cole DA, Martin JM, Powers B. A competency-based model of child depression: a longitudinal study of peer, parent, teacher, and self-evaluations. J Child Psychol Psychiatry 1997; 38:505–14.
8. Harter S. The Construction of the Self: A Developmental Perspective. New York: Guilford, 1999.
9. Horn WF, Wagner AE, Ialongo N. Sex differences in school-aged children with pervasive attention deficit hyperactivity disorder. J Abnorm Child Psychol 1989; 17:109–25.
10. Ialongo NS, Lopez M, Horn WF, Pascoe JM, Greenberg G. Effects of psychostimulant medication on self-perceptions of competence, control, and mood in children with attention deficit hyperactivity disorder. J Clin Child Adolesc 1994; 23:161–73.
11. Treuting JJ, Hinshaw SP. Depression and self-esteem in boys with attention-deficit/hyperactivity disorder: associations with comorbid aggression and explanatory attributional mechanisms. J Abnorm Child Psychol 2001; 29:23–39.
12. Diener MB, Milich R. Effects of positive feedback on the social interactions of boys with attention deficit hyperactivity disorder: A test of the self-protective hypothesis. J Clin Child Adolesc 1997; 26:256–65.

13. Hoza B, Pelham WE, Dobbs J, Owens JS, Pillow DR. Do boys with attention-deficit/hyperactivity disorder have positive illusory self-concepts? J Abnorm Psychol 2002; 111:268–78.
14. Hoza B, Pelham WE, Milich R, Pillow D, McBride K. The self-perceptions and attributions of attention deficit hyperactivity disordered and nonreferred boys. J Abnorm Child Psychol 1993; 21:271–86.
15. Hoza B, Pelham WE, Waschbusch DA, Kipp H, Owens JS. Academic task persistence of normally achieving ADHD and control boys: performance, self-evaluations, and attributions. J Consult Clin Psychol 2001; 69:271–83.
16. Hoza B, Waschbusch DA, Pelham WE, Molina BSG, Milich R. Attention-deficit/hyperactivity disordered and control boys' responses to social success and failure. Child Dev 2000; 71:432–46.
17. Edens JF. Aggressive children's self-systems and the quality of their relationships with significant others. Aggress Violent Beh 1999; 4:151–77.
18. Hoza B, Gerdes AC, Hinshaw SP, et al. Self-perceptions of competence in children with ADHD and comparison children. J Consult Clin Psychol 2004; 72:382–91.
19. Asarnow JR, Bates S. Depression in child psychiatric patients: cognitive and attributional patterns. J Abnorm Child Psychol 1988; 6:601–15.
20. Owens JS, Hoza B. The role of inattention and hyperactivity/impulsivity in the positive illusory bias. J Consult Clin Psychol 2003; 71:680–91.
21. Gresham FM, MacMillan DL, Bocian KM, Ward SL, Forness SR. Comorbidity of hyperactivity-impulsivity-inattention and conduct problems: risk factors in social, affective, and academic domains. J Abnorm Psychol 1998; 26:393–406.
22. Gresham FM, Lane KL, MacMillan DL, Bocian KM, Ward SL. Effects of positive and negative illusory biases: comparisons across social and academic self-concept domains. J School Psychol 2000; 38:151–75.
23. Patterson CJ, Kupersmidt JB, Griesler PC. Children's perceptions of self and of relationships with others as a function of sociometric status. Child Dev 1990; 61:1335–49.
24. Edens JF, Cavell TA, Hughes JN. The self-systems of aggressive children: a cluster-analytic investigation. J Child Psychol Psychiatry 1999; 40:441–53.
25. David CF, Kistner JA. Do positive self-perceptions have a "dark side"? Examination of the link between perceptual bias and aggression. J Abnorm Child Psychol 2000; 28:327–37.
26. Hess LE, Atkins MS. Victims and aggressors at school: teacher, self and peer perceptions of psychosocial functioning. Appl Dev Sci 1998; 2:75–89.
27. Hughes JN, Cavell TA, Grossman PB. A positive view of self: risk or protection for aggressive children? Dev Psychopathol 1997; 9:75–94.
28. Hymel S, Bowker A, Woody E. Aggressive versus withdrawn unpopular children: variations in peer and self-perceptions in multiple domains. Child Dev 1993; 64:879–96.
29. Schneider MJ, Leitenberg H. A comparison of aggressive and withdrawn children's self-esteem, optimism and pessimism, and causal attributions for success and failure. J Abnorm Child Psychol 1989; 17:133–44.

30. Webster-Stratton C, Lindsay DW. Social competence and conduct problems in young children: issues in assessment. J Clin Child Adolesc 1999; 28:25–43.
31. Hinshaw SP. On the distinction between attentional deficits/hyperactivity and conduct problems/aggression in child psychopathology. Psychol Bull 1987; 101: 443–63.
32. Barkley RA. Behavioral inhibition, sustained attention, and executive functions: constructing a unifying theory of ADHD. Psychol Bull 1997; 121:65–94.
33. Ownsworth TL, McFarland K, Young RM. The investigation of factors underlying deficits in self-awareness and self-regulation. Brain Inj 2002; 16: 291–309.
34. Abikoff H. Cognitive training in ADHD children: less to it than meets the eye. J Learn Disabil 1991; 24:205–9.
35. Pelham WE, Wheeler T, Chronis A. Empirically supported psychosocial treatments for attention deficit hyperactivity disorder. J Clin Child Adolesc 1998; 27:190–205.
36. Ohan JL, Johnston C. Are the performance over-estimates given by boys with ADHD self-protective? J Consult Clin Psychol 2002; 31:230–41.
37. Kruger J, Dunning D. Unskilled and unaware of it: How difficulties in recognizing one's own incompetence lead to inflated self-assessments. J Pers Soc Psychol 1999; 77:1121–34.
38. Kuhne M, Schachar R, Tannock R. Impact of comorbid oppositional or conduct problems on attention-deficit hyperactivity disorder. J Am Acad Child Adolesc Psychiatry 1997; 36:1715–25.
39. Lochman JE, Lampron LB, Burch PR, Curry JF. Client characteristics associated with behavior change for treated and untreated aggressive boys. J Abnorm Child Psychol 1985; 13:527–38.
40. Hoza B, Pelham WE. Social-cognitive predictors of treatment response in children with ADHD. J Soc Clin Psychol 1995; 14:23–5.

5

The Family Context of ADHD

Charlotte Johnston and Douglas Scoular
Department of Psychology, University of British Columbia, Vancouver, British Columbia, Canada

The families of children with attention deficit hyperactivity disorder (ADHD) have been the focus of investigations for more than a quarter of a century (1,2), with interest in areas such as parent–child interactions, parental characteristics, as well as marital relations and family involvement in the treatment process. This research, although largely descriptive in nature, has provided ample documentation of the areas in which these families are likely to face challenges, as well as areas of strength. Recently, research concerning families of children with ADHD has been characterized by a progressive understanding of the relation between family or parental characteristics and the conduct problems that commonly co-occur in children with ADHD. Given necessary space limitations, in this chapter we have chosen to highlight research in five domains of functioning within families of children with ADHD including parent–child interactions, parental psychopathology, parental cognitions, marital relationships, and the role of families in treatment.

As a background to this review, we note the need for a developmentally informed and interactive model for understanding how childhood ADHD interacts over time with the family context in which the child resides (3). Such a developmental psychopathology conceptualization is necessary to allow integration of what is known about the families of children with ADHD with new and increasing information concerning the characteristics of children with the disorder, including their biological or genetic make-up. Despite strong evidence for an underlying biological origin in ADHD (4), the heterogeneity of clinical presentations of ADHD suggests diverse pathways in the development of the disorder, and it is likely that this diversity reflects the interaction of cultural, social, and biological factors over time (5,6). Within such a framework, the child's behavior is understood to influence the functioning of the family, and at the same time, the behaviors of other family members exert an impact on the child. This approach encourages identification of risk and protective factors within the child and family context that, acting at different points in time across the child's development, might serve to accelerate or buffer the development of ADHD symptomatology or accompanying conduct problems. For example, a child's early difficult temperament may serve as a risk factor for emerging problems in parenting responsiveness and together these child and parent difficulties may exacerbate the child's inattentive or impulsive behavior. Alternately, a family's ability to respond to challenging child behaviors with sensitive modeling or teaching of effective self-regulation strategies may serve to protect the child from escalating difficulties with inattention/impulsivity, or alternately, to prevent the development of an oppositional pattern of behavior. Thus, we argue that conceptualizing the relations between family characteristics and child ADHD as interactive and constantly evolving is important in understanding, not only the development of ADHD, but also the co-occurrence of ADHD and oppositional or conduct problems (7,8).

PARENT–CHILD INTERACTIONS AND PARENTING BEHAVIORS

Numerous studies have identified high levels of both parent and child aversive behaviors in interactions in families of children with ADHD. Compared to families of nonproblem children, children with ADHD are more aversive and less compliant, and their parents are more negative, directive, and less socially engaging (9,10). Similar difficulties in parent-child interactions have been reported for both boys and girls with ADHD (11), from preschool through adolescent ages (12,13), and in father–child as well as mother–child interactions (14). Thus, parent–child interaction difficulties are a well-established characteristic of families of children with ADHD.

However, questions remain regarding the extent to which these difficulties are associated with ADHD versus with comorbid child conduct problems. Johnston (15) and Gomez and Sanson (16) both found higher levels of negative and noncompliant child behavior in children with comorbid ADHD and conduct problems compared to children with only ADHD or to nonproblem children. However, Gomez and Sanson observed more directive, negative, and less rewarding behaviors by mothers in a comorbid group as compared to the other two groups, whereas Johnston reported no differences in observed mother or father behavior among the three groups. Johnston did find, however, that parents in both the ADHD only and ADHD/conduct problems groups reported less optimal parenting strategies compared to the nonproblem group. Supporting the need to focus on positive as well as problematic aspects of parent–child interactions,

Lindahl (17) found that, although parent–child conflict distinguished both ADHD and comorbid children from nonproblem families, it was positive family interactions that best discriminated between families of children with only ADHD and families of children with conduct problems. Similarly, Johnston et al. (18) found that, among families of children with ADHD, maternal responsiveness in parent–child interactions was related to the child's level of conduct problems, but was not related to the child's level of ADHD symptomatology.

In general, across the range of child ages and a variety of dimensions of parenting or parent–child interactions, results from cross-sectional studies clearly suggest more difficulties in families of children with ADHD and co-occurring conduct problems in contrast to families of nonproblem children. However, whether parent–child interactions in families of children with only ADHD are most similar to nonproblem families or to the comorbid group, or fall between these groups varies across studies. Unfortunately, cross-sectional studies are unable to address issues related to how parenting and child characteristics may interact in the development of child problems or parent–child interaction difficulties over time. Longitudinal studies conducted in community samples have suggested that difficulties in parenting behavior are more strongly predictive of continuation of child conduct problems than of the continuation of ADHD symptoms (19) and that parenting problems may combine with child ADHD behaviors to predict the highest risk of child aggression (20). More such longitudinal, prospective studies measuring a range of parenting behaviors and styles and a range of child behavioral tendencies are needed to elucidate the development and course of these family problems and child outcomes.

PARENTAL PSYCHOPATHOLOGY

Elevations in a variety of forms of parental psychopathology have been found in families of both male and female children with ADHD, in both mothers and fathers, and across a range of child ages (11,21,22). However, as with the research into parent–child interactions, in many instances it appears that difficulties in parental psychological functioning may be linked more closely to conduct problems than to ADHD (13,23), although such findings are not entirely consistent (15,24).

One aspect of parental psychopathology that has received considerable attention, particularly among mothers of children with ADHD, is depression. Several studies have identified higher rates of depression in mothers of children with ADHD as compared to mothers of nonproblem children (11,22). Many, although not all, of these studies suggest that problems with depression are particularly likely among mothers of children with both ADHD and conduct problems, or in families with more than one child with

ADHD (25). Other studies have focused on parental antisocial behavior, particularly among fathers of children with ADHD. These studies quite clearly indicate that parental antisocial behavior is most closely related to the presence of comorbid child conduct problems rather than to ADHD per se (23,26). Still other studies have focused on parental alcohol problems and found higher rates of alcohol use in parents of children with ADHD as compared to parents of nonproblem children (22,27). Again, it seems clear that this elevation in parental alcohol abuse is more strongly associated with child conduct problems, including physical aggression, than with ADHD symptomatology (28). High rates of ADHD also have been reported among parents of children with ADHD (29). Here, in contrast to the findings for depression, antisocial behavior, and alcohol abuse, where the relation seems to be stronger with child conduct problems, ADHD among parents appears most closely related to the child's problems with ADHD (25,30).

As with the study of parent–child interactions, much more work is needed to understand how various aspects of parental psychological functioning interact with child characteristics in the development and maintenance of child ADHD and conduct problems. A few glimpses of the types of research that will inform this area can be found. For example, one can easily imagine how a parent's own difficulties with ADHD would interfere with his/her ability to monitor and manage challenging child behavior. So far, both case studies and more controlled studies have supported this speculation that impairment of parenting skills may play a role in mediating the association between parent and child ADHD symptoms (31,32,33). Another example of the type of work that is needed in this area comes from an interesting series of studies by Lang and colleagues (34,35). These studies demonstrated both that difficult child behavior can elicit increased alcohol consumption among parents, and that consumption of alcohol increases inappropriate parenting behaviors such as demandingness, indulgence, failure to attend to the child, and off-task comments.

PARENTAL COGNITIONS

The study of social cognitions among parents of children with ADHD is an emerging area of research. To date, focus has been on two primary types of cognitions: parenting efficacy and attributions for child behavior. Given the parent–child difficulties in families of children with ADHD, it is not surprising that several studies have reported diminished parenting satisfaction and efficacy among parents of children with ADHD, with children ranging from preschool to school age (36,37). Considering how parenting sense of efficacy relates to child conduct problems, Johnston (15) found that both mothers and fathers of ADHD children with comorbid conduct problems reported lower levels of parenting competence than parents of children with

ADHD alone, and both of these groups were lower than parents of nonproblem children. Thus, as with parent–child interactions, parents' thoughts about their parenting competence appear most at risk in those parents who must face the challenges of a child with both ADHD and conduct problems.

Other research has focused on the causal attributions that parents offer for the behavior of children with ADHD. Across a variety of assessment methods, compared to parents of nonproblem children, parents of children with ADHD see both the symptoms of ADHD and child conduct problems as caused by uncontrollable, stable factors within the child, but see children's positive behavior as less dispositional and see themselves as less responsible for child behaviors (38,39). A necessary next step in this research is to determine whether the differences found in attributions across parents of nonproblem children and children with ADHD are related to differences in parenting reactions to the children, and to subsequent differences in child behavior, and to map the mutual influences among child and parent behavior and parental cognitions in families of children with ADHD.

MARITAL RELATIONSHIPS

Studies examining marital relationships in families of children with ADHD have generated inconsistent findings. Some have reported more marital conflict and less satisfaction in couples with children with ADHD as compared to couples with nonproblem children (11,36); however, these results have not always been replicated (40). Although researchers have looked to comorbid conduct problems as an explanation for these mixed findings, here again the results are not entirely consistent. Reports of greater marital difficulties in parents of children with ADHD and comorbid conduct problems as compared to parents of children with only ADHD have been reported (17), but so have reports of no differences in martial functioning among the two groups of ADHD children (15,41). In sum, although disrupted martial relationships may characterize some families of children with ADHD, this is far from universal and much remains to be discovered about which child or parental characteristics are most closely linked to functioning within the marital system.

FAMILY INVOLVEMENT IN TREATMENT

Parents play essential roles in both the pharmacological and psychosocial treatments that have been shown to be efficacious for treating children with ADHD. Parents are central, not only in decisions regarding choice of treatment, but also in the implementation and maintenance of these treatments. For example, the efficacy of stimulant medication in reducing a child's ADHD symptoms has been suggested to vary depending upon the type of medication management support and advice received by the parents (42). Child attitudes and beliefs (43), as well as parental knowledge of ADHD (44) appear predictive of medication adherence. Greater research of the interplay of these factors as predictors of initial and ongoing treatment utilization will be important in advancing our knowledge of the role that families play in pharmacological treatments. Parents also play a crucial role in implementation of effective psychosocial treatments for children with ADHD (45), particularly behavioral parent training. Such programs are designed to alter parenting strategies so as to reduce disruptive child behaviors. The parents' willingness and ability to engage in psychosocial treatments, as well as their success in implementing the recommended strategies is a crucial determinant of the success of these treatments in improving child outcomes.

Not surprisingly, the elevated levels of intrapersonal or marital difficulties that often occur in parents of children with ADHD or ADHD and conduct problems can stand as significant obstacles to parents' effective involvement in the treatment of the child's ADHD. However, on a more optimistic note, and consistent with the interactional view of child ADHD and family functioning that we presented earlier, both pharmacological and behavioral treatments for ADHD have been demonstrated to hold promise in reducing parental distress, improving marital distress, and improving feelings of parenting competence (46,47).

CONCLUSION

We have presented a brief review of aspects of family functioning that are related to ADHD in children, and tried to elucidate the extent to which these associations between family and child characteristics are specific to the child's ADHD symptoms or to co-occurring conduct problems. We also have argued for a transactional approach as a method to conceptualize how dimensions of family functioning interact with child characteristics over time, and may function to influence, not only the severity but also the type of child problem. This approach recognizes that the vast majority of research is clear in ruling out the possibility that aspects of family functioning, such as parenting, are the primary cause of childhood ADHD. Instead, an interactive model argues that the characteristics of children (including biological predispositions to ADHD) are involved in a mutually influential dance through time with the environment of the family. Difficulties inherent in children are likely to serve as risk factors for a family's functioning, while at the same time aspects of the family context, such as less than optimal parenting, may exacerbate the nature and extent of the child's difficulties.

REFERENCES

1. Battle ES, Lacey B. A context for hyperactivity in children, over time. Child Develop 1972; 43:757–73.
2. Campbell SB. Mother–child interactions in reflective, impulsive, and hyperactive children. Develop Psychol 1973; 8:341–9.
3. Johnston C, Mash EJ. Families of children with Attention Deficit Hyperactivity Disorder: review and recommendations for future research. Clinl Child Fam Psychol Rev 2001; 43:183–207.
4. Kuntsi J, Stevenson J. Hyperactivity in children: a focus on genetic research and psychological theories. Clin Child Fam Psychol Rev 2000; 3:1–24.
5. Campbell SB. Attention-Deficit/Hyperactivity Disorder: a developmental view. In: Sameroff AJ, Lewis M, Miller SM, eds. Handbook of Developmental Psychopathology. 2nd ed. New York: Kluwer Academic/Plenum Publishers, 2000:383–401.
6. Rutter M, Sroufe LA. Developmental psychopathology: concepts and challenges. Develop Psychopathol 2000; 12:265–96.
7. Frick, PJ. Family dysfunction and the disruptive behavior disorders: a review of recent empirical findings. Adv Clin Child Psychol 1994; 16:203–26.
8. Taylor E, Chadwick O, Heptinstall E, Danckaerts M. Hyperactivity and conduct problems as risk factors for adolescent development. J Am Acad Child Adolesc Psychiatry 1996; 35:1213–26.
9. Cunningham CE, Barkley RA. The interactions of hyperactive and normal children with their mothers in free play and structured task. Child Develop 1979; 50:217–24.
10. Mash EJ, Johnston C. A comparison of the mother–child interactions of younger and older hyperactive and normal children. Child Develop 1982; 53: 1371–82.
11. Befera MS, Barkley RA. Hyperactive and normal girls and boys: mother child interaction parent psychiatric status and child psychopathology. J Child Psychol Psychiatry 1985; 26:439–52.
12. DuPaul GJ, McGoey KE, Eckert TL, VanBrakle J. Preschool children with Attention-Deficit/Hyperactivity Disorder: impairments in behavioral social and school functioning. J Am Acad Child Adolesc Psychiatry 2001; 40:508–15.
13. Barkley RA, Fischer M, Edelbrock C, Smallish L. The adolescent outcome of hyperactive children diagnosed by research criteria. III. Mother child interactions family conflicts and maternal psychopathology. J Child Psychol Psychiatry 1991; 32:233–55.
14. Tallmadge J, Barkley RA. The interactions of hyperactive and normal boys with their mothers and fathers. J Abnorm Child Psychol 1983; 11:565–79.
15. Johnston C. Parent characteristics and parent–child interactions in families of nonproblem children and ADHD children with higher and lower levels of oppositional-defiant behavior. J Abnorm Child Psychol 1996; 24:85–104.
16. Gomez R, Sanson AV. Mother child interactions and noncompliance in hyperactive boys with and without conduct problems. J Child Psychol Psychiatry 1994; 35:477–90.
17. Lindahl KM. Family process variables and children's disruptive behavior problems. J Fam Psychol 1998; 12:420–36.

18. Johnston C, Murray C, Hinshaw SP, Pelham WE, Hoza B. Responsiveness in interactions of mothers and sons with ADHD: relationships to maternal and child characteristics. J Abnorm Child Psychol 2002; 30:77–88.
19. August GJ, Realmuto GM, Joyce R, Hektner JM. Persistence and desistance of oppositional defiant disorder in a community sample of children with ADHD. J Am Acad Child Adolesc Psychiatry 1999; 38:1262–70.
20. Colder CR, Lochman JE, Wells KC. The moderating effects of children's fear and activity levels of relations between parenting practices and childhood symptomatology. J Abnorm Child Psychol 1997; 25:251–63.
21. Nigg JT, Hinshaw SP. Parent personality traits and psychopathology associated with antisocial behaviors in childhood attention deficit hyperactivity disorder. J Child Psychol Psychiatry 1998; 39:145–59.
22. Cunningham CE, Benness BB, Siegel LS. Family functioning time allocation and parental depression in the families of normal and ADHD children. J Clin Child Psychol 1988; 17:169–77.
23. Frick PJ, Kuper K, Silverthorn P, Cotter M. Antisocial behavior somatization and sensation-seeking behavior in mothers of clinic-referred children. J Am Acad Child Adolesc Psychiatry 1995; 34:805–12.
24. Faraone SV, Biederman J. Nature nurture and attention deficit hyperactivity disorder. Develop Rev 2000; 20:568–81.
25. Stormont-Spurgin M, Zentall SS. Contributing factors in the manifestation of aggression in preschoolers with hyperactivity. J Child Psychol Psychiatry 1995; 36:491–509.
26. Biederman J, Munir K, Knee D. Conduct and oppositional disorder in clinically referred children with attention deficit disorder: a controlled family study. J Am Acad Child Adolesc Psychiatry 1987; 26:724–7.
27. Gadow KD, Nolan EE, Litcher L, et al. Comparison of Attention-Deficit/Hyperactivity Disorder symptoms syndromes in Ukrainian schoolchildren. J Am Acad Child Adolesc Psychiatry 2000; 39:1520–7.
28. Carbonneau R, Tremblay RE, Vitaro F, Dobkin PL, Saucier JF, Pihl RO. Paternal alcoholism paternal absence and the development of problem behaviors in boys from age six to twelve years. J Stud Alcohol 1998; 59:387–98.
29. Biederman J, Faraone SV, Mick E, et al. High risk for attention deficit hyperactivity disorder among children of parents with childhood onset of the disorder: a pilot study. J Am Psychiatry 1995; 152:431–5.
30. Faraone SV, Biederman J, Chen W, Milberger S. Genetic heterogeneity in attention deficit hyperactivity disorder ADHD: gender psychiatric comorbidity and maternal ADHD. J Abnorm Psychol 1995; 104:334–45.
31. Evans SW, Vallano G, Pelham W. Treatment of parenting behavior with a psychostimulant: a case study of an adult with attention deficit hyperactivity disorder. J Child Adolesc Psychopharmacol 1994; 4:63–9.
32. Daly JM, Fritsch SL. Case study: maternal residual attention deficit disorder associated with failure to thrive in a two month old infant. J Am Acad Child Adolesc Psychiatry 1995; 34:55–7.
33. Murray C, Johnston C. Parenting in mothers with and without Attention-Deficit-Hyperactivity Disorder. J Abnorm Psychol 2006; 115:52–61.

34. Pelham WE, Lang AR, Atkeson B, et al. Effects of deviant child behavior on parental alcohol consumption: stress induced drinking in parents of ADHD children. Am J Addict 1998; 7:103–14.
35. Lang AR, Pelham WE, Atkeson BM, Murphy DA. Effects of alcohol intoxication on parenting behavior in interactions with child confederates exhibiting normal or deviant behaviors. J Abnorm Child Psychol 1999; 27: 177–89.
36. Shelton TL, Barkley RA, Crosswait C, et al. Psychiatric and psychological morbidity as a function of adaptive disability in preschool children with aggressive and hyperactive impulsive inattentive behavior. J Abnorm Child Psychol 1998; 26:475–94.
37. Mash EJ, Johnston C. Sibling interactions of hyperactive and normal children and their relationship to reports of maternal stress and self-esteem. J Clin Child Psychol 1983; 12:91–9.
38. Johnston C, Freeman WS. Attributions for child behavior in parents of children without behavior disorders and children with attention deficit hyperactivity disorder. J Consult Clin Psychol 1997; 65:636–45.
39. Johnston C, Reynolds S, Freeman WS, Geller J. Assessing parent attributions for child behavior using open-ended questions. J Clin Child Psychol 1998; 27: 87–97.
40. Szatmari P, Offord DR, Boyle MH. Correlates associated impairments and patterns of service utilization of children with attention deficit disorder: findings from the Ontario Child Health Study. J Child Psychol Psychiatry 1989; 30:205–17.
41. Stormont-Spurgin M, Zentall S. Child rearing practices associated with aggression in youth with and without ADHD: An exploratory study. Int J Disabil Develop Educ 1996; 43:135–46.
42. Jensen PS, Hinshaw SP, Swanson JM, et al. Findings from the NIMH Multimodal Treatment Study of ADHD MTA: implications and applications for primary care providers. J Develop Behav Pediatr 2001; 221:60–73.
43. Efron D, Jarman FC, Barker MJ. Child and parent perceptions of stimulant medication treatment in attention deficit hyperactivity disorder. J Pediatric Child Health 1998; 343:288–92.
44. Firestone P. Factors associated with children's adherence to stimulant medication. Am J Orthopsychiatry 1982; 52:447–57.
45. Pelham WE, Wheeler T, Chronis A. Empirically supported psychosocial treatments for attention deficit hyperactivity disorder. J Clin Child Psychol 1998; 272:190–205.
46. Pisterman S, Firestone P, McGrath P, Goodman J. The effects of parent training on parenting stress and sense of competence. Can J Behav Sci 1992; 241:41–58.
47. Anastopoulos A, Shelton T, DuPaul G, Guevremont D. Parent training for attention-deficit hyperactivity disorder: its impact on parent functioning. J Abnorm Child Psychol 1993; 215:581–96.

6

Comorbidity as an Organizing Principle

Linda J. Pfiffner

Department of Psychiatry, University of California San Francisco, San Francisco, California, U.S.A.

Most children presenting to clinics and meeting the diagnosis of ADHD also have one or more comorbid disruptive behavior or emotional disorders (1). It is increasingly clear that consideration of these disorders is critical to sharpen our conceptualization of ADHD and its etiologies, to the diagnostic process, and to treatment choice and outcome. This chapter discusses the impact and implications of comorbid disruptive behavior, anxiety, and depressive disorders.

OPPOSITIONAL DEFIANT DISORDER AND CONDUCT DISORDER

The two other disruptive behavior disorders, oppositional defiant disorder (ODD) and conduct disorder (CD), are commonly comorbid with ADHD. ODD, present in up to two-thirds or more of cases, is characterized by chronic argumentativeness, defiance, and anger (2). The more pernicious CD, involving serious violations of societal norms, is present in a quarter to half of all cases (2–4). ODD is generally considered a milder disorder than CD, but it is far from benign: it is associated with functional impairment and disturbed interpersonal relations, and in some cases it progresses to CD. Children having both ADHD and CD have more learning problems, neuropsychological deficits, and poorer prognosis with high rates of antisocial outcomes (1). The combination of ADHD and CD is associated with an earlier age of onset for CD and more persistent and serious conduct problems (5).

Multiple risk factors related to heredity and family environment have been linked to each of the disruptive behavior disorders (6). The association between paternal antisocial personality disorder (APD) and child CD in boys with ADHD has been replicated in several studies (7–9). Weaker associations have been reported for paternal APD and comorbid ODD in children with ADHD (8,10) with some studies showing no association (11). Parental depression also has been linked to disruptive behavior in children, perhaps via common familial vulnerabilities (2), via an association with parental antisocial behaviors (11), or due to the difficulty of raising children with a disruptive behavior disorder. There is less evidence for a specific association between parental anxiety and disruptive behavior disorders, particularly when comorbid anxiety in the child is controlled (2,10).

Parenting practices form a second set of family risk factors for comorbid externalizing disorders. Dysfunctional parenting is common in families with children having ADHD and may partly be a reaction to the difficulties of raising a child with ADHD; it may also serve an etiological role in the emergence of comorbid disruptive behavior disorders (6). Consistent with social learning theory, children with oppositional and conduct problems often have families characterized by coercive interaction styles, inconsistent discipline, lack of parental involvement, and lack of positive and warm interactions between parent and child (12–14). Recent studies with ADHD children suggest that certain kinds of dysfunctional parenting, including maternal lack of responsiveness (6,15), lack of warmth and positive involvement, overly negative discipline (16), lax and inconsistent parenting, and a lack of cohesion among family members (17), are related to comorbid oppositional or conduct problems rather than ADHD per se. Comorbid externalizing problems are also predictive of dysfunction in the sibling relationship with greater conflict and less warmth/closeness among siblings of children with these problems than those without (18).

Pfiffner et al. (11) compared parenting practices of parents of children with ADHD only versus ADHD+ODD versus ADHD+CD. Similarly negative and ineffective disciplinary styles were found among parents of children with either of these disruptive behaviour disorders (DBDs) relative to those of children without a comorbid DBD. In family process theories (14), negative/ineffective discipline is related to compliance problems and to negative, coercive interchanges. The results are consistent with a bidirectional model (6): the behavioral challenges exhibited by difficult children tax and degrade primary caregivers' limit-setting capabilities and in turn, caregivers' ineffective discipline reinforces children's oppositional and conduct problems.

On the other hand, Pfiffner et al. (11) found that mothers' lack of positive involvement (including warmth and interpersonal involvement) was associated with an increased risk that a child with ADHD would develop comorbid CD, but not comorbid ODD. The apparent risk posed by this factor is consistent with long-standing notions that antisocial personality development is often accompanied by impoverished attachment and affective development (19–21). Interestingly, dysfunctional parenting was related to CD primarily in families without paternal APD. If the odds of developing CD were already increased due to the presence of a father with APD symptoms, dysfunctional parenting was not strongly associated with further increase. A possible interpretation is that dysfunctional parenting can lead to failures of socialization and affective development, but that a similar outcome might occur if children inherit temperamental risks from APD fathers. In other words, this finding of moderator effects is consistent with the idea that CD can result from multiple causal pathways (22).

Treatments effective for ADHD are also useful for comorbid ODD and CD. Stimulant medication shows benefit for ODD and CD symptoms, decreasing ODD and overt and covert conduct disorder symptoms at dosages similar to those used to treat ADHD symptoms (23). Likewise, children with ADHD and comorbid ODD or CD show a similarly positive response to stimulant medication as those with only ADHD (24,25) and antisocial behaviors such as stealing and fighting can be reduced with stimulant medication (26). Behavioral interventions are also beneficial for addressing many of the associated impairments with ODD or CD including parent–child dysfunction (27) and social skills problems (28,29). Treatment implications of the parenting findings reviewed above include the need to target parenting skills on the part of mothers and fathers related to effective limit-setting and discipline as covered in parent training programs (30–32). Deficiencies in bonding, positive involvement, and attachment may be addressed by parent training components such as strategic activities to increase positive, nonjudgmental parent–child involvement (e.g., "Child's Game"), specific praise and positive reinforcement programs as well as effective communication strategies to enhance the quality of the positive relationship between parent and child. The child's sibling relationships should also be strengthened given the likelihood for conflict and lack of closeness. In more serious cases of comorbid CD and delinquency, multisystemic therapy (MST) may be indicated (33).

ANXIETY DISORDERS

As many as one-quarter to one-half of ADHD cases meet criteria for one or more anxiety disorders (1). Although, far less studied than comorbid disruptive behavior disorders, ADHD with comorbid anxiety appears to be associated with distinct correlates, outcomes, and response to treatment that have lead to consideration of ADHD plus anxiety as a distinct subgroup of ADHD (1). Children with ADHD and anxiety are less impulsive (34,35) but have impaired working memory (36), report more school and social difficulties (2) and experience more stressful life events and parental separations and divorce (2,37) relative to those with ADHD only.

Little is known about the origin of anxiety disorders in children with ADHD or about the underlying mechanisms for their differential response to treatment. However, genetic vulnerability is one possible etiological pathway given that genetic heritability of anxiety is estimated to be moderate (38). Several studies with ADHD children support family transmission. Biederman et al. (39) found through a familial risk analysis that relatives of children with ADHD plus an anxiety disorder had a greater risk for anxiety than relatives of children with ADHD but without an anxiety disorder, with risk for anxiety disorders being higher for mothers than for fathers. Pfiffner et al. (10) found a strong association between parental anxiety disorders and child comorbid (with ADHD) anxiety disorders, even while controlling for the significant association of parental depressive disorders and child comorbid anxiety disorders. This finding was replicated in a recent study by Pfiffner and McBurnett (40).

Parenting may also play a role in the development of anxiety. Pfiffner and McBurnett (40) report that positive contingent responsiveness and overprotectiveness/possessiveness are key parenting practices specifically associated with anxiety, rather than with disruptive behavior disorders or general psychopathology. These results are most consistent with a model specifying three family factors (maternal anxiety, overprotectiveness, and lack of positive parenting) as distinct correlates of child comorbid anxiety. The greatest risk for child anxiety occurs when all three of these factors are present. This outcome would be predicted by combining the ideas of Parker (41)—that it is the combination of inadequate care and excessive protectiveness (rather than either in isolation) that is particularly anxiogenic—with the findings of Moore et al. (42)—that child anxiety is related to parenting practices independent of any relationship to maternal anxiety. Using a community sample, Kepley and Ostrander (43) also reported that the family environment of children with ADHD and comorbid anxiety was more insular and discouraging of autonomy than that of children without anxiety. Based on patterns with anxious, non-ADHD youth, additional parenting factors to consider in the development of anxiety among ADHD youth include excessively high parental expectations, modeling of anxious behaviors, and parental support for avoidant solutions to problems.

It is noteworthy that comorbid anxiety in ADHD frequently co-occurs with CD (44) and there is evidence that doubly comorbid children are especially impaired (45). The association between anxiety and CD may have significance for understanding family factors associated with comorbid anxiety based on recent theorizing that anxiety in the presence of CD is quite different than in its absence. The former is reported to reflect negative affectivity resulting from perceptions that negative consequences are inevitable, perhaps due to repeated frustrations and failures. The latter is reported to be “classic” anxiety or fearfulness, resulting from sensitivity to cues of impending danger, and is the more traditional form of anxiety (46). In children with ADHD, anxiety has been described as being more like negative affectivity than fearfulness, perhaps due to the frequent co-occurrence of anxiety and CD in this group of children (44). It is possible that anxiety accompanied by CD may have family correlates that are more similar to those of CD (e.g., discipline problems) than those of fearfulness (e.g., overprotectiveness). However, the moderating role of CD in the associations between family factors and anxiety has been unexplored.

Based on the findings reported above, children with ADHD and an anxiety disorder will likely benefit from parenting programs that promote frequent, contingent, and specific positive feedback, but they could also benefit from specific strategies to encourage steps toward independence and developmentally appropriate risk-taking. The commonly found presence of anxiety in mothers of children with ADHD and comorbid anxiety is an important consideration, because unrecognized parental anxiety can be an impediment to full participation in the therapeutic process. Also, clinicians should be prepared to assess other likely targets for intervention (e.g., child cognitions, parent anxiety, family support of avoidance behaviors, etc.) based on the presence of comorbid anxiety. The additive benefit of including, for example, a cognitive behavior therapy component for children to the parenting component for parents seems to make clinical sense but has not been evaluated.

Several studies report that comorbid anxiety decreases response of children with ADHD to methylphenidate (47,48). However, more recent studies show similar response to stimulant medication in ADHD children with and without comorbid anxiety (24,49). In the NIMH collaborative MTA study, comorbid anxiety-moderated response to treatment such that those with anxiety responded equally well to medication and/or behavioral interventions while those without anxiety tended to benefit relatively more from medication. Those with comorbid anxiety and ODD or CD responded best to a combination of medication and behavioral interventions (24). While further study is needed, the preponderance of evidence suggests that comorbid anxiety is not a contraindication for stimulant treatment, although monitoring of possible side effects of increased anxiety and over-focusing has been recommended (50). Furthermore, evidence exists that among children with ADHD and anxiety who are being treated with a stimulant, the addition of an selective serotonin reuptake inhibitor (SSRI) does not provide added benefit (51).

DEPRESSIVE DISORDERS

Comorbid depressive disorders appear to be somewhat less common among youth with ADHD than either comorbid anxiety or disruptive behavior disorders during the early school years (24). However, rates of mood disorders are still estimated in the 10% to 30% range and are higher among those with ADHD than comparison children (2,50,52). Even in the absence of a clinical depressive disorder, demoralization and low self-esteem are very common among youth with ADHD, particularly among those who are also aggressive (53). The repeated social and academic failures experienced by those ADHD may indeed lead to depressive symptoms which usually follow onset of ADHD. Although there is likely an interrelationship between the two, evidence supports the notion that ADHD and major depression (MD) are independent and distinct disorders with their combination, particularly when also accompanied by CD (50), associated with significant long-term difficulties (54) including suicidality (55) and exacerbated and prolonged symptoms (56). The few studies conducted on psychosocial risk factors or correlates of comorbid MD have combined internalizing spectrum disorders and show higher levels of stress and depressive symptoms among parents and generally greater levels of family and psychosocial adversity (1). A later age of onset for ADHD has been reported to be correlated with a greater rate of parent-reported child anxious/depressive symptoms (57).

Ample evidence supports a linkage between parental and child depression (58). However, specificity of this relationship in an ADHD sample is not as clear. To investigate familial relationships between ADHD and affective disorders, Biederman et al. (59) compared rates of attention deficit disorder (ADD) and affective disorders among family members of youth with either ADHD only, ADHD plus an affective disorders or neither. They found higher rates of ADHD diagnoses among family members of those with ADHD relative to normal control children, however, rates of affective disorders were similar among the relatives of those with either ADHD or ADHD+ an affective disorder. These results lead the authors to conclude that ADD children with and without an affective disorder share familial etiological factors. However, other studies have failed to show such a strong relationship between ADHD and parental affective disorder (50). The role of comorbid conduct disorder in this relationship is also not clear, although it is possible that CD could account for at least part of the association between ADHD and parental depression given the strong association between ADHD and CD on the one hand and between CD and parental depression on the other.

Few studies exist to guide the medication decisions for youth with ADHD and comorbid MD. Beiderman et al. (60) reports that a tricyclic antidepressant may be particularly effective in addressing depressive symptoms among ADHD youth who also have ADHD, although direct comparison with stimulants was not made. Garfinkel et al. (61) found that tricyclic antidepressants (clomipramine, desipramine) were more effective in reducing affective symptoms among children with ADD than methylphenidate, but were less effective than methylphenidate in reducing ADHD symptoms. In a small sample of children with ADHD and comorbid depression, Emslie et al. (62) reported that most ($N = 9/15$) responded to stimulant treatment without need for subsequent medication for depression, but others who had more severe depressive symptoms were treated with either a combination of ADHD and a SSRI or an SSRI alone. In reviewing these and other studies, Pliszka et al. (63) favorably weighed stimulant treatment to antidepressant treatment when ADHD symptoms predominate and suicidal behavior and vegetative signs are minimal. However, for cases in which depressive symptoms are serious and predominate, antidepressants (SSRIs) were recommended as the initial medication choice.

Use of evidence-based behavioral treatments for ADHD may well improve self-esteem and other depressive symptoms due to improvements in school and social impairments. For example, the MTA study reports benefit for depressive symptoms from combined stimulant treatment and behavioral interventions relative to stimulant treatment alone (64). It is also possible that cognitive behavior therapy directed to the comorbid depression would be helpful, but this has yet to be evaluated empirically.

REFERENCES

1. Jensen PS, Martin D, Cantwell DP. Comorbidity in ADHD: implications for research, practice, and DSM-V. J Am Acad Child Adolesc Psychiatry 1997; 36: 1065–79.
2. Biederman J, Newcorn J, Sprich S. Comorbidity of attention deficit hyperactivity disorder with conduct, depressive, anxiety, and other disorders. Am J Psychiatry 1991; 148:564–77.
3. Barkley RA, DuPaul GJ, McMurray MB. Comprehensive evaluation of attention deficit disorder with and without hyperactivity as defined by research criteria. J Consult Clin Psychol 1990; 58:775–89.
4. Szatmari P, Boyle M, Offord DR. ADDH and conduct disorder: degree of diagnostic overlap and differences among correlates. J Am Acad Child Adolesc Psychiatry 1989; 28:865–72.
5. Lahey BB, McBurnett K, Loeber R. Are attention-deficit/hyperactivity disorder and oppositional defiant disorder developmental precursors to conduct disorder? In: Sameroff AJ, Lewis M, Miller SM, eds. Handbook of Developmental Psychopathology. 2nd ed. New York: Kluwer Academic/ Plenum, 2000.
6. Johnston C, Mash EJ. Families of children with attention-deficit/hyperactivity disorder: review and recommendations for future research. Clin Child Fam Psychol Rev 2001; 4:183–207.
7. Biederman J, Munir K, Knee D. Conduct and oppositional disorder in clinically referred children with attention deficit disorder: a controlled family study. J Am Acad Child Adolesc Psychiatry 1987; 26:724–7.
8. Frick PJ, Lahey BB, Loeber R, Stouthamer-Loeber M. Familial risk factors to oppositional defiant disorder and conduct disorder: parental psychopathology and maternal parenting. J Consult Clin Psychol 1992; 60:49–55.

9. Lahey BB, Piacentini JC, McBurnett K, Stone P, Hartdagen S, Hynd G. Psychopathology in the parents of children with conduct disorder and hyperactivity. J Am Acad Child Adolesc Psychiatry 1988; 27:163–70.
10. Pfiffner LJ, McBurnett K, Lahey BB, et al. Association of parental psychopathology to the comorbid disorders of boys with attention-deficit hyperactivity disorder. J Consult Clin Psychol 1999; 67:881–93.
11. Pfiffner LJ, McBurnett K, Rathouz PJ, Judice S. Family correlates of oppositional and conduct disorders in children with attention deficit hyperactivity disorder. J Abnorm Child Psychol 2005; 33:551–63.
12. Fletcher KE, Fischer M, Barkley RA, Smallish L. A sequential analysis of the mother-adolescent interactions of ADHD, ADHD/ODD, and normal teenagers during neutral and conflict discussions. J Abnorm Child Psychol 1996; 24:271–97.
13. Loeber R, Tengs T. The analysis of coercive chains between children, mothers, and siblings. J Family Violence 1986; 1:51–70.
14. Patterson GR, Reid JB, Dishion TJ. Antisocial Boys. Eugene, OR: Castalia Publishing Company, 1992.
15. Johnston C, Murray C, Hinshaw S, Pelham W, Hoza B. Responsiveness in interactions of mothers and sons with ADHD: relations to maternal and child characteristics. J Abnorm Child Psychol 2002; 30:77–88.
16. Kashdan TB, Jacob R, Pelham W, et al. Depression and anxiety in parents of children with ADHD and varying levels of oppositional defiant behaviors: modeling relationships with family functioning. J Clin Child Adolesc Psychol 2004; 33:169–81.
17. Lindahl K. Family process variables and children's disruptive behavior problems. J Fam Psychol 1998; 12:420–36.
18. Mikami A, Pfiffner L. Sibling relationships among children with ADHD. J Attent Disord. In press.
19. Cleckley HM. The mask of sanity. Postgrad Med 1951; 9:193–7.
20. Greenberg MT, Speltz ML, DeKlyen M. The role of attachment in the early development of disruptive behavior problems. Dev Psychopathol 1993; 5: 191–213.
21. Kochanska G. Toward a synthesis of parental socialization and child temperament in early development of conscience. Child Dev 1993; 64:325–47.
22. Frick PJ, Loney BR. Understanding the association between parent and child antisocial behavior. In: McMahon RJ, Peters RD, eds. The Effects of Parental Dysfunction on Children. New York: Plenum, 2002:105–26.
23. Greenhill LL. Stimulant medication treatment of children with attention deficit hyperactivity disorder. In: Jensen P, Cooper JR, eds. Attention Deficit Hyperactivity Disorder: State of the Science, Best Practices. Kingston, NJ: Civic Research Institute, 2002:9-1–9-27.
24. Jensen P, Hinshaw S, Kraemer HC, et al. ADHD comorbidity findings from the MTA study: comparing comorbid subgroups. J Am Acad Child Adolesc Psychiatry 2001; 40:147–58.
25. McBurnett K, Pfiffner L, Elliott G, Cooper K. Effectiveness of OROS methylphenidate in patients with or without comorbid oppositional defiant disorder and conduct disorder. In: 17th Annual International Conference of CHADD, Dallas, TX, 2005.

26. Connor DE, Glatt SJ, Lopez M, Jackson D, Melloni RH. Psychopharmacology and aggression. I. A meta-analysis of stimulant effects on overt/covert aggression-related behaviors in ADHD. J Am Acad Child Adolesc Psychiatry 2002; 41:253–61.
27. Wells KC, Epstein JN, Hinshaw S, et al. parenting and family stress treatment outcomes in attention deficit hyperactivity disorder (ADHD): an empirical analysis in the MTA study. J Abnorm Child Psychol 2000; 28: 543–53.
28. Hinshaw S, Owens EB, Wells KC, et al. Family processes and treatment outcome in the MTA: negative/ineffective parenting practices in relation to multimodal treatment. J Abnorm Child Psychol 2000; 28:555–68.
29. Pfiffner LJ, McBurnett K. Social skills training with parent generalization: treatment effects for children with attention deficit disorder. J Consult Clin Psychol 1997; 65:749–57.
30. Barkley RA. Defiant Children: A Clinician's Manual for Parent Training. New York: Guilford Press, 1987.
31. Kazdin AE. Parent Management Training: Treatment for Oppositional, Aggressive, and Antisocial Behavior in Children and Adolescents. New York: Oxford University Press, 2005.
32. Patterson GR. The next generation of PMTO models. Behav Ther 2005; 28: 27–33.
33. Henggeler S, Borduin C. Family Therapy and Beyond: A Multisystemic Approach to Treating the Behavior Problems of Children and Adolescents. Pacific Grove, CA: Brooks/Cole, 1990.
34. Newcorn JH, Halperin JM, Jensen PS, et al. Symptom profiles in children with ADHD: effects of comorbidity and gender. J Am Acad Child Adolesc Psychiatry 2001; 40:137–46.
35. Pliszka SR. Comorbidity of attention-deficit hyperactivity disorder and overanxious disorder. J Am Acad Child Adolesc Psychiatry 1992; 31: 197–203.
36. Tannock R, Ickowicz A, Schachar R. Differential effects of methylphenidate on working memory in ADHD children with and without comorbid anxiety. J Am Acad Child Adolesc Psychiatry 1995; 34:886–96.
37. Jensen PS, Shervette RE III, Xenakis SN, Richters J. Anxiety and depressive disorders in attention deficit disorder with hyperactivity: new findings. Am J Psychiatry 1993; 150:1203–9.
38. Kendler KS, Neale MC, Kessler RC, Heath AC. Generalized anxiety disorder in women: a population-based twin study. Arch Gen Psychiatry 1992; 49: 267–272.
39. Biederman J, Faraone SV, Keenan K, Steingard R, Tsuang T. Familial association between attention deficit disorder and anxiety disorders. Am J Psychiatry 1991; 148:251–6.
40. Pfiffner L, McBurnett K. Family correlates of comorbid anxiety disorders in children with attention deficit/hyperactivity disorder. J Abnorm Child Psychol 2006; 34:719–29.
41. Parker G. Parental Overprotection: A Risk Factor in Psychosocial Development. New York: Grune & Stratton, 1983.

42. Moore PS, Whaley SE, Sigman M. Interactions between mothers and children: impacts of maternal and child anxiety. J Abnorm Child Psychol 2004; 113: 471–6.
43. Kepley HO, Ostrander R. Family characteristics of anxious ADHD children: preliminary results. J Attent Disord 2007; 10:317–23.
44. March JS, Swanson JM, Arnold LE, et al. Anxiety as a predictor and outcome variable in the multimodal treatment study of children with ADHD (MTA). J Abnorm Child Psychol 2000; 28:527–41.
45. Livingston RL, Dykman R, Ackerman PT. The frequency and significance of additional self-reported psychiatric diagnoses in children with attention deficit disorder. J Abnorm Child Psychol 1990; 18:465–78.
46. Frick P, Lilienfeld S, Ellis M, Loney B, Silverthorn P. The association between anxiety and psychopathy dimensions in children. J Abnorm Child Psychol 1999; 27:383–92.
47. DuPaul GJ, Barkley RA, McMurray MB. Response of children with ADHD to methylphenidate: interaction with internalizing symptoms. J Am Acad Child Adolesc Psychiatry 1994; 33:894–903.
48. Pliszka SR. Effect of anxiety on cognition, behavior, and stimulant response in ADHD. J Am Acad Child Adolesc Psychiatry 1989; 28:882–7.
49. Diamond IR, Tannock R, Schachar R. Response to methylphenidate in children with ADHD and comorbid anxiety. J Am Acad Child Adolesc Psychiatry 1999; 38:402–9.
50. Pliszka SR, Carlson CL, Swanson JM. ADHD with Comorbid Disorders: Clinical Assessment and Management New York: Guilford Press, 1999.
51. Abikoff H, McGough J, Vitiello B, et al. Sequential pharmacotherapy for children with comorbid attention-deficit/hyperactivity and anxiety disorders. J Am Acad Child Adolesc Psychiatry 2005; 44:418–27.
52. Munir K, Biederman J, Knee D. Psychiatric comorbidity in patients with attention deficit disorder: a controlled study. J Am Acad Child Adolesc Psychiatry 1987; 26:844–8.
53. Treuting JJ, Hinshaw SP. Depression and self-esteem in boys with attention-deficit/hyperactivity disorder: associations with comorbid aggression and explanatory attributional mechanisms. J Abnorm Child Psychol 2001; 29: 23–39.
54. Biederman J, Mick E, Faraone SV. Depression in attention deficit hyperactivity disorder (ADHD) children: "True" depression or demoralization? J Affect Disord 1998; 47:113–22.
55. Lewinsohn PM, Rohde P, Seeley JR. Psychosocial characteristics of adolescents with a history of suicide attempt. J Am Acad Child Adolesc Psychiatry 1993; 32:60–8.
56. Renouf AG, Kovacs M, Mukerji P. Relationship of depressive, conduct, and comorbid disorders and social functioning in childhood. J Am Acad Child Adolesc Psychiatry 1997; 36:998–1004.
57. Connor DE, Edwards G, Fletcher K, Baird J, Barkley RA, Steingard R. Correlates of comorbid psychopathology in children with ADHD. J Am Acad Child Adolesc Psychiatry 2003; 42:193–200.

58. Beardslee WR, Versage VM, Gladstone T. Children of affectively ill parents: a review of the past 10 years. J Am Acad Child Adolesc Psychiatry 1998; 37: 1134–41.
59. Biederman J, Faraone SV, Keenan K, Tsuang M. Evidence of familial association between attention deficit disorder and major affective disorders. Arch Gen Psychiatry 1991; 48:633–42.
60. Biederman J, Baldessarini R, Wright V, Knee D, Harmatz J. A double-blind placebo-controlled study of desipramine in the treatment of ADD. I. Efficacy. J Am Acad Child Adolesc Psychiatry 1989; 28:777–84.
61. Garfinkel B, Wender P, Sloman L, O'Neill I. Tricyclic antidepressant and methylphenidate treatment of attention deficit disorder in children. J Am Acad Child Psychiatry 1983; 22:343–8.
62. Emslie G, Hughes CW, Crismon ML, Lopez M, Pliszka SR, Toprac MG. A feasibility study of the childhood depression medication algorithm: The Texas Children's Medication Algorithm Project (CMAP). J Am Acad Child Adolesc Psychiatry 2004; 43:519–27.
63. Pliszka SR, Crismon ML, Hughes CW, et al. The Texas Children's Medication Algorithm Project: revision of the algorithm for pharmacotherapy of attention-deficit/hyperactivity disorder. J Am Acad Child Adolesc Psychiatry 2006; 45: 642–57.
64. Jensen PS, Hinshaw SP, Swanson JM, et al. Findings from the NIMH Multimodal Treatment Study of ADHD (MTA): implications and applications for primary care providers. J Dev Behav Pediatr 2001; 22:60–73.

7

Dysfunctions of Attention, Learning, and Central Auditory Processing: What's the Difference?

Juliana Sanchez Bloom
The Children's Hospital of Philadelphia, Philadelphia, Pennsylvania, U.S.A.

George W. Hynd
Purdue University, West Lafayette, Indiana, U.S.A.

INTRODUCTION

Central auditory processing disorder (CAPD) is a developmental disorder involving dysfunction of the auditory perceptual system that is not due to a peripheral hearing loss (1). Children diagnosed with CAPD typically have poor listening skills, difficulty hearing in background noise, difficulty following oral instructions, academic difficulties, poor auditory association skills, distractibility/inattentiveness, and require increased time to complete tasks (6). This disorder, which is typically diagnosed by an audiologist, was conceptualized in the last 40 years (2). Conceptual and diagnostic concepts surrounding the disorder are typically taught in speech-language pathology and audiology training programs, leaving physicians and psychologists with a paucity of knowledge on the subject (2). Furthermore, CAPD is not a disorder listed in the DSM-IV (8), which provides a framework for diagnosis for many professionals. However, CAPD is an important disorder to understand due to the fact that it shares symptomatology with attention deficit hyperactivity disorder (ADHD) and language-based learning disabilities (language-based LD), which can make accurate differential diagnosis difficult.

The overlapping symptomatology between CAPD, ADHD, and LD has led many researchers to question if CAPD is in fact a separate and distinct disorder from ADHD, and to a lesser degree, language-based LD such as developmental dyslexia (2). Diagnostic criteria for these disorders overlap significantly (1,2,5), as does behavioral presentation (6). This overlapping symptomatology has led to the assertion that differential diagnosis is extremely difficult, and may depend on whether the child is evaluated by a psychologist, physician, or an audiologist (2,7).

DEFINITION

In 1993, The American Speech-Language-Hearing Association (ASHA) formed a task force on central auditory processing consensus development to provide a definition, assessment strategies, and treatment parameters for CAPD (3). This task force, whose consensus was published in 1995, defined CAPD as an observed deficiency in one or more of the central auditory processes, which include sound localization and lateralization, auditory discrimination and pattern recognition, temporal resolution, masking, integration, and ordering, auditory performance decrements with competing acoustic signals, and auditory performance decrements with degrading acoustic signals (3). These central auditory processes occur after hearing processes but before conscious awareness, and the deficits in CAPD are presumed to apply to both verbal and nonverbal acoustic information (3). Furthermore, the ASHA task force stated that while CAPD is presumed to result from deficits in audition, but it may also result from a more widespread dysfunction, such as difficulties with attention. Despite the efforts of the ASHA task force, there remains little consensus as to the definition, appropriate assessment and treatment of CAPD, and some suggest that research has not supported the idea that there is a specific auditory deficit in CAPD (4). Reflective of this perspective, Cacace and McFarland (1) assert that CAPD, in definition, assessment, and intervention, is "vague and loosely defined."

CAPD AND ADHD

Overlapping Symptomatology

Many symptoms of CAPD overlap with those associated with ADHD, including auditory attention problems, distractibility, and inattentiveness. Children with ADHD demonstrate significant difficulty on tasks used to assess central auditory processing skills (2), and children with CAPD demonstrate difficulties with attention, particularly auditory attention (6). Thus, differential diagnosis between the two disorders can be challenging. Furthermore, there has been a debate in the literature as to whether CAPD and ADHD reflect a single developmental disorder (7) or comorbid disorders (6).

CAPD/ADHD: Evidence for Discrete Disorders

In order to explore the question of whether or not ADHD and CAPD represent independent disorders, Riccio and colleagues (2) explored the incidence of ADHD in children who met criteria for CAPD. Half of the CAPD sample also met criteria for ADHD, which is higher than expected based on the population base rates. Within the comorbid ADHD/CAPD group, some children were experiencing difficulties with attention alone, while others were experiencing difficulty with attention, hyperactivity, and impulsivity. Impaired language abilities were found in the entire sample, but no significant between-group differences were found in the cognitive, auditory, or language measures. The authors concluded that, for children who were experiencing comorbid ADHD/CAPD, the "inattention, hyperactivity, and impulsivity may be resulting from auditory-linguistic problems rather than the ADHD syndrome per se." Strengthening this argument was the fact that no behavioral disorders associated with ADHD [such as oppositional-defiant disorder (ODD)] were found in this sample.

Chermak and colleagues (6) compared ranking by psychiatrists, audiologists, teachers, and pediatricians of the behaviors related to ADHD and CAPD. Overall, professionals described exclusive sets of behaviors that characterize each disorder. They tended to characterize children with ADHD as inattentive, distractible, impulsive, and as having a heightened activity level. Children with CAPD were described as having difficulty hearing background noise, difficulty following directions, poor listening skills, and academic problems. Only two symptoms were endorsed as falling into both categories: inattention and distractibility. However, these symptoms were ranked ordered first and second for ADHD and ranked seventh and sixth for children with CAPD, showing that the majority of behaviors were seen as unique to one disorder or the other. Thus, it appears that children with ADHD, particularly those children that present with hyperactivity and impulsivity, and children with CAPD have distinguishable clinical presentations (6). While children with CAPD demonstrate inattention and distractibility, these symptoms do not define the disorder as in ADHD; rather, difficulties in listening, hearing, following oral directions, and experiencing difficulty in academic settings are defining characteristics of CAPD (Table 1).

Table 1 Rank Order of Behavioral Means Greater than One Standard Deviation Above the Respective Grand Mean

ADHD	CAPD
Inattentive	Difficulty hearing in background noise
Distracted	Difficulty following oral instructions
Hyperactive	Poor listening skills
Fidgety/restless	Academic difficulties
Impulsive	Poor auditory association skills
Interrupts or intrudes	Distracted
	Inattentive

Source: Adapted from Ref. 6.

Strengthening the argument that ADHD and CAPD represent discrete disorders is a recent shift in the conceptualization of ADHD, led by Barkley and colleagues (9,15). While ADHD has traditionally been viewed as solely a dysfunction of attention, the last decade has seen the disorder characterized primarily as a deficit in impulse control and behavioral regulation (9). Some researchers suggest that hyperactivity is the hallmark of ADHD as opposed to dysfunction of attention, and the use of hyperactivity alone for diagnostic criteria has been proposed (15). CAPD, by contrast, is not characterized by hyperactivity and deficits in impulse control. This suggests that CAPD and ADHD are discrete disorders when criteria beyond auditory inattentiveness are used (15).

CAPD AND LANGUAGE-BASED LEARNING DISABILITIES

As ADHD and CAPD are highly comorbid disorders (2), ADHD and language-based LD are highly comorbid disorders (10), so, not surprisingly, CAPD and language-based LD share significant symptomatology. Disorders of auditory perception have been suggested as the underlying cause of language-based LD such as developmental dyslexia (11). Phonological processing in particular has been well documented as the core deficit in dyslexia (12). The disorders of auditory perception found in language-based LD, such as phonological processing, are very similar to the central auditory processing dysfunctions in CAPD (4) as they involve difficulty in the discrimination and manipulation of auditory stimuli (3). In addition, many children with CAPD have learning problems (4). This overlap has led to difficulty distinguishing between the two disorders and questions as to whether the disorders are distinct (1). However, some have suggested that the auditory processing problems associated with developmental dyslexia are specific to the encoding of speech and are not a more general dysfunction of the encoding of all auditory stimuli (1), which would suggest distinct etiologies of CAPD and dyslexia.

CONCEPTUAL DIFFERENCES BETWEEN CAPD, ADHD, AND LANGUAGE-BASED LD

Cacace and McFarland (1) introduced the idea that modality specificity is the primary way to differentiate CAPD from LD and ADHD. The authors posit that the primary deficit of CAPD is the processing of acoustic information, and that people with CAPD should display impairments during the processing of information in other sensory modalities. This definition of CAPD as a unimodal dysfunction contrasts with the current state of knowledge surrounding ADHD and LD, which are multimodal in nature (1).

There is considerable evidence that supports the idea that developmental dyslexia is associated with a sensory processing deficit that is not restricted to a single sensory modality (1). Although there is a great deal of evidence that anomalies in the auditory cortex of the left temporal lobe may result in dyslexia, there is also evidence that correlates the cognitive and behavioral symptoms of dyslexia with executive symptoms in the frontal lobes (13) and the thalamic nuclei of the visual system (14). Furthermore, neurobiological evidence suggests that variations within brain regions associated with auditory processing, visual processing, and interhemispheric processing exist in developmental dyslexia (15), suggesting multimodal deficits of language-based LD. Thus, dyslexia can have a complex neurological basis involving multiple sensory areas and behavioral deficits are observed across modalities. The multimodal nature of dyslexia differentiates it from CAPD, which is conceptualized as a disorder of only one modality (1).

Both functional and structural imaging studies support neurobiological anomalies in a biological basis of ADHD in the frontal lobe and basal ganglia, areas not related to auditory processing (16). Furthermore, children with ADHD show impaired performance on neuropsychological tasks across modalities, whereas children with CAPD show inattentiveness solely in response to auditory stimuli (1). Cacace and McFarland (1) conclude that children with ADHD have multimodal attentional problems. Again, the multimodal nature of the deficits in ADHD separate ADHD from the unimodal conceptualization of CAPD.

While the Cacace and McFarland model of conceptualizing CAPD and how it differs from other disorders is compelling, the fact remains that research has not shown clearly that a specific auditory deficit exists in CAPD (1,4). The modality-specific model of differentiating CAPD from disorders with overlapping symptomatology is a useful tool provided that research has documented clearly the existence of children who have this specific deficit. A child with ADHD or language-based LD would be likely to present as having a deficit in one or more of the central auditory processes if evaluated by an audiologist, and would likely been diagnosed with CAPD despite the multimodal nature of the child's deficits. Thus, a multimodal assessment is necessary in both clinical practice and research on CAPD.

CLINICAL IMPLICATIONS

Implications for Differential Diagnosis

Although a significant amount of overlapping symptomatology exists between CAPD, ADHD, and language-based LD, evidence suggests that the three disorders are conceptually distinct. When overlapping symptoms exist, the modality/ies of the deficits must be thoroughly assessed for accurate differential diagnosis (1,7). Collaboration among speech-language pathologists, audiologists, neuropsychologists, physicians, and school psychologists may be necessary to ensure accurate differential diagnosis because these professionals may need to collaborate assess thoroughly across modalities (4,7). If auditory attention problems exist but visual attention is not impaired, there is a family history of hearing problems, and there is evidence of five or more ear infections in the first 2 years of life, a referral to an audiologist for a CAPD evaluation is certainly warranted.

Implications for Pharmacological Intervention

While there is substantial evidence that methylphenidate enhances attention in children with ADHD, the effect of stimulant medication on auditory processing is not fully understood. Some research has found stimulant medication to be effective in both CAPD and ADHD (7,14), while some research has found mixed effectiveness depending on symptomatology. Research has shown that, in a comorbid group, auditory processing improved with the use of stimulant medication (15). In a recent study of a comorbid population, however, Ritalin reduced impulsivity and inattention but did not result in improved auditory functioning (5). Further research is necessary to determine the effects of stimulant medication on the auditory processing and attention of children with CAPD and the comorbid condition. This will allow for appropriate interventions to be designed.

INCONSISTENT FINDINGS AND UNDERSTUDIED AREAS

Future research on CAPD should also focus on the developmental trajectory of children with CAPD into adulthood. It is not clear at this time if the problems remediate as one gets older, if children with CAPD are able to compensate for their dysfunctions in central auditory processing, and what factors may affect remediation and compensation. Furthermore, does the developmental trajectory change if the children with CAPD also have comorbid ADHD or language-based LD? Understanding the developmental trajectory of children with CAPD would pinpoint important areas for intervention.

Finally, there is a dearth of research on the possible biological basis of CAPD. The question remains as to whether or not there are genes that may predispose or cause an individual to develop CAPD. Family and genetic studies are necessary to answer this question. In addition, structural and functional neuroimaging studies would provide valuable information as to what neuroanatomical areas are affected, if any, in children with CAPD. This information would aid researchers in understanding the neurobiological basis of the central auditory processes and how the biological substrate underlying these processes may be altered in children with CAPD.

Although Cacace and McFarland's definition of CAPD as unimodal disorder is extremely useful in the conceptualization of this disorder, the existence of CAPD as a disorder that is separate and distinct from language-based LD and ADHD has not been well-documented in the literature (1). CAPD may be a solitary disorder with a high comorbidity with ADHD and language-based LD, or it may be an associated feature of those well-defined disorders. Furthermore, the fact that CAPD does not appear in the DSM-IV (8) as a distinct diagnosis makes any such diagnosis questionable in terms of qualifying a child for clinical- or school-related services. Thus, research should attempt to elucidate if in fact CAPD exists as a unitary and distinct disorder as an understanding of the nature of CAPD is essential for communication among professionals, the development or appropriate intervention, and the delivery of services to children.

ACKNOWLEDGMENT

Preparation of this chapter was supported in part by a grant to the second author (GWH) from the National Institute for Child Health and Human Developmental, National Institutes of Health (NICHD/NIH #26890-06).

REFERENCES

1. Cacace AT, McFarland DJ. Central auditory processing disorder in school-aged children: a critical review. J Speech Lang Hear Res 1998; 41:355–74.
2. Riccio CA, Hynd GW, Cohen MJ, Hall J, Molt L. Central auditory processing disorder and attention-deficit hyperactivity. J Am Acad Child Adolesc Psychiatry 1994; 33:849–57.
3. American Speech, Language, and Hearing Association. Central auditory processing: current status of research and implications for clinical practice. Am J Audiol 1996; 5:41–54.
4. Bellis TJ, Ferre JM. Multidimensional approach to the differential diagnosis of central auditory processing disorders in children. J Am Acad Audiol 1999; 10: 319–28.
5. Tillery KL, Katz J, Keller WD. Effects of methylphenidate (Ritalin) on auditory performance in children with attention and auditory processing disorders. J Speech Lang Hear Res 2000; 43:893–900.
6. Chermak GD, Somers EK, Seikel JA. Behavioral signs of central auditory processing disorder and attention deficit hyperactivity disorder. J Am Acad Audiol 1998; 9:78–84.
7. Riccio CA, Hynd GW. Relationship between ADHD and central auditory processing disorder: a review of the literature. School Psychol Int 1996; 17: 235–51.

8. American Psychiatric Association. Diagnostic and Statistical Manual of Mental Disorders. 4th ed., revised. Washington, D.C.: American Psychiatric Association.
9. Barkley RA. Attention deficit hyperactivity disorder. In: Mash EJ, Barkley RA, eds. Child Psychopathology. New York: Guilford Press, 1996:390–435.
10. Morgan AE, Hynd GW. Dyslexia, neurolinguistic ability, and anatomical variation of the planum temporale. Neuropsychol Rev 1998; 8:79–93.
11. Lombardino LJ, Riccio C, Hynd GW, Pinheiro SB. Linguistic deficits in children with reading disabilities. Am J Speech-Lang Pathol 1997; 6:71–8.
12. Hynd GW, Semrud-Clikeman M. Dyslexia and brain morphology. Psychol Bull 1989; 106:447–82.
13. Eden GF, VanMeter JW, Rumsey JM, Zeffiro TA. The visual deficit theory of developmental dyslexia. Neuroimage 1996; 4:S108–17.
14. Miller CJ, Sanchez J, Hynd GW. Neurological correlates of reading disabilities. In: Swanson HL, Harris KR, Graham S, eds. Handbook of Learning Disabilities. New York: Guilford Press, 2003:242–55.
15. Barkley RA. Attention-Deficit Hyperactivity Disorder. 2nd ed. New York: Guilford Press, 1998.
16. Riccio CA, Hynd GW, Cohen MJ, Gonzalez JJ. Neurological basis of attention deficit hyperactivity disorder. Except Child 1993; 60:118–24.

Section III: Clinical Neuroscience

8

Neuroanatomy of ADHD

F. Xavier Castellanos and Eleanor Ainslie
Institute for Pediatric Neuroscience, NYU Child Study Center, New York University School of Medicine, New York, New York, U.S.A.

The third edition of the *Diagnostic and Statistical Manual of Mental Disorders* (DSM-III) marked a paradigm shift from psychoanalysis toward an empirically based classification of disorders, with the implicit goal that psychiatric disorders would eventually be referenced to specific enumerable brain dysfunctions. Although this goal has not yet been achieved for any psychiatric disorder, recent advances in brain imaging could assist in this process. Anatomic magnetic resonance imaging (MRI) is the principal technology used to examine the pediatric brain, mainly because it does not use ionizing radiation, in contrast to methods like computed axial tomography, positron emission tomography, and single-photon emission computed tomography. Therefore, although those approaches will also inevitably contribute to our understanding of the pathophysiology of attention deficit hyperactivity disorder (ADHD), we will limit ourselves to recent MRI studies of children and adolescents (roughly ages 5–18) diagnosed with this common psychiatric condition.

As valuable as MRI can be, we must precede our review with a word about the technique's limitations. Depending on the viewpoint, the neuroanatomical literature on ADHD presents either a reasonable degree of concordance (1), or a distressing absence of truly confirmed findings (2). Early studies, which have been reviewed in detail elsewhere (3–5), had several limitations, some of which continue to represent obstacles in current work. The high cost of obtaining MRI scans results in small sample sizes, which tend to yield insufficient statistical power. As Rossi and coworkers have pointed out, when most studies in a field only have statistical power in the range of 50%, then inconsistent results are to be expected (6).

Comparison of results across studies is also hampered by variability in subject selection, which is driven by factors that are idiosyncratic to each setting and study. Another source of inconsistencies in the anatomical literature has been derived from a focus on lateralization and indices of asymmetry (7), which, perhaps are biologically interesting, but intrinsically much less reliable than the volumetric measures from which they are constructed (8,9). Lastly, the field has not yet adopted standard quantitative analytical methods which would improve comparisons across studies. Current methods include hand-tracing of individual regions of interest, which tends to optimize validity at the expense of reliability; fully automated methods, which maximize test–retest reliability but can still only be applied to a few large regions; and semiautomated methods, which combine the strengths and weaknesses of the other two alternatives. Despite these concerns, progress continues in delineating the brain anatomy of ADHD.

NORMAL BRAIN DEVELOPMENT

ADHD cannot be considered without taking into account developmental factors; likewise, an examination of the brain anatomy of ADHD must be referenced to healthy brain development. Since the late 1980s, converging studies have shown that over 90% of total brain volume of a young adult is attained by age 5 (10,11), though the apparent stability of total brain volume during childhood and adolescence masks complex changes in gray and white matter and subcortical compartments (12). Increasing myelination is reflected in linear increases of white matter volumes during the pediatric age range, which are statistically greater in males (13). Heterogeneity of white matter development has been noted in the corpus callosum, the anterior cross-sectional area of which increases first, followed by posterior growth through late adolescence (14). Gray matter also shows a heterogeneous overall growth pattern: volumes peak at about age 12 in frontal and parietal lobes and at about age 16 for the temporal lobe (12). (In the cerebellum, considered as the sum of both white and gray matter, volumes peak at around age 18.) Total gray matter volume increases until early-to-mid adolescence before decreasing during late adolescence (12), probably reflecting selective pruning of neuronal connections (15). Similarly, the caudate reaches its maximum volume before 10 years of age.

One of the pivotal achievements of pediatric medicine was the derivation of norms for the expected developmental trajectories of weight, height, and head circumference from birth to adulthood. Such growth charts, which have long been commonplace in every pediatrician's office, facilitate the early detection of growth deficits and make possible timely interventions. The availability of noninvasive high-resolution MRI scans now makes it feasible to begin to develop growth charts for the human brain. While such potentially clinically useful tools are not yet at hand, a multisite project, contracted by three of the U.S. National Institutes of Health with seven sites in the United States and Canada continues to advance toward this goal.

NEUROANATOMICAL ABNORMALITIES IN ADHD

The brains of children with ADHD are significantly smaller, on average, than the brains of healthy comparison children throughout childhood and adolescence (16). Beyond this globally decreased volume, there is more conflicting evidence in support of a distributed circuit, the disruption of which likely underlies ADHD symptoms. At least in boys, this circuit appears to include right prefrontal brain regions, the basal ganglia, the cerebellar hemispheres, and a subregion of the cerebellar vermis. Lastly, the distribution of gray and white matter may be altered in ADHD. We will discuss these abnormalities in turn.

Decreased Global Brain Volume

As Table 1 shows, most studies have found overall reductions in total brain volume in children with ADHD compared to age- and sex-matched controls. In a meta-analysis of published volumetric studies in ADHD, we found a highly significant overall effect ($Z = 19.84$; $P < .0001$; 95% CI: 8.79 to 30.90), which remained significant even when the largest study (16) or the study with the largest effect size (17) were excluded. In the largest study, Castellanos et al. examined 152 children and adolescents with ADHD and 139 controls, and analyzed the results using fully automated methods. Children with ADHD showed overall cerebral volumes that were 3.2% smaller than controls, adjusted for significant covariates ($P = .004$; Fig. 1). All four major lobes were comparably affected, but after adjustment for total brain volume, these differences were statistically subsumed; however, the decreased volume of the cerebellum (−3.5%) remained statistically significant (16). The volumetric abnormalities were at least as pronounced in the 49 medication-naïve children with ADHD as in the 103 children with ADHD who were being treated with stimulants. This finding supports the conclusion that volume reductions in ADHD do not arise from stimulant treatment.

Prefrontal Brain

Anatomic hypotheses of the substrates of ADHD have generally focused on the role of the prefrontal cortex (PFC) in the disorder, which is known to be involved in executive functioning, a group of high-order mental abilities including behavioral planning and response inhibition, selective attention, and the organization of information in problem-solving tasks. Normally, the right PFC is slightly larger than the left (18), but the region is more

Table 1 Meta-Analysis of Total Brain Volume in ADHD

Study	Measure	Mean NC	SD NC	*N* NC	Mean ADHD	SD ADHD	*N* ADHD	Total *N*	% change	Effect size	Estimated difference[b]	95% CI
Aylward et al. (1996)	Representative brain volume	305.6	14.5	11	295.9	17.9	10	21	3.2%	0.60		
Filipek et al. (1997)	Right hemisphere volume	659.4	47.1	15	627.9	47.4	15	30	4.8%	0.67		
Bullmore (1999)[a]	Gray and white matter voxels	1342.1	129.11	16	1302.3	142.5	18	34	3.0%	0.29		
Bussing (2002)	Cerebral hemispheres	1172	89	19	1182.5	93.1	12	31	−0.9%	−0.12		
Hesslinger et al. (2002)	Total brain volume	1075	118.5	17	1174.3	187.8	8	25	−9.2%	−0.69		
Mostofsky et al. (2002)	Gray and white matter voxels	1241.4	54.7	12	1138.0	101.7	12	24	8.3%	1.27		
Castellanos et al. (2002)	Gray and white matter voxels	1104.5	111.3	139	1059.4	117.5	152	291	4.1%	0.39		
	Totals/average			229			227	456	1.9%	0.34	19.84	(8.79–30.90)

[a] Variance estimated.
[b] Estimated true difference in SD units.
Abbreviations: ADHD, attention-deficit/hyperactivity disorder; CI, confidence interval; NC, normal control; SD, standard deviation.

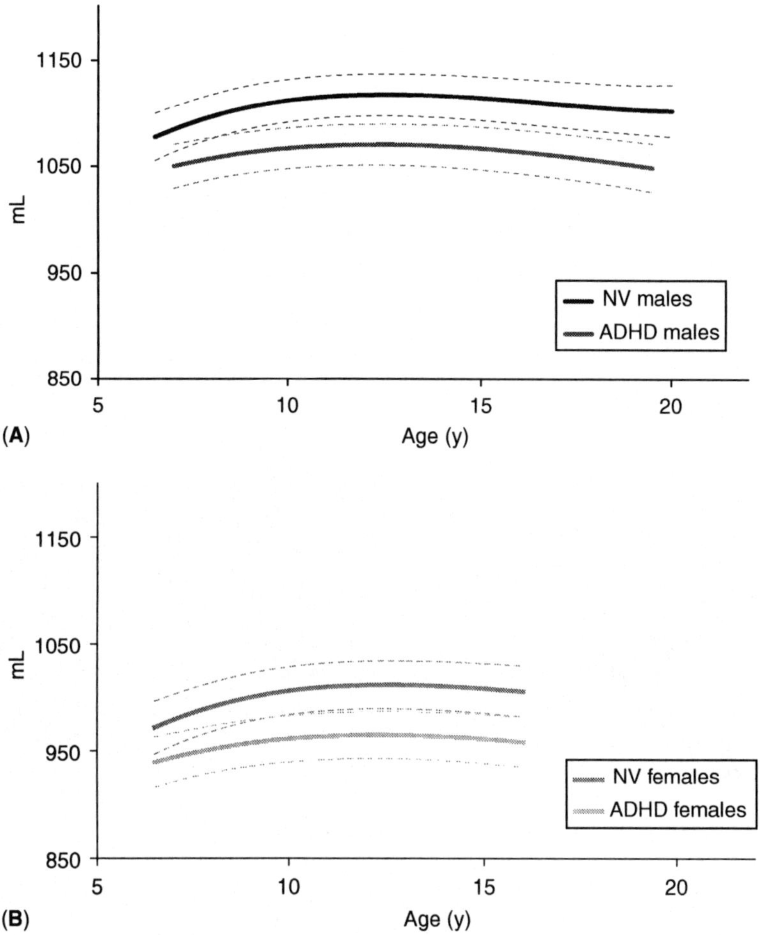

Figure 1 Predicted unadjusted longitudinal growth curves for total cerebral volumes for male (**A**) and female (**B**) patients with ADHD and controls. *Abbreviation*: ADHD, attention deficit hyperactivity disorder. *Source*: From Ref. 16.

symmetrical in ADHD (13,19–21). Also, reduced size of the right PFC was correlated with response inhibition problems in boys with ADHD (22).

While these studies have examined overall volumetric differences in the PFC, other recent studies have differentiated frontal gray and white matter volumes. Reductions in both gray and white matter were reported for the right PFC (23,24), but Kates et al. (25) reported similar reductions in the left PFC. These latter findings were confirmed recently by Mostofsky et al. (17) who reported significant white matter reduction confined to the left PFC, with gray matter reduced in both hemispheres but more so in the right.

Another recent development has been the quantification of PFC subregions. Hesslinger and colleagues (26) found that eight adult patients with ADHD who had never been medicated had significantly smaller left orbital-frontal cortical gray and white matter volumes than did 17 comparison subjects (−12%, $P = .04$). Investigators are also studying the dorsolateral PFC; Yeo et al. reported that right dorsolateral prefrontal volume, measured as a block, was significantly smaller in 23 children with non-comorbid ADHD as compared to 24 controls (27). While these reports are currently difficult to integrate because of many differences in methods and subjects, automated image analysis techniques should alleviate this problem in future studies.

Basal Ganglia

Along with the PFC, the caudate nucleus and its associated circuits have long been implicated in ADHD (28). The caudate nucleus and the putamen serve as the entry point to the basal ganglia, and abnormalities of both structures have been reported in this disorder. Researchers have noted both volumetric differences (most studies have reported a decrease, with one exception) (21,23) and loss of asymmetry (21,29,30) in ADHD—although it is still unclear whether the normal caudate is asymmetric, and if so, whether this asymmetry normally favors the right (21) or the left side (12,23,29–31). When total caudate volume was analyzed in a mixed cross-sectional/longitudinal design, decreased volumes were detected in the group with ADHD for ages below 16 (Fig. 2), but not beyond that age (16). Such transient

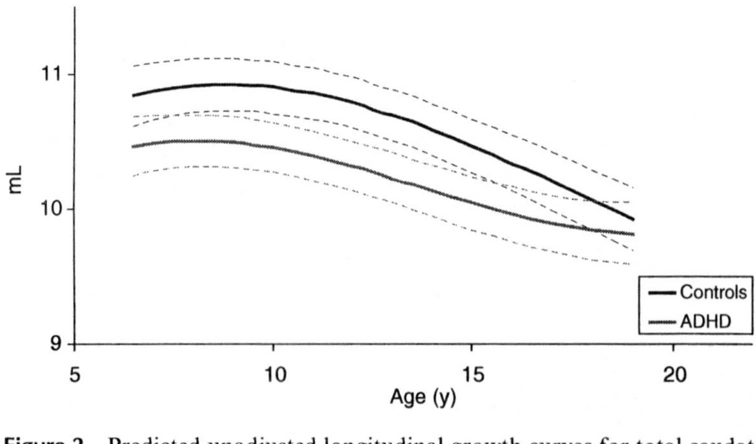

Figure 2 Predicted unadjusted longitudinal growth curves for total caudate volume for patients with ADHD and controls. *Abbreviation*: ADHD, attention deficit hyperactivity disorder. *Source*: From Ref. 16.

abnormalities may relate to the diminishment of motoric symptoms in ADHD with increasing age, but this speculation should be tested directly.

Studies of the putamen, a region associated with primary and supplementary motor areas that may contribute to the motoric symptoms of ADHD, have yielded equally ambiguous results. Investigators who examined putamen volumes as regions of interest did not detect significant differences (21,32). On the other hand, a recent preliminary functional imaging study detected decreased blood flow in the putamen of objectively hyperactive boys with ADHD compared to those boys whose activity level resembled that of controls (33). Putamen lesions are also associated with greater likelihood of ADHD. Two instructive cases of severe ADHD associated with a traumatic amniocentesis at 17 weeks gestation revealed complete elimination of the right basal ganglia (34). In addition, lesions of the right putamen and posterior ventral putamen have been associated with higher incidence of secondary ADHD (S-ADHD) and ADHD, respectively (35,36). The relationship between injury and the disorder's symptoms will be further explored below. Lastly, the globus pallidus, which receives input from caudate and putamen, has been examined; although it is difficult to measure reliably, it was found to be significantly smaller in boys with ADHD (21,32). However, the two studies differed as to whether the size reduction was greater in the left or right side.

Cerebellum

The cerebellum is associated with coordination of motor movements, but functional neuroimaging studies have clearly demonstrated cerebellar involvement in nonmotor functions (37–43). MRI studies of the cerebellum in ADHD have detected smaller cerebellar hemispheric volumes (21) which are sustained throughout adolescence (Fig. 3) (16). Within the cerebellum, the posterior-inferior vermal lobules (VIII-X) were particularly smaller compared to the contrast group of right-handed boys (44). This finding has been independently replicated in both boys (45) and girls with ADHD (31). Consequently, the cerebellar hemispheres and the posterior-inferior cerebellar vermis are becoming increasingly incorporated into hypotheses of ADHD (46).

ASSOCIATION OF HEAD TRAUMA AND ADHD

In addition to comparisons between children with ADHD and controls, several investigators have begun focusing on the effects of early brain lesions or head trauma on the secondary development of ADHD. The disorder is associated with increased pre- or perinatal adverse events (47) and with closed head injury (48). ADHD is the most common psychiatric disorder to develop after brain injury (49) or stroke (50) in childhood, and its

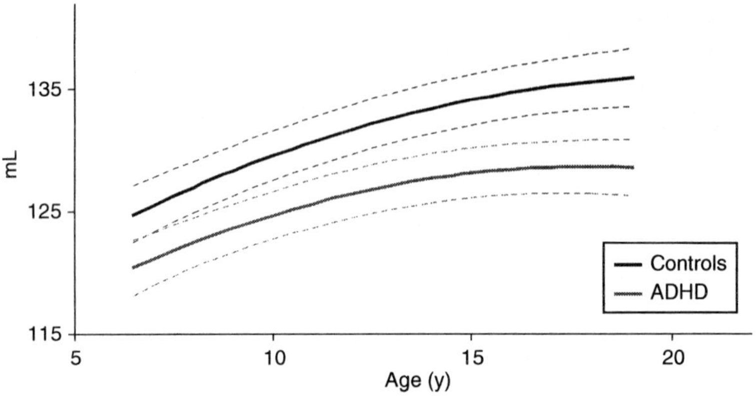

Figure 3 Predicted unadjusted longitudinal growth curves for cerebellar volumes for patients with ADHD and controls. *Abbreviation*: ADHD, attention deficit hyperactivity disorder. *Source*: From Ref. 16.

occurrence is correlated with severity of injury (51). The most common form of head trauma in childhood and adolescence is closed head injury, which can particularly affect inhibitory capacity (52) and executive function, deficits of which are symptomatic of ADHD, and can result in personality changes (e.g., increased aggression). In the interest of delineating a potential circuit underlying ADHD, MRI has been used to identify the specific sites of injury, which have then been correlated with the emergence of S-ADHD, in which symptoms can appear after age 7 (48). When 99 children who suffered closed head injury, ranging in age from 4 to19 years, were followed for a year, the odds of developing S-ADHD were 3.6 times higher among children with thalamus injury and 3.2 times higher in children with basal ganglia injury (53). Further brain injury studies, especially those using imaging techniques, should shed further light on neurodevelopmental susceptibilities.

CONCLUSIONS

Although methodological inconsistencies and low statistical power are still important limiting factors, there is increasing evidence that ADHD is associated with globally decreased brain volumes which appear to represent a nonprogressive deficit presumably resulting from early genetic and/or environmental factors. Putative sex differences are probably best understood as the result of sampling variations; referred samples of boys and girls with ADHD differ from community-based samples (54), but when patient samples have been recruited to meet equivalent severity criteria (55), results have been comparable, though slightly less prominent, for girls (16).

Beyond global volumetric differences in the brain, there is more evidence for right prefrontal deficits, although there are also several findings of decreases on the left. The same sort of inconsistency is reported for findings in basal ganglia structures. The safest conclusion, supported by cases of head trauma, is that basal ganglia are an important link in the circuits implicated in ADHD, but that we cannot specify whether such deficits are truly lateralized. At least for the caudate nucleus, the volumetric abnormalities seem to be age-dependent, as they are no longer detected after mid-adolescence (7,16).

The most robustly deviant region in brain associated with ADHD is the cerebellum, both when measured algorithmically as a single unit, which is mostly composed of the hemispheres (16), and even more so in hand-traced measurements of the posterior-inferior cerebellar vermis (31,44,45). Thus, one of the most promising and unexpected frontiers of ADHD research is the exploration of the cerebellum's influence on cortico-striatal-thalamo-cortical (CSTC) circuits (56), which choose, initiate, and carry out complex motor and cognitive responses (57). The posterior-inferior lobules of the cerebellar vermis appear to differ from the remaining cerebellar hemispheres and vermis in selectively containing dopamine-transporter-like immunoreactive axons (58).

Despite the suboptimal variability of recent results, the current literature has begun to reveal several key brain structures involved in ADHD. The increasing availability of neuroimaging, along with growing interest in developing convergent methods and standards, will facilitate the elaboration of testable models of the disorder's pathophysiology.

REFERENCES

1. Swanson J, Castellanos FX, Murias M, LaHoste GJ, Kennedy J. Cognitive neuroscience of attention deficit hyperactivity disorder and hyperkinetic disorder. Curr Opin Neurobiol 1998; 8:263–71.
2. Baumeister AA, Hawkins MF. Incoherence of neuroimaging studies of attention deficit/hyperactivity disorder. Clin Neuropharmacol 2001; 24:2–10.
3. Tannock R. Attention deficit hyperactivity disorder: advances in cognitive, neurobiological, and genetic research. J Child Psychol Psychiatry 1998; 39: 65–99.
4. Castellanos FX. Neuroimaging of attention-deficit hyperactivity disorder. Child Adoles Psychiatr Clin N Am 1997; 6:383–411.
5. Faraone SV, Biederman J. Neurobiology of attention-deficit hyperactivity disorder. Biol Psychiatry 1998; 44:951–8.
6. Rossi JS. Statistical power of psychological research: what have we gained in 20 years? J Consult Clin Psychol 1990; 58:646–56.
7. Castellanos FX, Giedd JN, Eckburg P, et al. Quantitative morphology of the caudate nucleus in attention deficit hyperactivity disorder. Am J Psychiatry 1994; 151:1791–6.

8. Arndt S, Cohen G, Alliger RJ, Swayze VW II, Andreasen NC. Problems with ratio and proportion measures of imaged cerebral structures. Psychiatry Res 1991; 40:79–89.
9. Bullmore E, Brammer M, Harvey I, Ron M. Against the laterality index as a measure of cerebral asymmetry. Psychiatry Res Neuroimag 1995; 61:121–4.
10. Jernigan TL, Tallal P. Late childhood changes in brain morphology observable with MRI. Dev Med Child Neurol 1990; 32:379–85.
11. Jernigan TL, Trauner DA, Hesselink JR, Tallal PA. Maturation of human cerebrum observed in vivo during adolescence. Brain 1991; 114:2037–49.
12. Giedd JN, Blumenthal J, Jeffries NO, et al. Brain development during childhood and adolescence: a longitudinal MRI study. Nat Neurosci 1999; 2: 861–3.
13. Reiss AL, Abrams MT, Singer HS, Ross JL, Denckla MB. Brain development, gender and IQ in children. A volumetric imaging study. Brain 1996; 119: 1763–74.
14. Giedd JN, Blumenthal J, Jeffries NO, et al. Development of the human corpus callosum during childhood and adolescence: a longitudinal MRI study. Prog Neuropsychopharmacol Biol Psychiatry 1999; 23:571–88.
15. Huttenlocher PR. Synaptic density in human frontal cortex—developmental changes and effects of aging. Brain Res 1979; 163:195–205.
16. Castellanos FX, Lee PP, Sharp W, et al. Developmental trajectories of brain volume abnormalities in children and adolescents with attention-deficit/ hyperactivity disorder. JAMA 2002; 288:1740–8.
17. Mostofsky SH, Cooper KL, Kates WR, Denckla MB, Kaufmann WE. Smaller prefrontal and premotor volumes in boys with attention-deficit/hyperactivity disorder. Biol Psychiatry 2002; 52:785–94.
18. Weinberger DR, Luchins DJ, Morihisa J, Wyatt RJ. Asymmetrical volumes of the right and left frontal and occipital regions of the human brain. Neurology 1982; 11:97–100.
19. Shaywitz BA, Shaywitz SE, Byrne T, Cohen DJ, Rothman S. Attention deficit disorder: quantitative analysis of CT. Neurology 1983; 33:1500–3.
20. Hynd GW, Semrud-Clikeman M, Lorys AR, Novey ES, Eliopulos D. Brain morphology in developmental dyslexia and attention deficit disorder/hyperactivity. Arch Neurol 1990; 47:919–26.
21. Castellanos FX, Giedd JN, Marsh WL, et al. Quantitative brain magnetic resonance imaging in attention-deficit/hyperactivity disorder. Arch Gen Psychiatry 1996; 53:607–16.
22. Casey BJ, Castellanos FX, Giedd JN, et al. Implication of right frontostriatal circuitry in response inhibition and attention-deficit/hyperactivity disorder. J Am Acad Child Adolesc Psychiatry 1997; 36:374–83.
23. Filipek PA, Semrud-Clikeman M, Steingard RJ, Renshaw PF, Kennedy DN, Biederman J. Volumetric MRI analysis comparing subjects having attention-deficit hyperactivity disorder and normal controls. Neurology 1997; 48: 589–601.
24. Overmeyer S, Bullmore ET, Suckling J, et al. Distributed grey and white matter deficits in hyperkinetic disorder: MRI evidence for anatomical abnormality in an attentional network. Psychol Med 2001; 31:1425–35.

25. Kates WR, Frederikse M, Mostofsky SH, et al. MRI parcellation of the frontal lobe in boys with attention deficit hyperactivity disorder or Tourette syndrome. Psychiatry Res 2002; 116:63–81.
26. Hesslinger B, Tebartz van E, Thiel T, Haegele K, Hennig J, Ebert D. Frontoorbital volume reductions in adult patients with attention deficit hyperactivity disorder. Neurosci Lett 2002; 328:319–21.
27. Yeo RA, Hill DE, Campbell RA, et al. Proton magnetic resonance spectroscopy investigation of the right frontal lobe in children with attention-deficit/hyperactivity disorder. J Am Acad Child Adolesc Psychiatry 2003; 42:303–10.
28. Pontius AA. Dysfunction patterns analogous to frontal lobe system and caudate nucleus syndromes in some groups of minimal brain dysfunction. J Am Med Wom Assoc 1973; 28:285–92.
29. Hynd GW, Hern KL, Novey ES, et al. Attention deficit hyperactivity disorder and asymmetry of the caudate nucleus. J Child Neurol 1993; 8:339–47.
30. Mataró M, García-Sánchez C, Junqué C, Estévez-González A, Pujol J. Magnetic resonance imaging measurement of the caudate nucleus in adolescents with attention-deficit hyperactivity disorder and its relationship with neuropsychological and behavioral measures. Arch Neurol 1997; 54: 963–8.
31. Castellanos FX, Giedd JN, Berquin PC, et al. Quantitative brain magnetic resonance imaging in girls with attention-deficit/hyperactivity disorder. Arch Gen Psychiatry 2001; 58:289–95.
32. Aylward EH, Reiss AL, Reader MJ, Singer HS, Brown JE, Denckla MB. Basal ganglia volumes in children with attention-deficit hyperactivity disorder. J Child Neurol 1996; 11:112–5.
33. Teicher MH, Anderson CM, Polcari A, Glod CA, Maas LC, Renshaw PF. Functional deficits in basal ganglia of children with attention-deficit/hyperactivity disorder shown with functional magnetic resonance imaging relaxometry. Nat Med 2000; 6:470–3.
34. DeLong GR. Mid-gestation right basal ganglia lesion: clinical observations in two children. Neurology 2002; 59:54–8.
35. Herskovits EH, Megalooikonomou V, Davatzikos C, Chen A, Bryan RN, Gerring JP. Is the spatial distribution of brain lesions associated with closed-head injury predictive of subsequent development of attention-deficit/hyperactivity disorder? Analysis with brain-image database. Radiology 1999; 213: 389–94.
36. Max JE, Fox PT, Lancaster JL, et al. Putamen lesions and the development of attention-deficit/hyperactivity symptomatology. J Am Acad Child Adolesc Psychiatry 2002; 41:563–71.
37. Allen G, Buxton RB, Wong EC, Courchesne E. Attentional activation of the cerebellum independent of motor movement. Science 1997; 275:1940–3.
38. de Zubicaray GI, Zelaya FO, Andrew C, Williams SC, Bullmore ET. Cerebral regions associated with verbal response initiation, suppression and strategy use. Neuropsychologia 2000; 38:1292–304.
39. Desmond JE, Gabrieli JD, Glover GH. Dissociation of frontal and cerebellar activity in a cognitive task: evidence for a distinction between selection and search. Neuroimage 1998; 7:368–76.

40. Desmond JE, Gabrieli JD, Wagner AD, Ginier BL, Glover GH. Lobular patterns of cerebellar activation in verbal working-memory and finger-tapping tasks as revealed by functional MRI. J Neurosci 1997; 17:9675–85.
41. Rao SM, Bobholz JA, Hammeke TA, et al. Functional MRI evidence for subcortical participation in conceptual reasoning skills. NeuroReport 1997; 8: 1987–93.
42. Thomas KM, King SW, Franzen PL, et al. A developmental functional MRI study of spatial working memory. Neuroimage 1999; 10(3 Pt. 1):327–38.
43. Tracy JI, Faro SH, Mohamed FB, Pinsk M, Pinus A. Functional localization of a "Time Keeper" function separate from attentional resources and task strategy. Neuroimage 2000; 11:228–42.
44. Berquin PC, Giedd JN, Jacobsen LK, et al. The cerebellum in attention-deficit/ hyperactivity disorder: a morphometric study. Neurology 1998; 50:1087–93.
45. Mostofsky SH, Reiss AL, Lockhart P, Denckla MB. Evaluation of cerebellar size in attention-deficit hyperactivity disorder. J Child Neurol 1998; 13:434–9.
46. Anderson CM, Polcari AM, Lowen SB, Renshaw PF, Teicher MH. Effects of methylphenidate on functional magnetic resonance relaxometry of the cerebellar vermis in children with ADHD. Am J Psychiatry 2002; 159:1322–8.
47. Milberger S, Biederman J, Faraone SV, Guite J, Tsuang MT. Pregnancy, delivery and infancy complications and attention deficit hyperactivity disorder: issues of gene–environment interaction. Biol Psychiatry 1997; 41:65–75.
48. Gerring JP, Brady KD, Chen A, et al. Premorbid prevalence of ADHD and development of secondary ADHD after closed head injury. J Am Acad Child Adolesc Psychiatry 1998; 37:647–54.
49. Max JE, Lindgren SD, Knutson C, Pearson CS, Ihrig D, Welborn A. Child and adolescent traumatic brain injury: psychiatric findings from a paediatric outpatient specialty clinic. Brain Inj 1997; 11:699–711.
50. Max JE, Mathews K, Lansing AE, et al. Psychiatric disorders after childhood stroke. J Am Acad Child Adolesc Psychiatry 2002; 41:555–62.
51. Max JE, Arndt S, Castillo CS, et al. Attention-deficit hyperactivity symptomatology after traumatic brain injury: a prospective study. J Am Acad Child Adolesc Psychiatry 1998; 37:841–7.
52. Simpson A, Schmitter-Edgecombe M. Intactness of inhibitory attentional mechanisms following severe closed-head injury. Neuropsychology 2000; 14: 310–9.
53. Gerring J, Brady K, Chen A, et al. Neuroimaging variables related to development of secondary attention deficit hyperactivity disorder after closed head injury in children and adolescents. Brain Inj 2000; 14:205–18.
54. Gaub M, Carlson CL. Gender differences in ADHD: a meta-analysis and critical review. J Am Acad Child Adolesc Psychiatry 1997; 36:1036–45.
55. Sharp WS, Walter JM, Marsh WL, Ritchie GF, Hamburger SD, Castellanos FX. ADHD in girls: clinical comparability of a research sample. J Am Acad Child Adolesc Psychiatry 1999; 38:40–7.
56. Alexander GE, DeLong MR, Strick PL. Parallel organization of functionally segregated circuits linking basal ganglia and cortex. Annu Rev Neurosci 1986; 9:357–81.

57. Graybiel AM. The basal ganglia and chunking of action repertoires. Neurobiol Learn Mem 1998; 70:119–36.
58. Melchitzky DS, Lewis DA. Tyrosine hydroxylase- and dopamine transporter-immunoreactive axons in the primate cerebellum. Evidence for a lobular- and laminar-specific dopamine innervation. Neuropsychopharmacology 2000; 22: 466–72.
59. Bullmore ET, Suckling J, Overmeyer S, Rabe-Hesketh S, Taylor E, Brammer MJ. Global, Voxel, and cluster tests, by theory and permutation, for a difference between two groups of structural MR images of the brain. IEEE Trans Med Imaging 1999; 18:32–42.
60. Bussing R, Grudnik J, Mason D, Wasiak M, Leonard C. ADHD and conduct disorder: an MRI study in a community sample. World J Biol Psychiatry 2002; 3:216–20.

9

Interactions Among Motivation and Attention Systems: Implications for Theories of ADHD

Douglas Derryberry and Marjorie A. Reed
Department of Psychology, Oregon State University, Corvallis, Oregon, U.S.A.

Temperament models approach attention deficit hyperactivity disorder (ADHD) in terms of neural systems involved in motivation, emotion, arousal, and attention. This chapter emphasizes individual differences in two motivational systems that are activated in appetitive and defensive situations, along with an attentional system related to voluntary or effortful control. The basic framework suggests that the two motivational systems exert relatively reactive or involuntary effects on behavior and attention. With the development of frontal circuits, however, the motivational systems become capable of recruiting executive attentional systems that allow for more refined and voluntary motivational functions. Individual differences across these systems leave some children vulnerable to impulsive disorders such as ADHD, as characterized by hyperactivity, attentional deficits, and impulsive behavior.

In the following sections we briefly discuss the various systems, emphasizing their effects on both behavior and attention. We then discuss interactions between the systems, illustrating how some profiles might increase vulnerability whereas others serve a more protective function. Our approach suggests that symptoms of ADHD can arise from several different developmental pathways. For some children, the problem may involve only a single system, such as an overly strong approach system or a weak frontal attentional capacity. In others, two or more systems might be involved, such as strong approach accompanied by weak inhibitory capacities. An important theme is that the three systems are highly interactive, with reciprocal influences upon one another. In some cases interactive influences may prove beneficial for voluntary control, but in others, the interactive effects may constrain the child's ability for self-control. Thus, it is essential to consider the various ways in which these systems influence one another.

REWARD-RELATED APPETITIVE MOTIVATION

An initial neural system relevant to ADHD is responsible for producing approach behavior in response to expected rewards (1–3). Although the precise formulations vary, this appetitive system is thought to be focused within subcortical limbic regions and to receive reward-related inputs from the cortex. Upon detecting a potential reward, the system recruits dopaminergic projections to facilitate approach behavior and emotional states such as "hope" and "anticipatory eagerness". In addition, some have suggested that strong appetitive systems may produce frustrative reactions when a reward is blocked (3–5). Individual differences in this system are thought to underlie personality dimensions related to extraversion (or neurotic extraversion). For example, as one moves from the "introverted" to the "extraverted" pole of this dimension, the person becomes more sensitive to potential rewards, shows faster and more vigorous approach behavior, and greater hope and eagerness. In terms of psychopathology, this system may contribute to the hyperkinetic and impulsive behaviors evident in ADHD, as well as the proneness to emotions such as hope and frustration.

In addition to these behavioral and emotional effects, the appetitive system also exerts effects on attention. In many cases these are reflexive or involuntary effects, mediated by projections from the motivational system to the "posterior attentional system" described by Posner (6). The posterior system is a distributed system that produces reactive orienting through operations of "disengaging," "moving," and "engaging" attention. Our research with college students suggests that appetitive motivation makes it more difficult for individuals to disengage attention from a reward-related spatial location, with the effect strongest in neurotic extraverts (7). Such a bias may also occur in ADHD, causing such children to have difficulty shifting from a salient rewarding activity in favor of less-rewarding tasks.

Another attentional process influenced by motivational and emotional states involves adjustments in the breadth of attention. Relevant neural mechanisms appear lateralized, with posterior left hemisphere circuits supporting a "focusing" or "narrowing" of attention, and posterior right hemisphere circuits promoting a "broadening" or more global attentional scope. In emotional terms, evidence suggest that negative states such as anxiety promote a narrowing of attention while positive or appetitive states promote a broadening of attention (8). If an ADHD child is subject to strong appetitive motivation, they may often show a relatively broad attentional focus. As a result, they may have more difficulty focusing on the details of the situation, and may be more responsive to task-irrelevant information sources.

In addition to these reactive influences, the approach system can also access frontal attentional mechanisms that allow for voluntary control. As discussed in more detail below, voluntary attentional mechanisms allow the individual to access additional information (rules, beliefs, feelings) that helps in selecting, planning, and controlling approach responses. In delaying gratification, for example, the child may be able to access knowledge that a delayed reward will be greater than an immediate reward, and voluntarily shift attention away from cues that intensify the immediately rewarding aspects of the situation (9).

Unfortunately, evidence relating individual differences in approach motivation to ADHD remains inconsistent. Early concept identification studies suggested that children with ADHD may be overly sensitive to rewards, to the loss of reward, and to the failure of expected rewards to appear (10). More recent studies suggest that ADHD children are especially sensitive to individual instances of reward, which bias their responses in relation to more frequently rewarded stimuli (11). In addition, ADHD children may have particular difficulty in delaying reward, with a strong preference for immediate over delayed rewards (12,13). While these studies suggest an oversensitivity to salient rewards in ADHD children, other findings are more difficult to interpret. For example, children with ADHD slowed down more dramatically in the reward condition on a stop task than normal controls, and this slowing was interpreted as a strategy to increase the chance of being rewarded (14). Also problematic are findings that ADHD children make more errors of commission in a go/no-go task, regardless of whether the conditions involved reward or response costs (15).

Also supportive of strong appetitive motivation are findings suggesting that ADHD children are prone to frustration. It is worth noting that our view linking frustration to reward and appetitive motivation differs from models such as Gray's, which view frustration as an output of the anxiety-related behavioral inhibition system. Along with others (3,4), we suggest that it makes more functional sense to link frustration to a general appetitive motivational system that responds to nonreward as well as reward. In any event, Douglas and Parry (16) found ADHD children to show more frustrative behavior (i.e., more vigorous lever pulling) under conditions of low reward probability and reward extinction. ADHD children have been found to show greater frustration than controls in a nonsense word spelling task under partial reinforcement (17). In a more general model of impulsive problems, Newman and his colleagues have suggested that disorders such as ADHD may involve a facilitation of a dominant response set (e.g., approach) by the nonspecific arousal resulting from a negative outcome (e.g., frustration) (18,19).

PUNISHMENT-RELATED INHIBITORY MOTIVATION

A second motivational system often related to ADHD is Gray's "behavioral inhibition system." Relevant circuitry is distributed across the orbital cortex, hippocampus, amygdala, hypothalamus, and periqueductal gray, with different stations responsible for generating different forms of fear-related behavior (20). In Gray's formulation, the system responds to signals of punishment by inhibiting ongoing behavior and producing an emotional state of fear or anxiety. It also increases cortical arousal and enhances attention, thereby facilitating the processing of the threatening signal. Individual differences in the reactivity of the behavioral inhibition system are thought to underlie dimensions related to neuroticism and neurotic introversion.

Theorists have suggested that children with ADHD may possess relatively weak inhibition systems (21,22). As a result, they are relatively insensitive to signals of punishment, and are less able to inhibit approach responses. At a behavioral level, deficits in inhibition could lead to the same types of problems as those arising from an overactive approach system; i.e., impulsive, short latency approach responses that are difficult to stop. In this case, however, the approach behavior would not necessarily be accompanied by positive emotion, but rather, by a relative absence of fear and anxiety.

Like the approach system, the anxiety-related system exerts influences upon attention that complement its behavioral functions. One influence is on orienting, with increased attention allocated to threatening stimuli so that they can be effectively evaluated. Our studies with college students indicate that anxious individuals have difficulty shifting from a threatening stimulus (7). Assuming that ADHD kids possess weak anxiety/inhibition systems, it would be relatively easy for them to disengage from signals of punishment or nonreward, thereby lessening the capacity for these stimuli to constrain their behavior. At conceptual levels, children with a weak anxiety system may also find it easy to shift attention and avoid ruminating on the negative consequences of their behavior.

The second reactive influence is on attentional focusing, with anxiety serving to concentrate attention on dominant or central perceptual stimuli. Presumably, such narrowing serves to facilitate the processing of local details that may be important in evaluating the stimulus and situation (8). If the anxiety system is weak, then important details that could constrain behavior may be overlooked. For example, the child may overlook certain aspects of another's facial expression or tone of voice, and thus continue with inappropriate behavior. At a more conceptual level, the child may have difficulty maintaining the "self-focused" attention related to anxiety, and may thus have difficulty evaluating the appropriateness of their own behavior.

Many studies suggest that ADHD children are deficient in inhibiting responses. For example, they have difficulty inhibiting the initiation of response go/no-go tasks (15), suppressing an already-selected response in the stop-signal task (23,24), and stopping and changing a response in the change task (25). However, evidence that such inhibitory problems may be linked to an underreactive behavioral inhibition system (BIS) is lacking. For example, studies that manipulate incentives have not found insensitivity to punishment cues in ADHD children (15,26). In addition, the prediction that ADHD children should be low in anxiety is problematic. ADHD is often comorbid with anxiety disorders, suggesting an overreactive rather than underreactive BIS. Tannock (27) estimates that ADHD and anxiety disorders occur together in approximately 25% of cases. These and other problems for the weak-BIS approach to ADHD are well discussed by Nigg (28).

It may turn out that the individual differences in BIS reactivity will prove helpful in understanding the comorbid disorders accompanying ADHD. A weak BIS may exist in children where ADHD combines with conduct problems or undersocialized aggressive problems (21). Such children may have considerable difficulty in withholding approach responses because they fail to anticipate negative consequences. They may also fail to learn from their inappropriate behavior because their inattention to punishment makes it difficult to link it to their own behavior. In contrast, other ADHD children may possess a relatively strong BIS, making them vulnerable to comorbid anxiety. Compared to ADHD children with less anxiety, the more anxious children should show attenuated impulsive symptoms (29). They should be more attentive to potential punishments. Attentional orienting and focusing on threat should also make it easier for them to link actual punishments to their own inappropriate behaviors. As a result, anxious ADHD children should show better learning related to social and moral development.

So far we have described two types of motivational systems, one related to approach and the other to inhibition, which may contribute to ADHD. Both systems are capable of explaining some of the behavioral and attentional symptoms related to ADHD. These effects are primarily involuntary, a more or less reactive component of the overall pattern (i.e., behavioral, autonomic, attentional) of the motivational state. To better understand ADHD, however, it is necessary to consider a third system that allows for more voluntary control.

EXECUTIVE ATTENTIONAL PROCESSES

The systems responsible for voluntary control are thought to arise from "executive" attentional systems within the frontal lobe. Two of the most influential models include Posner's "anterior attentional system" (6) and Shallice's "supervisory attentional system" (30). In addition, other theorists have discussed executive processes that go beyond attention, such as working memory and various forms of emotion regulation (31). Although much can be gained by studying these additional processes, we limit our present discussion to processes specified by Posner's "anterior attentional system." This circuitry is focused in the anterior cingulate cortex where it receives extensive inputs from motivational, perceptual, conceptual, response, and arousal systems. Based on this input, the anterior system provides voluntary control across the course of processing. For example, it regulates the posterior orienting system, thereby providing more flexible control over incoming perceptual content. When conceptual content is activated, the anterior system inhibits dominant conceptual associations, allowing control over highly automatized patterns of thought. It also inhibits dominant response tendencies, allowing more flexible response evaluation and selection. Finally, the anterior system is involved in detecting errors, allowing for corrections of responses and plans that go wrong (6,32). Children's differences in anterior system function have been investigated through Rothbart's construct of "effortful control" (33,34). Children scoring high on measures of effort control tend to show less negative emotion, which is consistent with the ideas that they can employ their attentional skills to cope with the impact of negative stimuli. In addition, effortful control is related to moral emotions such as empathy and guilt, and moreover, to the internalization of moral principles and the development of social competence (35–37).

Many symptoms related to ADHD may result from frontal deficits related to effortful control. Focusing on voluntary control of information access during response processing, we suggest that it involves attention to sensory events, alternative response options, and the affective outcomes associated with these responses. If the child's flexibility in attending to these three forms of information is impaired, then they will be at a disadvantage in controlling their behavior. Such inflexibility may in part arise from difficulties in disengaging attention of certain information in order to attend to other important sources (38).

During the initial selection of a response, children must often inhibit the dominant tendency and replace it with an alternative response. Rather than immediately reaching for a food item, for example, the child must suppress this tendency and obtain permission from the parent. This situation can be modeled as a simple conflict situation, where alternative responses have been associated with alternative outcomes. The impulsive act of reaching may be related to an immediate reward along with potential disapproval from the parents, whereas the alternative response of asking may be related to a slightly delayed reward along with potential approval from the parent. To the extent that the child is able to disengage attention from stimuli that support the dominant tendency, such as the rewarding visual and taste cues, they should be better able to also attend to other information regarding the various outcomes. They can then weigh these outcomes and select the more optimal response. Such attentional flexibility may be impaired in ADHD children, leaving them at a disadvantage in inhibiting the dominant response. In many situations, effective behavior involves not only selecting a response, but setting up a plan or strategy involving a sequential set of responses. Although planning involves additional executive functions, attentional flexibility will play an important role. The most effective plans will be those that build with conditional response options, such that alternative actions can be executed depending on changing environmental events. Constructing such a plan requires that attention move flexibly among anticipated events, various response options, and their associated outcomes. If such flexibility is lacking, then the plan is likely to prove deficient. Recent studies have found deficits in strategy generation to be particularly severe in children with ADHD (39,40).

In other situations, a response or plan may be relatively easy to select, but must then be delayed in order to obtain a more optimal reward. Much research suggests that ADHD children have an aversion to delay. Although problems in delaying approach may reflect underlying motivational processes (41), they may also arise from attentional limitations. Mischel and his colleagues have shown that when presented with an attractive object and instructed to wait before approaching it, children who are successful in delaying gratification rely on a variety of attentional strategies (9,42). In general, these strategies involve disengaging from the rewarding aspects of the object (e.g., how good it might taste), and attending instead to "cooler" properties of the object (e.g., its color or shape) or to peripheral stimuli in the room. An inability to execute these types of distraction strategies may leave the ADHD child vulnerable to increased frustration as they attempt to wait, leading to a shorter period of delay.

Beyond distraction strategies, children acquire more complex cognitive strategies that support their self-control. We have recently suggested that children develop strategies of attending to conceptual and affective information that support their efforts for self-control (43). At a conceptual level, for example, the child can employ executive attention to engage various beliefs about what they "should" do (e.g., "I should be patient and calm") and what they "can" do (e.g., "I can resist this temptation"). At an affective level, the child may attend to representations of affective outcomes that might result from success (e.g., feelings of pride or self-satisfaction) and failure (e.g., feelings of guilt) in their attempts to control their behavior. As can be seen, these strategies can be complex and require considerable flexibility in shifting attention among different perceptual, conceptual, and affective content. If their executive attentional capacity is limited, children with ADHD may have difficulty in taking advantage of these strategies.

Once a response is initiated, another important executive function involves monitoring responses and correcting errors (32). Children with good attention may initiate a relatively impulsive response, but can still monitor the response and make adjustments if they are not getting closer to their goal. In addition, the child's impulsive responses may elicit negative responses from others, but they can shift to more acceptable responses. To the extent that executive attention is deficient in ADHD children, they may often lack the attentional flexibility to track rapidly changing outcomes and response options. Thus, their responses may tend to be ballistic and perseverative, and they may often find themselves frustrated or faced with disapproval from others.

After a response has failed, children with good attention are able to reflect on their failure and form a representation of the problematic behaviors and outcomes. Again, such reflection requires attentional flexibility in disengaging from the experienced frustration and reconsidering the individual actions and their relation to the unfolding negative events. A child with weak executive attention may have difficulty with such reflection, lacking the flexibility required for replaying, isolating, and linking the causal effects. In more extreme cases, some children may be virtually unable to disengage from their frustration, which functions to invigorate a dominant and ineffective follow-up response (18,19).

We have focused our discussion of executive functions primarily on limitations in attentional flexibility. The basic point is that the processing involved in selecting, executing, and reflecting on responses is complex, requiring attentional flexibility. If this flexibility is impaired, then the more dominant and often ineffective responses will tend to be favored, as is often the case in children with ADHD. It is important to understand, however, that this inflexibility may not always be solely due to the problems with executive attention. Rather, it may emerge from interactions between the voluntary attentional and more reactive motivational influences. In the final section, we consider several interactions between systems that seem relevant to ADHD.

INTERACTIONS BETWEEN MOTIVATIONAL AND ATTENTIONAL SYSTEMS

Perhaps the most obvious interaction involves children with a strong approach system accompanied by a relatively weak voluntary attentional capacity. There are several ways in which the strong approach system may tend to constrain the regulatory effects of voluntary attention. For example, some of the voluntary functions mentioned above (e.g., planning, reflection on failure) require time. If the approach motivation is too strong, then the child's impulse to act tends to short circuit the voluntary processes. In addition, with strong approach motivation, approach responses, especially those associated with immediate reward, will be strongly potentiated and would be difficult to inhibit even with strong attentional capacity. Moreover, if the effect of strong approach motivation is to delay disengagement from a source of reward (7), then crucial attentional flexibility will be impaired. As can be seen, these reactive influences arising from strong approach motivation will only be controllable by strong executive abilities.

Similar, but not identical, effects might come about with another combination of temperamental characteristics, when strong approach is combined with low fear motivation. The lack of reactive behavioral inhibition would tend to disinhibit approach responses, often leaving insufficient time for more effortful processing (31). These children's thoughts could be dominated by immediate reward, along with a relative absence of information related to potential punishment. Because of this absence, it may prove difficult for such a child to voluntarily engage affective content that might support self-control (e.g., anticipated feelings of guilt or empathy), because such feelings are uncommon and thus not strongly stored as representations (44,45). In addition, the overly broad scope of their attention, resulting from an approach-related expansion in the absence of an anxiety-related narrowing, may make it difficult for them to focus on important details involved in planning and evaluating responses. Presumably, these limitations can be to some extent overcome if the child has good attentional control, but more effort and flexibility will be required.

As mentioned earlier, ADHD children with comorbid anxiety may actually benefit in several ways. For example, the strong anxiety may provide reactive control over dominant approach tendencies by inhibiting the selected response and allocating attention in favor of potential punishment. These reactive influences may actually prove beneficial to some executive functions. For example, increased attention to negative information may make it easier for the child to anticipate potential negative outcomes during planning, to detect and correct these outcomes during the execution phase, and to take better account of their mistakes in reflecting on their problematic behavior. At the same time, however, anxiety has other reactive effects that may impair executive functions. In particular, anxiety elicits an attentional narrowing along with enhanced attention to threat, both of which could easily undermine the flexibility required in controlling responses. The anxious ADHD child's strategies may prove effective in fairly simple situations, but in more complex situations substantial rigidity may characterize their behavior.

CONCLUSIONS

In this chapter we have considered ADHD as an outcome of reactive motivational processes and voluntary attentional processes. Although much evidence suggests an important role for executive processes, we have tried to emphasize that the executive capacity will depend not only on frontal systems, but also on the subcortical motivational systems with which they interact. These subcortical systems exert reactive influences on behavior and attention, and it is within this reactive context that the executive mechanisms must operate. Thus, research needs to consider both types of processes. This can be most readily done by considering different types of executive processes set within motivational contexts that manipulate the child's reward- and punishment-related systems. Such an approach promises a broader and more integrated view of the functional deficits accomp anying ADHD.

REFERENCES

1. Depue RA, Collins PF. Neurobiology of the structure of personality: dopamine, facilitation of incentive motivation, and extraversion. Behav Brain Sci 1999; 22:491–555.
2. Gray JA. The Psychology of Fear and Stress. 2nd ed. New York: McGraw-Hill, 1987.
3. Panksepp J. Affective Neuroscience. New York: Oxford, 1998.
4. Depue RA, Iacono WG. Neurobehavioral aspects of affective disorders. Ann Rev Psychol 1989; 40:457–92.
5. Derryberry D, Rothbart MK. Reactive and effortful processes in the organization of temperament. Dev Psychopathol 1997; 9:633–52.
6. Posner MI, Raichle ME. Images of Mind. New York: Scientific American Library, 1994.
7. Derryberry D, Reed MA. Temperament and attention: orienting toward and away from positive and negative signals. J Pers Soc Psychol 1994; 66:1128–39.
8. Derryberry D, Tucker DM. Motivating the focus of attention. In: Niedenthal P, Kitayama S, eds. The Heart's Eye: Emotional Influences in Perception and Attention. San Diego, CA: Academic Press, 1993:170–96.
9. Metcalfe J, Mischel W. A hot/cool-system analysis of delay of gratification: dynamics of willpower. Psychol Rev 1999; 106:3–19.
10. Parry P, Douglas VI. Effects of reinforcement on concept identification in hyperactive children. J Abnorm Child Psychol 1983; 11:327–40.
11. Tripp G, Alsop B. Sensitivity to reward frequency in boys with attention deficit hyperactivity disorder. J Clin Child Psychol 1999; 28:366–75.
12. Barkley RA, Edwards G, Laneri M, Fletcher K, Metevia L. Executive functioning, temporal discounting, and sense of time in adolescents with attention deficit hyperactivity disorder (ADHD) and oppositional defiant disorder (ODD). J Abnorm Child Psychol 2001; 29:541–56.
13. Tripp G, Alsop B. Sensitivity to reward delay in children with attention deficit hyperactivity disorder (ADHD). J Child Psychol Psychiatry 2001; 42:691–8.
14. Scheres A, Oosterlaan J, Sergeant J. Response inhibition in children with DSM-IV subtypes of AD/HD and related disruptive disorders: the role of reward. Child Neuropsychol 2001; 7:172–89.

15. Iaboni F, Douglas VI, Baker AG. Effects of reward and response costs on inhibition in ADHD children. J Abnorm Psychol 1995; 104:232–40.
16. Douglas VI, Parry PA. Effects of reward and nonreward on frustration and attention in attention deficit disorder. J Abnorm Child Psychol 1994; 22:281–302.
17. Wigal T, Swanson JM, Douglas VI, Wigal SB, Wippler CM, Cavoto KF. Effect of reinforcement on facial responsivity and persistence in children with attention-deficit hyperactivity disorder. Behav Modif 1998; 1998:143–66.
18. Wallace JF, Newman JP, Bachorowski J. Failures of response modulation: impulsive behavior in anxious and impulsive individuals. J Res Person 1991; 25: 23–44.
19. Newman JP, Wallace JF. Diverse pathways to deficient self-regulation: implications for disinhibitory psychopathology in children. Clin Psychol Rev 1993; 13:699–720.
20. Gray JA, McNaughton N. The neuropsychology of anxiety: reprise. In: Hope DA, ed. Nebraska Symposium on Motivation: Perspectives on Anxiety, Panic, and Fear, Vol 43. Lincoln, Nebraska: University of Nebraska Press, 1996:61–134.
21. Quay HC. The psychobiology of undersocialized aggressive conduct disorder: a theoretical perspective. Dev Psychopathol 1993; 5:165–80.
22. Quay HC. Inhibition and attention deficit hyperactivity disorder. J Abnorm Child Psychol 1997; 27:7–13.
23. Schachar R, Logan GD. Impulsivity and inhibitory control in normal development and childhood psychopathology. Dev Psychol 1990; 26:710–20.
24. Stevens J, Quittner AL, Zuckerman JB, Moore S. Behavioral inhibition, self-regulation of motivation, and working memory in children with attention deficit hyperactivity disorder. Dev Neuropsychol 2002; 21:117–39.
25. Serjeant J. The cognitive-energetic model: an empirical approach to attention-deficit hyperactivity disorder. Neurosci Biobehav Rev 2000:7–12.
26. Oosterlaan J, Sergeant JA. Effects of reward and response cost on response inhibition in AD/HD, disruptive, anxious, and normal children. J Abnorm Child Psychol 1998; 26:161–74.
27. Tannock R. Attention-deficit/hyper activity disorder with anxiety disorders. In: Brown TE, ed. Attention-Deficit Disorders and Comorbidities in Children, Adolescents, and Adults. Washington, D.C.: American Psychiatric Publishing, 2000:125–70.
28. Nigg JT. Is ADHD a disinhibitory disorder? Psychol Bull 2001; 127:571–98.
29. Pliszka SR. Effect of anxiety on cognition, behavior, and stimulant response in ADHD. J Am Acad Child Adolesc Psychiatry 1989; 28:882–7.
30. Stuss DT, Shallice T, Alexander MP, Picton TW. A multidisciplinary approach to anterior attentional functions. In: Grafman J, Holyoak KJ, Boller F, eds. Structure and Functions of the Human Prefrontal Cortex (Annals of the New York Academy of Sciences), Vol 769. New York: The New York Academy of Sciences, 1995.
31. Barkley RA. Behavioral inhibition, sustained attention, and executive functions: constructing a unifying theory of ADHD. Psychol Bull 1997; 121:65–94.

32. Posner MI, DiGirolamo GJ. Executive attention: conflict, target detection and cognitive control. In: Parasuraman R, ed. The Attentive Brain. Cambridge, MA: MIT Press, 1998:401–23.
33. Rothbart MK, Derryberry D, Posner MI. A psychobiological approach to the development of temperament. In: Bates JE, Wachs TD, eds. Temperament: Individual Differences at the Interface of Biology and Behavior. Washington, D.C.: American Psychological Association, 1994:83–116.
34. Rothbart MK, Bates JE. Temperament. In: Damon WSE, Eisenberg NVE, eds. Handbook of Child Psychology, Vol 3. Social, Emotional and Personality Development. 5th ed. New York: Wiley, 1998:105–76.
35. Eisenberg N, Fabes RA, Bernzweig J, Karbon M, Poulin R, Hanish L. The relations of emotionality and regulation to preschoolers' social skills and sociometric status. Child Dev 1993; 64:1418–38.
36. Kochanska G, Murray K, Jacques TY, Koenig AL, Vandegeest KA. Inhibitory control in young children and its role in emerging internalization. Child Dev 1996; 67:490–507.
37. Rothbart MK, Ahadi SA, Hershey KL. Temperament and social behavior in childhood. Merrill-Palmer Q 1994; 40:21–39.
38. Wood C, Maruff P, Levy F, Farrow M, Hay D. Covert orienting of visual spatial attention in attention deficit hyperactivity disorder: does comorbidity make a difference? Arch Clin Neuropsychol 1999; 14:179–89.
39. Nigg JT, Butler KM, Huang-Pollock CL, Henderson JM. Inhibitory processes in adults with persistent childhood onset ADHD. J Consult Clin Psychol 2002; 70:153–7.
40. Shallice T, Marzocchi GM, Coser S, Del Savio M, Meuter RF, Rumiati RI. Executive function profile of children with attention deficit hyperactivity disorder. Dev Neuropsychol 2002; 21:43–71.
41. Sonuga-Barke E. Psychological heterogeneity in AD/HD—a dual pathway model of behaviour and cognition. Behav Brain Res 2002; 130:29–36.
42. Mischel W. Delay of gratification as process and as person variable in development. In: Magnusson D, Allen VP, eds. Human Development: An Interactional Perspective. New York: Academic Press, 1983:149–65.
43. Derryberry D, Reed MA, Pilkenton-Taylor C. Temperament and coping: advantages of an individual differences perspective. Dev Psychopathol, 2003; 15:1049–66.
44. Braaten EB, Rosen LA. Self-regulation of affect in Attention Deficit-Hyperactivity Disorder (ADHD) and non-ADHD Boys: differences in emapthic responding. J Consult Clin Psychol 2000; 68:313–21.
45. Derryberry D, Reed MA. Regulatory processes and the development of cognitive representations. Dev Psychopathol 1996; 8:215–34.

10

Where is the "Attention Deficit" in ADHD? Perspectives from Cognitive Neuroscience and Recommendations for Future Research

Cynthia L. Huang-Pollock

Department of Psychology, Pennsylvania State University, University Park, Pennsylvania, U.S.A.

INTRODUCTION

The suggestion that individuals with attention deficit hyperactivity disorder (ADHD) suffer from a subtle neurological dysfunction has existed throughout the history of modern clinical observations. However, after 100 years of observation and research, the identity of the primary mechanism(s) underlying this childhood disorder has yet to be conclusively resolved, as illustrated by the variety of neuropsychological theories covered in this edition. Whereas behavioral observations of "inattention" reliably distinguish children with ADHD from non-ADHD children (1), determination of whether inattention is a cognitive hallmark that identifies ADHD children from their non-ADHD counterparts has been more elusive. Clarification of this issue would allow for the development of more complete and accurate theoretical models of ADHD, aide in the etiological determination of the disorder, and inform cognitive neuroscience of the structure of attentional processes in normal and abnormal development. Clinically, such information would allow for more objective diagnostic procedures, earlier detection, and targeted therapies for rehabilitation.

The largest challenge to clinical research in this respect is to clearly define and accurately measure the multiple constructs of attention. Prior to the advent of modern technologies that allow for improved control and measurement of component processes, clinical research more frequently relied upon face-valid definitions of "attention" and tasks of attention, rather than methodologies that tapped theoretically based and empirically supported attention structures. However, recent advances in cognitive neuroscience are providing new opportunities to examine the status of attention in ADHD. Due to the vast literature to be covered, this chapter will focus on only two of the more recent approaches to the study of attention in ADHD. The first of these is a distributed network model of visuospatial attentional orienting that Posner (2) and others' have extensively developed, and which has been applied to a variety of clinical populations. The second is a perceptual load model of selective attention that has garnered increasing excitement among cognitive neuroscientists since the mid-1990s (3). This model provides a unique perspective into the nature of selective attention, and may prove useful to the critique of previous findings and to the development of future studies of selective attention deficits in ADHD.

VISUOSPATIAL ATTENTIONAL ORIENTING

Although there is great variation in methodologies, the basic task is a simple target detection task in which reaction time (RT) is the main dependent variable. Participants are instructed to maintain fixation at a central point, and are cued to the location of a future target (i.e., right or left visual field) by an exogenous or endogenous cue. Figure 1 presents a schematic diagram of the paradigm. Exogenous cues orient attention automatically and appear

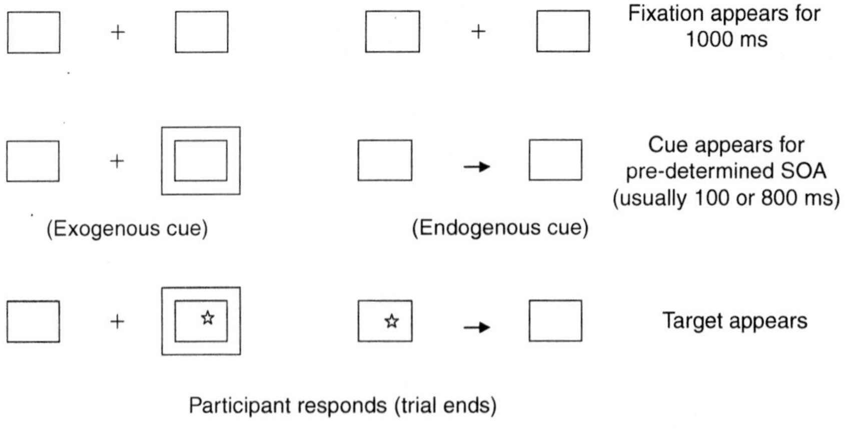

Figure 1 Diagram of the covert-orienting procedures for exogenous (right valid target) and endogenous (left invalid target) cueing conditions.

as a peripheral "brightening" in the right or left visual field. They are nonprobabilistic, that is only 50% of targets appear in a previously cued position. Endogenous cues, which are centrally located arrows, are probabilistic (typically 80% of targets appear in a previously cued location). Participants are therefore able to take advantage of the cueing probabilities to orient attention voluntarily for improved performance. Both cues decrease RT to detection at the cued location (benefits), with an accompanying increase in RT to targets appearing at the noncued position (costs).

Using this framework, Posner and colleagues have demonstrated that attentional control is derived from a network of at least three systems working together to orient visuospatial attention in a top-down goal-oriented manner, as well as a more data-driven automatic fashion. The posterior attention system (PAS), comprised of the superior parietal cortex, pulvinar, and superior colliculus, is responsible for automatically engaging, disengaging, and shifting attention in space. Thus, orientation to exogenous cues is believed to access the PAS. In contrast, the anterior attention system (AAS) is responsible for bringing targets into conscious awareness, for voluntary shifts of attention, and for decision-making. PET studies have found that midline frontal areas including the anterior cingulated gyrus and areas of the supplementary motor cortex are involved in detection (4–6). Orientation to endogenous cues accesses the AAS. The third network, the vigilance network, is responsible for maintaining sustained attention as well as for phasic alertness. This system is comprised of the noradrenergic system of the locus coeruleus, the cholinergic system of the basal forebrain, the intralaminar thalamic nuclei, and the right prefrontal cortex (7,8). The orienting paradigm was not optimally designed to evaluate the functioning of the vigilance network, but evidence for such a dysfunction could include slower RTs, increased variability of response, or specific performance deficits following neutral versus uncued targets in the experimental group (7,9,10).

This model has been validated by evidence from neuroimaging studies and studies of brain injured individuals (11–13). Accordingly, it has received extensive usage within clinical research for a wide range of disorders including Alzheimer's (14), Parkinson's disease (15), schizophrenia (16–18), brain injury, and collosotomy patients (19,20). Between 1990 and 2007, there have been 17 published studies of attentional orienting in ADHD utilizing Posner's model.

A review of that literature (21) found mixed evidence for a PAS deficit. That is, only 4 of 11 studies (22–25) found slower RTs for ADHD children (or their biological parents, as was the case in Nigg et al. (23)) to invalidly cued targets following exogenous cues. However, the affected visual field, and thus the affected hemisphere, did not replicate among the four. Poorer performance following invalid cues is associated with a deficit in the disengage operation, and has been found in individuals with documented right parietal lobe lesions. Despite qualitative replication, quantitative meta-analytic review (of the nine studies providing enough data to be included in analyses) found homogeneously small effect sizes across studies (average $D = 0.26$), suggesting that any observed effects were too small for clinical relevance (21). Assuming population effects of that size, sample sizes of at least 112 for both the ADHD and non-ADHD controls would be needed for power $= 0.80$ in a two-way repeated measures design. None of the studies approached that *n*, which may help to explain the inconsistency in results among studies.

With respect to voluntary AAS processes, all four studies using endogenous cues found significant group differences, but no study finding replicated another (21). Due to incomplete data reporting, only two of the four endogenous studies could be analyzed quantitatively (26,27). However, their reported effect sizes were significantly heterogeneous to prevent an accurate summary of findings. That is, the average effect size for McDonald et al. (26) was 2.44 (due to atypically small standard deviation of RTs) in comparison to Pearson et al.'s (27) 0.13. Error rates, which may be indicators of AAS functioning, were modestly supportive of an AAS deficit. Seven of eight studies found more errors of commission in their ADHD group, but only three were significantly so (28–30). Two of four studies found greater omission errors, but only Swanson et al. (24) found significant group differences in the number of such errors.

And finally with respect to the vigilance network, 7 of 12 studies found slower RTs in the ADHD group, but only four of these were significant (23,25,26,31). Oberlin et al. (32), published after the 2003 meta-analysis, used a paradigm similar to the visuospatial cueing task (Attention Network Task), and found that adults with ADHD-C (but not ADHD-I) were generally slower to target detection following both spatial and alerting cues. The generalized slowness was corrected following administration of stimulant medications and results were interpreted as indicative of deficits in phasic alerting (32). As another potential index of vigilance system functionality, Huang-Pollock et al. (33), but not Novak et al. (29), found greater variability in RT for the combined but not inattentive subtype. However, effect sizes calculated from group mean RTs and standard deviations collapsed across cueing conditions were homogenous and small (average $D = 0.18$; Ref. 21).

None of the three studies that examined performance over time found performance to deteriorate at a greater rate than controls, supporting previous arguments against a sustained attention deficit in ADHD (34,35). However, the orienting paradigm was not optimally designed to measure sustained attention. To address this concern, Huang-Pollock et al. (36) collected data from 135 children with ADHD-C, ADHD-I, and non-ADHD controls using exogenous and endogenous cueing conditions to assess PAS and AAS functionality, respectively, but also evaluated the vigilance system directly using a sustained attention paradigm (i.e., an A–X Continuous Performance test, CPT). There was no evidence of either PAS or AAS dysfunction in either ADHD subtype, but clear vigilance system deficits on the CPT emerged. Children with ADHD, regardless of subtype, had lower sensitivity (d'), a highly activated response style ($\ln \beta$), and performance that decreased over time in a manner consistent with a sustained attention deficit. In a smaller ($N = 30$) sample of children with ADHD and non-ADHD controls, Barry et al. (37) found similar results that favored vigilance system involvement in the form of sustained attention deficits, but not AAS or PAS deficits.

Suggestions that ADHD may represent a right-lateralized deficit have been widely discussed (38–40). However, with respect to the orienting paradigm, five studies found evidence broadly consistent with right hemisphere dysfunction, one found evidence for a left hemisphere involvement, while four found no significant visual field effects. Thus, lateralized effects also did not strongly or consistently replicate across studies.

SUMMARY

Despite qualitative replication in favor for a PAS disengage deficit, suggestions of a nonspecific AAS deficit, and a possible alerting dysfunction in the vigilance system, quantitative meta-analytic review failed to find evidence for a clinically significant deficit in either the AAS or PAS attentional-orienting systems, or in the phasic response processes of the vigilance system. Of the three articles utilizing the Posner paradigm not included in the original 2003 meta-analytic review (36,37,41), none found significant group differences in performance that would indicate deficits in the PAS or AAS, supporting those initial interpretations. Sustained attention deficits as a function of the vigilance system remain an open possibility, but the orienting paradigm itself is not the best tool to test this hypothesis.

There are several reasons for the lack of strong findings, aside from the obvious interpretation that children with ADHD may not have deficits in the basic, low-level attentional processes needed to shift spatial attention. Comorbidity within study groups is one, but there were no consistent differences among studies that did (eight) or did not (five) control for comorbidity (21). Lack of homogeneity due to use of DSM-IIIR (42) criteria for the majority of studies reviewed, is another. However, consistent cognitive differences have yet to be demonstrated between the two subtypes (43), and some research suggests that it is the presence of inattention, rather than hyperactivity or impulsivity, which is associated with neuropsychological deficits in processing speed, vigilance, and inhibitory control (44). Huang-Pollock et al. (33,36) used DSM-IV (45) criteria to examine orienting in both the inattentive and the combined subtype of ADHD, and found no group differences in performance. Although Huang-Pollock et al. (33,36) excluded children with either five symptoms of hyperactivity or inattention from analysis because subtype is difficult to determine in those cases (46), the issue of within-group heterogeneity even using DSM-IV criteria remains a general problem within the field of clinical research. Thus, subtle cognitive distinctions between subtypes may be obscured. Clarification of this question may require stricter control over groups (e.g., children presenting with fewer than four hyperactive symptoms, and who do not have comorbid oppositional or conduct problems), or consideration of additional symptoms (e.g., sluggish cognitive tempo, SCT) (47).

Low power due to small sample sizes may be another reason cumulative evidence for an orienting deficit has been elusive. The average group effect size across studies using exogenous cues was small, and required a total *N* of 224 for power to equal 0.80. Furthermore, the potential confounding effects of eye movements were not always controlled, and the paradigm itself may simply be less reliable in children than in adults.

Due to the large variability in methodologies (e.g., presence or absence of a "neutral" condition, forced-choice vs. simple detection tasks, and differences in visual angle or cue-target delays), it is recommended that future studies carefully weigh the potential benefits of information obtained from novel-orienting designs against the need for closer replication attempts. The common use of mixed cue types (e.g., predictive exogenous cues, or simultaneously appearing endogenous and exogenous cues) is also problematic. Such designs prevent clear interpretation of any group deficits as evidence for an AAS or PAS dysfunction. Due to the limited space available here, interested readers are directed to Huang-Pollock and Nigg (21) for a more thorough discussion of all these issues.

Although an accumulation of these methodological problems may contribute to the lack of significant findings for an orienting deficit, it is difficult to be persuaded that at least in the combined subtype of ADHD, an attentional-orienting dysfunction could be of sufficient magnitude to be of clinical relevance. However, further examination of performance in the primarily inattentive subtype, and of children with SCT, would be of interest given theoretical considerations of the disorder. Future investigators who want to pursue this are advised to attend to the issues of methodology specific to orienting outlined above, as well as to more general issues including attention to subtyping, comorbidity, and sample size. They are also advised to publish full tables of RT and standard deviations for each group in order to enable better estimation of meta-analytic effects.

The distributed network model of attention has gained wide usage not only because the neural structures it taps are well validated, but also because the computer-generated paradigm is well suited for research into cognitive processes. More generally, however, its popularity is evidence of a growing interest among clinical researchers in the application of cognitive neuroscience's theoretical advances for use in the study of clinical populations.

Such advances not only offer new avenues of research, but also provide a way to critique previous methods and results for their validity of approach. For example, there has long been the question of whether ADHD is represented by a *selective* attention deficit, and a recent model of selective attention may help address this issue.

PERCEPTUAL LOAD MODEL OF SELECTIVE ATTENTION

The perceptual load model of selective attention, like other capacity-based theories of attention, is founded on the assumption that humans possess a limited capacity for processing information. As such, it is necessary for an act of selection to occur so that only relevant items present in the perceptual world are selected for further processing, and irrelevant items are discarded. Whether this act of selection occurs early (48), prior to a full analysis of features, or late (49), after a considerable amount of processing has already taken place, has long been a matter of debate. Lavie (3) proposed that the locus of selection (i.e., early vs. late in the stream of information processing) is a function of the perceptual load on the attentional system. This model has been demonstrated in adults (3,50–52) as well as in children (53). When perceptual load is high, selection occurs "early," on the basis of the perceptual features such as color, form, and movement. In this situation, distracting task-irrelevant information is never processed, and the distractor's potential interference effect is small. However, when perceptual load is low, all stimuli are processed automatically regardless of their task relevance until capacity is exhausted. Selection in this case occurs "late," and is made on the basis of semantic identity. Thus, irrelevant distractors can subsequently cause significant interference in performance.

Lavie and Tsal (52) define perceptual load as consisting of two separate components: (i) the number of potentially task-relevant items in a display and (ii) the nature of the processing required for each item. High loads are those in which there are more task-relevant items on display, or when the display requires greater effort to process. Figure 2 presents examples of low and high loads. Early selection of perceptual features involves a posterior network of brain structures including regions of parietal and temporoparietal cortex (54–57). Late selection of semantic information (e.g., Stroop-like tasks; Ref. 58), involves a largely anterior network including the anterior cingulate gyrus and various regions of prefrontal cortex (59,60). Thus, when perceptual load is low, selective attention relies on anterior processes. But, when perceptual load is high, selective attention shifts and comes under the control of posterior network processes. Table 1 summarizes the perceptual load model of selective attention.

Readers will recognize that the neuroanatomical structures described here are similar to those associated with attentional orientation. Thus, a brief clarification of the relationship between selection and orientation is

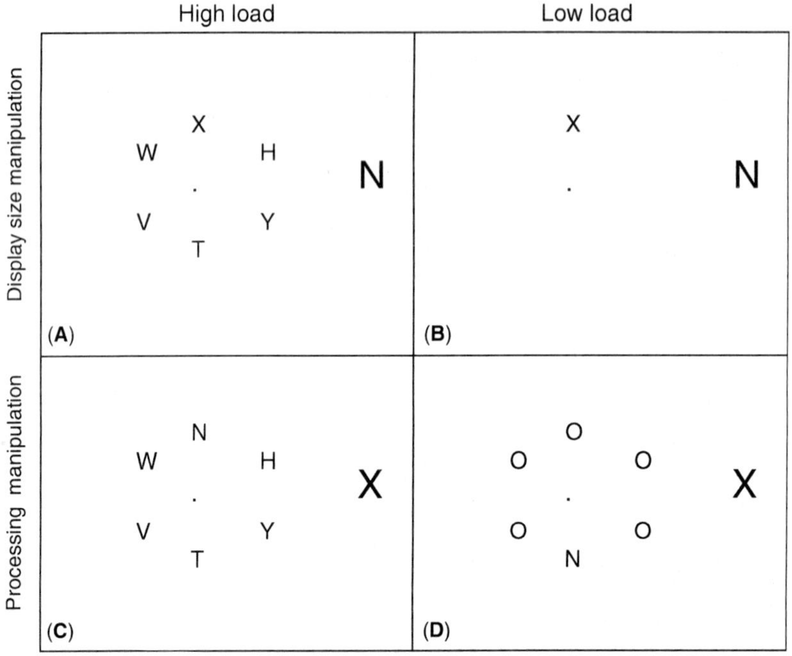

Figure 2 Example stimulus displays with high- and low-perceptual loads. The target, located in the circle of letters, can be either an "X" or and "N," thus requiring subjects to make a forced-choice response. The larger, peripheral letter represents the competing distractor. (**A**), (**B**): Manipulations of load by changing display sizes, with (**A**) representing a high load and (**B**) representing a low load. (**C**), (**D**): Manipulations of load by changing processing demands, with (**C**) representing a high load and (**D**) representing a low load.

required at this time. At its most basic, attentional orientation following an exogenous cue would be one example of an early selection process, because selection of a to-be-processed object is based on spatial location (i.e., the cue). In the orienting task, participants are instructed to maintain fixation at a central point. Automatic orientation to the peripheral cue occurs because the demands of maintaining fixation contribute only a low load to perceptual processes. Thus, there remains "extra" capacity available for the processing of the cue. Once oriented, information located within the cued region will receive facilitated processing in comparison to areas that are not selected, although automatic processing of irrelevant information would not be ruled out, assuming available capacity to process that information exists. Given that a particular spatial location will be attended, Lavie's (3) perceptual load model can be construed to ask: what determines future processing in that area? If the load is high, irrelevant information is more likely

Table 1 Summary of the Perceptual Load Model of Selective Attention

Locus of selection	Early	Late
Level of selection	External world	Internal representation
Selection based on	Perceptual features	Task demands
Perceptual load	High	Low
Automaticity	Automatic	Effortful
Neuroanatomical region	Largely posterior	Largely anterior

to be selected out of the stream of processing. If perceptual load is low, such information would continue to be processed along with relevant information.

One limitation to Lavie's (3) argument is that, at least in young adults, when participants are motivated to focus their attention to a discreet location in space, they are able to ignore distractors (i.e., abrupt visual onsets) (61). This occurs even when the perceptual load at the attended location is not sufficient to induce early selection. It may be that Lavie's (3) model of selection is optimal for situations in which individuals adopt a diffuse span of attention, or when they are unable to produce sufficient attentional focus (as in young children). That is, younger children whose anterior systems have not yet developed to sufficiently focus and maintain attention at fixed locations may depend more on older children or adults upon the automatic induction of early selection from heightened perceptual loads to limit interference from irrelevant information (53).

From the point of view of Lavie's (3) model, children with ADHD may be unable to shift from "late" to "early" selection to filter incoming stimuli from the environment, or, like younger children (53), they may require a greater perceptual load from their environment to engage this shift. Thus, the "beneficial" effects of high perceptual load to protect against distractor effects may be less evident in these children. Huang-Pollock et al. (62) examined both early and late selective attention using the perceptual load paradigm in children with DSM-IV ADHD combined and inattentive types, compared against non-ADHD controls. There were no significant differences in selective attention in either subtype. However, a subset of children with SCT demonstrated abnormal early selective attention deficits, and were unable to make the switch from late to early selection. Thus, it remains vitally important that future studies of selective attention or other cognitive processes in ADHD carefully attend to and reduce the group heterogeneity that arise from our current taxonomic classification. Consideration of SCT as well as stricter control over assignment to diagnostic subtypes is necessary to move the field forward in this respect.

Previous research has inconsistently supported a selective attention deficit in children with ADHD (63,64). However, when reinterpreted using Lavie's criteria, negative findings may be due to use of tasks that were not ideally suited to optimize the study of selective attention. That is, in order for early selective attention processes to be observed, a task must have (i) sufficient perceptual load to induce early selection (34,65,66) and (ii) the presence of a competing distractor that participants must suppress (67–70). Based on this model, future studies of selective attention in ADHD are also advised to attend to these two issues.

SUMMARY AND RECOMMENDATIONS FOR FUTURE RESEARCH

This chapter has reviewed and made specific recommendations for studies of visuospatial orienting and selective attention in ADHD. In summary, there appears to be little evidence for clinically significant deficits in the PAS or AAS as indexed by Posner's covert-orienting paradigm, in children with either the combined or primarily inattentive subtype of ADHD. Although lack of findings for PAS deficits is not entirely surprising, lack of evidence for AAS abnormalities is somewhat curious given theoretical explanations of the disorder. However, the executive construct is multicomponential (71), and these low-level early-developing voluntary attention processes may not be as impaired as those needed for higher level later-developing functions such as skill learning and attentional control. Some evidence for vigilance system deficits were found, but findings require replication among both of the primary DSM-IV subtypes. Only one study (62) has taken advantage of the perceptual load model of selective attention to examine early and late selective attention in ADHD. Results from that study found that children with ADHD and SCT demonstrated early selective attention deficits compared to children with ADHD without SCT or non-ADHD controls.

Regardless of the model of attention under investigation, future studies are advised to utilize models of attention processes that (i) target empirically validated attention structures and (ii) are capable of isolating component operations. Less-optimal functioning among a set of cognitive processes may in the end best describe the cognitive mechanisms that underlie ADHD. However, identifying which processes will require improved attempts at isolating and systematically combining component operations, allowing investigators to more accurately model, test, and describe the sequelae of such interactions.

REFERENCES

1. McBurnett K, Pfiffner L, Willcutt E, et al. Experimental cross-validation of DSM-IV types of ADHD. J Am Acad Child Adolesc Psychiatry 1999; 38:17–24.

2. Posner M. Orienting of attention. Quant J Exp Psychol 1980; 32:3–25.
3. Lavie N. Perceptual load as a necessary condition for selective attention. J Exp Psychol: Hum Percept Perform 1995; 21:451–68.
4. Jackson S, Marrocco R, Posner M. Networks of anatomical areas controlling visuospatial attention. Neural Netw 1994; 7:925–44.
5. Mirsky A. Disorders of attention: a neuropsychological perspective. In: Lyon GR, Krasnegor NA, eds. Attention, Memory, and Executive Function. Baltimore: Paul H. Brooks, 1996:71–95.
6. Posner M, Petersen S. The attention system of the human brain. Annu Rev Neurosci 1990; 13:25–42.
7. Parasuraman R, Warm J, See J. Brain systems of vigilance. In: Parasuraman R. ed. The Attentive Brain. Cambridge: MIT Press, 1998:221–56.
8. Rothbart M, Posner M, Rosicky J. Orienting in normal and pathological development. Dev Psychopathol 1994; 6:635–52.
9. Fan J, McCandliss B, Sommer T, Raz A, Posner M. Testing the efficiency and independence of attentional networks. J Cogn Neurosci 2002; 14:340–7.
10. Rueda M, Fan J, McCandliss B, et al. Development of attentional networks in childhood. Neuropsychologia 2004; 42:1029–40.
11. Posner M, Raichle M. Networks of attention. In: Images of Mind. New York: Scientific American Library, 1994:152–79.
12. Posner M, Walker J, Friederich F, Rafal R. How do the parietal lobes direct covert attention? Neuropsychologia 1987; 25:135–45.
13. Rafal R, Posner M. Deficits in human visual spatial attention following thalamic lesions. Proc Natl Acad Sci U S A 1987; 84:7349–53.
14. Parasuraman R, Greenwood P, Alexander G. Selective impairment of spatial attention during visual search in Alzheimer's disease. Neuroreport 1995; 6: 1861–4.
15. Flowers KA, Robertson C. Perceptual abnormalities in Parkinson's disease: top-down or bottom-up processes? Perception 1995; 24:1201–21.
16. Moran M, Thaker G, Smith D, et al. Shifts in covert visual attention in schizophrenic patients and normal controls. Biol Psychiatry 1992; 32:617–20.
17. Øie M, Rund B, Sundet K. Covert visual attention in patients with early-onset schizophrenia. Schizophr Res 1998; 34:195–205.
18. Strauss M, Novakovic T, Tien A, et al. Disengagement of attention in schizophrenia. Psychiatry Res 1991; 37:139–46.
19. Cremona-Meteyard S, Geffen G. Persistent visuospatial attention deficits following mild head injury in Australian rules football players. Neuropsychologia 1994; 32:649–62.
20. Mangun G, Luck S, Plager R, Loftus W, Hillyard S, Handy T. Monitoring the visual world: hemispheric asymmetries and subcortical processes in attention. J Cogn Neurosci 1994; 6:267–75.
21. Huang-Pollock CL, Nigg JT. Searching for the Attention Deficit in Attention Deficit Hyperactivity Disorder: the Case of Visuospatial Orienting. Clin Psychol Rev 2003; 23:801–30.
22. Epstein J, Conners K, Erhardt D, March J, Swanson J. Asymmetric hemispheric control of visual-spatial attention in adults with ADHD. Neuropsychology 1997; 11:467–73.

23. Nigg J, Swanson J, Hinshaw S. Covert visual attention in boys with ADHD: lateral effects, methylphenidate response, and results for parents. Neuropsychologia 1997; 35:165–76.
24. Swanson J, Posner M, Potkin S, Bonforte S, Youpa D, Fiore C. Activating tasks for the study of visual-spatial attention in ADHD children: a cognitive anatomic approach. J Child Neurol 1991; 6:S119–27.
25. Wood C, Maruff P, Levy F, Farrow M, Hay D. Covert orienting of visual spatial attention in ADHD: does comorbidity make a difference? Arch Clin Neuropsychol 1999; 14:179–89.
26. McDonald S, Bennett K, Chambers H, Castiello U. Covert orienting and focusing of attention in children with ADHD. Neuropsychologia 1999; 37: 345–56.
27. Pearson D, Yaffee L, Loveland K, Norton M. Covert visual attention in children with ADHD: evidence for developmental immaturity? Dev Psychopathol 1995; 7:351–67.
28. Carter C, Krener P, Chaderjian M, Northcutt C, Wolfe V. Abnormal processing of irrelevant information in ADHD. Psychiatry Res 1995; 56:59–70.
29. Novak G, Solanto M, Abikoff H. Spatial orienting and focused attention in ADHD. Psychophysiology 1995; 32:546–59.
30. Perchet C, Revol O, Fourneret P, Maguire F, Garcia-Larrea L. Attention shifts and anticipatory mechanisms in hyperactive children: an ERP study using the Posner paradigm. Biol Psychiatry 2001; 40:44–57.
31. Tomporowski P, Tinsley V, Hager L. Visuospatial attentional shifts and choice responses of adults and ADHD and non-ADHD children. Percept Mot Skills 1994; 79:1479–90.
32. Oberlin B, Alford J, Marrocco R. Normal attention orienting but abnormal stimulus alerting and conflict effect in combined subtype of ADHD. Behav Brain Res 2005; 165:1–11.
33. Huang-Pollock CL, Nigg JT, Henderson JM, Carr TH. Covert attention in children with ADHD. Poster Presented at the Annual Meeting of the American Psychological Society, Miami, FL, 2000. [For full report of data, see Huang-Pollock and Nigg, 2003].
34. van der Meere J, Sergeant J. Controlled processing and vigilance in hyperactivity: time will tell. J Abnorm Child Psychol 1988; 16:641–55.
35. Sergeant J, Oosterlaan J, van der Meere J. Information processing and energetic factors in ADHD. In: Quay H, Hogan A, eds. Handbook of Disruptive Behavior Disorders. New York: Kluwer Academic, 1999:75–103.
36. Huang-Pollock CL, Nigg JT, Halperin, JM. Single dissociation findings of ADHD deficits in vigilance but not anterior or posterior attention systems. Neuropsychology 2006; 20:420–9.
37. Barry T, Klinger LG, Lyman R, Hawkins L. Visual selective attention versus sustained attention in boys with Attention-Deficit/Hyperactivity Disorder. J Atten Disord 2001; 4:193–606.
38. Casey B, Castellanos F, Giedd J, Marsh W, Hamburger S, Schubert A. Implication of right frontostriatal circuitry in response inhibition and attention-deficit/hyperactivity disorder. J Am Acad Child Adolesc Psychiatry 1997; 36: 374–83.

39. Castellanos F, Giedd J, Marsh W, Hamburger S, Vaituzis A, Dickstein D. Quantitative brain magnetic resonance imaging in attention-deficit hyperactivity disorder. Arch Gen Psychiatry 1996; 53:607–16.
40. Lou H, Henrikson L, Bruhn P. Focal cerebral hypoperfusion in children with dysphasia and/or attention deficit disorder. Arch Neurol 1984; 41:825–9.
41. Collings R, Kwasman A. Visual orienting deficits among boys with ADHD-inattentive type. Individual Diff Res 2006; 4:111–22.
42. American Psychiatric Association. Diagnostic and Statistical Manual of Mental Disorders. 3rd ed., revised. Washington, D.C.: American Psychiatric Association, 1987.
43. Milich R, Balentine AC, Lynam DR. ADHD combined type and ADHD predominantly inattentive type are distinct and unrelated disorders. Clin Psychol: Sci Pract 2001; 8:463–88.
44. Chhabildas N, Pennington B, Willcutt E. A comparison of the neuropsychological profiles of the DSM-IV subtypes of ADHD. J Abnorm Child Psychol 2001; 29:529–40.
45. American Psychiatric Association. Diagnostic and Statistical Manual of Mental Disorders. 4th ed. Washington, D.C.: American Psychiatric Association, 1994.
46. McBurnett K, Pfiffner L, Frick P. Symptom properties as a function of ADHD type: an argument for continued study of sluggish cognitive tempo. J Abnorm Child Psychol 2001; 29:207–13.
47. Lahey B, Applegate B, McBurnett K, et al. DSM-IV field trials for attention deficit/hyperactivity disorder in children and adolescents. Am J Psychiatry 1994; 151:1673–85.
48. Broadbent D. Percept Communication. London: Pergamon Press, 1958.
49. Deutch J, Deutch D. Attention: some theoretical considerations. Psychol Rev 1963; 70:80–90.
50. Lavie N, Cox S. On the efficiency of attentional selection: efficient visual search results in inefficient rejection of distraction. Psychol Sci 1997; 8:395–8.
51. Lavie N, Fox E. The role of perceptual load in negative priming. J Exp Psychol: Hum Percept Perform 2000; 26:1038–52.
52. Lavie N, Tsal Y. Perceptual load as a major determinant of the locus of selection in visual attention. Percept Psychophys 1994; 56:183–97.
53. Huang-Pollock CL, Carr TH, Nigg JT. Perceptual load influences late versus early selection in child and adult selective attention. Dev Psychol 2002; 38: 363–75.
54. Arrington CM, Meyer AR, Carr TH, Rao SM. Neural mechanisms of visual attention: deploying and reorienting attention in space. J Cogn Neurosci 2000; 12(Suppl. 2):106–17.
55. Corbetta M. Frontoparietal cortical networks for directing attention and the eye to visual locations: identical, independent, or overlapping neural systems? Proc Natl Acad Sci U S A 1998; 95:831–8.
56. Friedrich FJ, Egly R, Rafal RD, Beck D. Spatial attention deficits in humans: a comparison of superior parietal and temporal-parietal junction lesions. Neuropsychology 1998; 12:193–207.
57. MacLeod CM. Fifty years of the Stroop effect: an integrative review and reinterpretation of effects. Psychol Bull 1991; 114:376–90.

58. Gitelman DR, Nobre AC, Parrish TB, et al. A large-scale distributed network for covert spatial attention: further anatomical delineation based on stringent behavioral and cognitive controls. Brain 1999; 122:1093–106.
59. Barch DM, Braver TS, Sabb FW, Noll DC. Anterior cingulate and the monitoring of response conflict: evidence from an fMRI study of overt verb generation. J Cogn Neurosci 2000; 12:298–311.
60. Ziegler J, Besson M, Jacobs A, Nazir TA, Carr TH. Neural correlates of orthographic and semantic processing: a multitask comparison using event-related potentials. J Cogn Neurosci 1997; 9:758–75.
61. Yantis S, Jonides J. Abrupt visual onsets and selective attention: voluntary versus automatic allocation. J Exp Psychol 1990; 16:121–34.
62. Huang-Pollock CL, Nigg JT, Carr TH. Deficient attention is hard to find: applying the perceptual load model of selective attention to attention deficit hyperactivity disorder subtypes. J Child Psychol Psychiatry 2005; 46:1211–8.
63. Douglas V. Attentional and cognitive problems. In: Rutter M, ed. Developmental Neuropsychiatry. New York: Gilford, 1983:280–329.
64. Taylor E, Sandberg S, Thorley G, Giles S. Developmental and cognitive contrasts. Inst Psychiatry Maudsley Monogr 1991; 33:51–65.
65. de Sonneville L, Njiokiktjien C, Hilhorst R. Methylphenidate-induced changes in ADDH information processors. J Child Psychol Psychiatry 1991; 32:285–95.
66. Barkley R, Anastopoulos A, Guveremont D, Fletcher K. Adolescents with ADHD: patterns of behavioral adjustment, academic functioning, and treatment utilization. J Am Acad Child Adolesc Psychiatry 1991; 30:752–76.
67. McIntyre C, Blackwell S, Denton C. Effect of noise distractibility on the spans of apprehension of hyperactive boys. J Abnorm Psychol 1978; 6:483–92.
68. Sharma V, Halperin J, Newcorn J, Wolf L. The dimension of focussed attention: relationship to behavior and cognitive functioning in children. Percept Mot Skills 1991; 72:787–93.
69. Tarnowski K, Prinz R, Nay S. Comparative analysis of attentional deficits in hyperactive and learning-disabled children. J Abnorm Psychol 1986; 95:341–5.
70. Hooks K, Milich R, Lorch E. Sustained and selective attention in boys with attention deficit hyperactivity disorder. J Clin Child Psychol 1994; 23:69–77.
71. Miyake A, Friedman N, Emeson M, Witzki A, Howerter A. The unity and diversity of executive functions and their contributions to complex frontal lobe tasks: a latent variable analysis. Cogn Psychol 2000; 41:49–100.

11

The Dual Pathway Hypothesis of ADHD: Retrospect and Prospect

Edmund J. S. Sonuga-Barke

Institute for Disorders of Impulse and Attention, University of Southampton, Southampton, U.K.

INTRODUCTION

The study of the psychopathophysiology of attention deficit hyperactivity disorder (ADHD) is at a wonderfully exciting phase in its development. Established ways of thinking about the condition are giving way to new ones: A paradigm shift is underway. We call it a paradigm shift because these changes relate to more than just a replacement of just one theory with another, but rather a fundamental shift in perspective—with one way of thinking about ADHD as a disorder giving way to another. Traditionally, ADHD researchers, influenced by assumptions within the classical disease model of psychiatric disorders (1), have attempted to isolate a common core deficit at the heart of ADHD. More recently there has been a growing acceptance that ADHD is a psychopathopsychologically heterogeneous disorder; with no particular pattern of impairment representing a necessary condition for the presence of the condition and with subgroups of children recognized each with a distinctive pattern of impairment (2). This has been a response to the inconclusive pattern found in studies of ADHD psychopathophysiology which are often contradictory and inconsistent and where replicated results are found, meta-analyses give pooled effect sizes in only the moderate range (i.e., Cohen's *d* .4–.6) (3). This shift in perspective has led to a different set of research questions being asked. Rather than asking; where is the core deficit responsible for ADHD? The question becomes: How many different profiles of impairment can be dissociated within the broader ADHD syndrome (4)?

In this chapter we give a brief overview of the development of the dual pathway model, first published in 2002. This model provides a useful starting point when thinking about heterogeneity in ADHD. The working hypothesis is that there are at least two dissociable pathways to ADHD which affect different subgroups of ADHD children. One pathway is predominantly cognitive and associated with executive/inhibitory dysfunction, and a second one predominantly motivational associated with a broad-based motivational style, delay aversion (5). Furthermore, we propose that (*i*) these pathways are underpinned at the neurobiological level by two functionally distinct, though anatomically proximate, dopamine modulated corticobasal-ganglia circuits (6) and (*ii*) follow different developmental pathways (7). In this chapter we review these developments and identify key question for future research and implications for clinical practice.

COGNITION AND MOTIVATION IN MODELS OF ADHD

Executive Dysfunction in ADHD

In the recent past ADHD has been seen as a disorder of dysregulation of cognition, action (8–10), and cognitive-energetic state (11,12) associated with the disruption of neurocognitive control systems (13–19). While nonexecutive processes have been implicated in the disorder (20), the most influential models could be called strong executive dysfunction models, in that they view brain-behavior relations as fully mediated by neuropsychological deficits in executive functions (8). Executive functions are higher order, top-down, cognitive processes that allow appropriate set maintenance and shift that facilitate the flexible pursuit of future goals. Deficits within the executive system in ADHD (21) have been consistently found with the strongest evidence existing in the area of response inhibition (8). Problems with working memory (15), planning, and set shift have also been identified (22). Executive dysfunction also disrupts the distribution of cognitive-energetic resources (i.e., effort) to those activation and arousal processes required to meet the changing demands of different situations and settings (9,11,12,23). Barkley (8) has argued that the general pattern of executive impairment associated with ADHD is grounded in more specific early appearing deficits in inhibition (24,25). Response inhibition refers to that ability to inhibit an inappropriate prepotent or dominant response in favor of a more appropriate alternative. Response inhibition is regarded as a necessary precondition for the establishment of self-control (26), emotional regulation (27), and cognitive flexibility (28). As a domain of competence, response inhibition appears to be fractionated into conceptually related clusters of functions with each cluster sharing elements of this common definition but being measured by different neuropsychological tests (29). The most commonly used tests of children's inhibitory control include measures of response-conflict resolution such as the Stroop test (30) and the speed of inhibitory processes such as the stop signal paradigm (31).

At a neurobiological level, inhibitory control and other executive functions appear to be underpinned by one of a number of functionally segregated but neuroanatomically proximate brain circuits connecting cortical foci, basal ganglia, and thalamic nuclei (32–34). This circuit (i.e., the executive circuit) links the prefrontal cortex to the dorsal neostriatum (preferentially the caudate nucleus) with reciprocal excitatory connections back up to cortical regions via the dorsomedial sections of the thalamus. Data from neuroimaging studies (structural and functional) give some support to the idea that executive dysfunction in ADHD is associated with disturbances in this circuit (35–40). Dopamine, widely implicated in ADHD, is a key neuromodulator of the executive loop (41–44) with two branches specifically implicated. The mesocorticol branch originates in the ventral tegmental area of the rostral portion of the brainstem and terminates in the prefrontal cortex while the nigrastriatal branch originates in the substantia nigra and terminates in the dorsal striatum.

Despite the broad pattern of evidence linking ADHD to executive dysfunction it is becoming increasingly clear that executive dysfunction models of ADHD are only partially supported by empirical evidence. For instance, Nigg et al. (45) found that only a subpopulation of ADHD children had significant impairment on any one executive task and that the pattern of severe and pervasive impairment predicted by the sorts of strong executive theories of ADHD influential during the last 10 or so years (8), was present in only a very small minority of ADHD cases. This and other recent analyses have led to the question; If not executive dysfunction what is "causing" ADHD in these unaffected children?

Delay Aversion in ADHD

Motivationally based models, which shift the focus from inhibitory deficits to suboptimal reward processes, offer an alternative to inhibitory-based executive deficits as a basis for ADHD (46–48). The literature has been reviewed by Luman et al. (49). The review highlights the sheer range of motivational hypotheses that have been proposed. For instance, it has been hypothesized at different times by different people that ADHD children are undersensitive to rewards (50); have an underactive behavioral inhibition system and, are insensitive to nonreward or punishment (51) (52). Kollins et al. (53) and Tripp and Alsop (54) have hypothesized that ADHD children are less sensitive to changes in reinforcement contingencies and reinforcement history, respectively. Another promising domain relates to the so-called "hot" executive processes implicated in decision-making about reward, risk, and punishment (55).

The most striking thing about the review is that despite the very broad range of deficits proposed, the evidence in support of any one is inconclusive—with initial positive findings followed by serial nonreplication. The one area that may be the exception relates to ADHD children's apparent sensitivity to delayed rewards. This is confirmed in a recent review (56). This phenomenon is at the heart of a number of models of ADHD (57) and can be seen most clearly in relation to ADHD children's choice of small immediate rewards (58–66; E. Willcutt, personal communication).

We have argued in the past that this pattern of preference is a hallmark of a broader motivational style called delay aversion (62). In one model (7) delay aversion is driven by fundamental impairments in the neural signaling of delayed rewards and associated increased reward discounting of delayed rewards (57); compounded by a pattern of delay-related negative affect acquired during development as the delay-impaired child learns to associate delay settings with censure and failure (5) and, expressed in different settings in different ways as a function of whether delay can be escaped or has to be tolerated and modified (5). Evidence for this broader motivational style comes from studies of ADHD children's levels of activity during delay (67); their response to the unexpected imposition of delay (68); the impact of delay on attention and perception (69,70); their performance on long and challenging tasks (71); their degree of reward discounting (72,73); their relative preference for reward immediacy over other reward parameters (74); and their response to slow event rates/sparse schedules (75,76). According to the delay aversion framework choices of small immediate rewards overlarge delayed rewards are motivated by two processes: (a) an unconditional preference for immediacy linked to deficits in signaling future rewards and (b) the desire to escape or avoid the negative delay-related affect. These effects add to each other to cause preference for immediacy over delay.

Interestingly the neurobiology of delay aversion and inhibitory deficits may share some common elements. It is likely that delay aversion is also related to alterations in one of the cortiobasal-ganglia circuits modulated by dopamine. However, in this case it is the reward circuit that is likely to play the dominant role. This links the ventral striatum (in particular the nucleus accumbens) to frontal regions (especially the anterior cingulate and orbitofrontal cortex), reciprocated via the ventral pallidum and related structures through the thalamus (77). The amygdala is also implicated in this system possibly playing a role in defining the motivational significance of incentives. Once again dopamine is a key neuromodulator. On this occasion, however, it is the mesolimbic branch of the dopamine system, originating in the ventral tegmental area and terminating in the nucleus accumbens and associated limbic foci, which is important. Studies point to a specific role for this circuit in signaling rewards, coding incentive value and regulating other behavioral processes involved in the maintenance of responding under conditions of delayed reward (78–84). Lesions in the core of the accumbens reduced the ability of rats to wait for large delayed reward in a self-control paradigm (82). Animal models have highlighted the way in which alterations of dopamine activity within this structure may distort or reduce signals of delayed rewards (46,47,85–87).

Understanding the Relationship Between Delay Aversion and Inhibitory-Based Executive Dysfunction; Competing or Complimentary: Additive or Synergistic

In trying to understand the nature of psychopathophysiological heterogeneity in ADHD we have attempted to model the relationship between delay aversion and inhibitory-based executive deficits in ADHD. The first possibility, which can be dismissed on the basis of recent studies, is that delay aversion and inhibitory deficits in ADHD represent different facets of the same underlying impairment construct. That is they affect the same ADHD children. A head-to-head study (44) of delay aversion and inhibitory deficits in ADHD set out to provide a direct comparison of these two models. School-aged children with a diagnosis of combined-type ADHD performed the stop signal task (where a dominant response already initiated is inhibited following a "stop" signal) and a choice delay task in which children had to choose between a large delayed reward and a small immediate reward. There was no association between choices of the small immediate reward (delay aversion) and stop signal reaction time. This suggested that inhibitory deficits and delay aversion were independent characteristics. Furthermore, performance on both tasks was strongly associated with ADHD group membership—in combination the two measures allowed nearly 90% of ADHD children to be correctly classified. A subsequent reanalysis suggested that different subgroups of ADHD children with inhibitory deficits, delay aversion, both impairments and neither could be identified. In suggesting that delay aversion and inhibitory deficits were independently associated with ADHD, this study was consistent with a dual pathway model of ADHD. A similar pattern of associations has recently been found in a study of executive function and delay aversion in preschoolers (88). The independent association inhibitory-based executive dysfunction and delay aversion has been extended to other motivational systems such as "hot" cognition (55) and validated in animal models of impulsiveness and aggression (89).

On the basis of this data we have proposed a dual pathway hypothesis of ADHD (90). This hypothesis builds on the idea that alterations within the executive circuit modulated by mesocortical dopamine and the reward circuit modulated by mesolimbic dopamine constitute more or less discrete neuropsychological bases for dissociable psychological processes leading to executive/inhibitory deficits and delay aversion, respectively. In initial models the two pathways were presented as independent factors acting additively (5) but more recent accounts have recognized the likelihood of synergistic interactions between motivational and cognitive factors. First, there is the suggestion that during development delay aversion can create the context for the development of executive dysfunction as this motivational style limits the opportunity for children to consolidate delay exploiting higher cognitive skills. At the same time executive dysfunction can lead to a learned helplessness and a motivation to avoid difficult and demanding and delay-rich tasks (6,7). At the same time there are likely to be synergies at the neurobiological level with cascading frontostriatal loops linking reward and cognitive processes (91). Taking a developmental perspective also highlights the possibility of the operation of compensatory mechanisms (7).

Finally, it must be recognized that a substantial minority of ADHD children may not be affected by either inhibitory-based executive dysfunction or delay aversion and that there are likely to be other operative pathways to ADHD (92). Candidate domains of dysfunction include: basic memory and perceptual deficits (2), state regulation and cognitive-energetic dysregulation (93), and altered timing processes operating in the millisecond range (94). Each represents a plausible putative ADHD psychopathophysiology and therefore may account for the condition in those ADHD children unaffected by executive dysfunction or delay aversion.

FUTURE DIRECTIONS FOR RESEARCH

While initial results are suggestive of the existence of independent delay aversion and executive pathways into ADHD further study of the relationship between these, and other candidate processes, is required to properly test this hypothesis. This research should employ multivariate approaches with large samples of children of different ages in longitudinal, genetically, and neurobiologically informative designs that would allow continuities and discontinuities between motivational and cognitive components of the disorder to be studied. It should also explore the interactions between motivational and cognitive features of the disorder, including at the neurobiological level and the possibility that ADHD children might develop compensatory skills and strategies. The implications for ADHD nosology and diagnosis need to be addressed. First, we need to identify the most diagnostically efficient and cost-effective test measures of delay aversion, executive dysfunction, and other key pathophysiologic markers. Second, the stability of these markers as dysfunctional traits needs to be established over time and context. Third, population norms for these markers need to be established and algorithms for establishing clinical thresholds need to be determined. Fourth, the relationship between the markers and other disorders needs to be tested. Fifth, perhaps most significantly, the clinical significance of delay aversion, inhibitory deficits, and other markers need to be investigated in terms of comorbidity, long-term outcome, treatment response, and how this varies by disorder type. Finally, the significance of these markers needs to be validated by studying their functional neuroanatomy.

CLINICAL IMPLICATIONS

Multiple pathway models could alter the way we think about ADHD clinically. First, they will encourage the identification of different psychological subgroups, with different impairment profiles. These subgroupings may be specific to ADHD and meet the criteria for clinical subtypes—e.g., ADHD–EF type. Alternatively, they may be seen rather in terms of comorbidity between ADHD and a neuropsychological impairment—e.g., ADHD and comorbid executive dysfunction. In this latter case such comorbidities could be shared with children with other conditions such as oppositional-defiant disorder or pervasive developmental disorder. Either way this would encourage a move away from current phenomenological symptom-based approaches to diagnosis toward more theoretically informed models. Information about the context for symptom expression would become more significant with diagnostic criteria making increasing reference to contextual factors in order to distinguish between delay averse and disinhibited type ADHD children. For instance, symptoms of inattention and overactivity only displayed in delay-rich settings may be indicative of a delay averse type of problem while more pervasive expressions might reflect more fundamental cognitive deficits associated with inhibitory deficits. Neuropsychological testing may also take on a greater significance. While at present evidence for the diagnostic value of laboratory tests is lacking it is possible that tests of inhibitory deficits and delay aversion may play a key role in the more precise definition of the clinical phenotype. Second, once the psychological subtypes have been identified it may be possible to better match them to particular treatment options. This applies equally to pharmacological and nonpharmacological interventions. Agents that target specific frontostriatal circuits are likely to be differentially effective in treating the inhibitory and delay averse subtypes. There may also be potential to tailor nonpharmacological treatments to psychological subtypes. For instance, shaping and fading of delay tolerance leading to desensitization to delay may be useful for the delay averse children while attention and cognitive training may be valuable for dysexecutive children.

REFERENCES

1. Sonuga-Barke EJS, Saxton T, Hall M. The role of interval underestimation in hyperactive children's failure to suppress responses over time. Behav Brain Res 1998; 94:45–50.
2. Rhodes SM, Coghill DR, Matthews K. Neuropsychological functioning in stimulant-naive boys with hyperkinetic disorder. Psychol Med 2005; 35: 1109–20.
3. Willcutt EG, Doyle AE, Nigg JT, Faraone SV, Pennington BF. Validity of the executive function theory of attention-deficit/hyperactivity disorder: a meta-analytic review. Biol Psychiatry 2005; 57:1336–46.
4. Nutt DJ, Fone K, Asherson P, et al. Evidence-based guidelines for management of attention-deficit/hyperactivity disorder in adolescents in transition to adult services and in adults: recommendations from the British Association for Psychopharmacology. J Psychopharmacol 2007; 21:10–41.
5. Sonuga-Barke EJS. Psychological heterogeneity in AD/HD; a dual pathway model of behaviour and cognition. Behav Brain Res 2002; 130:29–36.
6. Sonuga-Barke EJS. The dual pathway model of AD/HD; an elaboration of neuro-developmental characteristics. Neurosci Biobehav Rev; 2003; 27: 593–604.
7. Sonuga-Barke EJS. Causal models of ADHD: from simple single deficits to multiple developmental pathways. Biol Psychiatry 2005; 57:1231–8.
8. Barkley RA. Behavioural inhibition, sustained attention and executive functions: constructing a unified theory of AD/HD. Psychol Bull 1997; 121:65–94.
9. Douglas VI. Attentional and cognitive problems. In: Rutter M, ed. Developmental Neuro-psychiatry. New York: Guilford, 1983.
10. Douglas VI, Peters KG. Towards a clearer definition of attentional deficit in hyperactive children. In: Hale GA, Lewis M, eds. Attention and the Development of Cognitive Skills. New York: Plenum Press, 1979.
11. Van der Meere JJ. The role of inattention in hyperactivity disorders. In: Sandberg S, ed. Monographs on Child and Adolescent Psychiatry: Hyperactivity Disorders. Cambridge: Cambridge University Press, 1996.
12. Van der Meere J, Gunning B, Stemerdink N. The effect of methylphenidate and clonodine on response inhibition and state regulation in children with AD/HD. J Child Psychol Psychiatry 1998; 40:291–8.
13. Barnett R, Maruff P, Vance A, et al. Abnormal executive function in attention deficit hyperactivity disorder: the effect of stimulant medication and age on spatial working memory. Psychol Med 2001; 31:1107–15.
14. Bayliss DM, Roodenrys S. Executive processing and attention deficit hyperactivity disorder: an application of the supervisory attentional system. Dev Neuropsychol 2000; 17:161–80.
15. Cornoldi C, Barbieri A, Gaiani C, Zocchi S. Strategic memory deficits in attention deficit disorder with hyperactivity participants: the role of executive processes. Dev Neuropsychol 1999; 15:53–71.
16. Karatekin C, Asarnow, RF. Working memory in childhood onset schizophrenia and attention deficit/hyperactivity disorder. Psychiatry Res 1998; 80: 165–76.

17. Pennington BF, Ozonoff S. Executive functions and developmental psychopathology. J Child Psychol Psychiatry 1996; 37:51–87.
18. Seidman LJ, Beiderman J, Faraone SV, Wever W, Ouellette C. Toward defining a neuropsychology of attention deficit-hyperactivity disorder: performance of children and adolescents from a large clinically referred sample. J Consult Clin Psychol 1997; 65:150–60.
19. Sergeant JA, Geurts H, Oosterlaan J. How specific is a deficit of executive functioning for attention deficit/hyperactivity disorder? Behav Brain Res 2002; 130:3–28.
20. Rhodes SM, Coghill DR, Matthews K. Neuropsychological functioning in stimulant-naive boys with hyperkinetic disorder. Psychol Med 2005; 35: 1109–20.
21. Clark C, Prior M, Kinsella GJ. Do executive function deficits differentiate between adolescents with AD/HD and Oppositional Defiant/Conduct Disorder? A neuropsychological study using the Six Elements Test and Hayling Sentence Completion Test. J Abnormal Child Psychol 2000; 28:403–14.
22. Nigg JT, Hinshaw SP, Carte ET, Treuting JJ. Neuro-psychological correlates of childhood Attention Deficit/Hyperactivity Disorder: explainable by co-morbid disruptive behaviour and reading problems. J Abnorm Psychol 1998; 107: 468–80.
23. Sergeant J. The cognitive-energetic model: an empirical approach to Attention-Deficit Hyperactivity Disorder. Neurosci Biobehav Rev 2000; 24:7–12.
24. Nigg J. Is AD/HD a disinhibitory disorder? Psychol Bull 2001; 127:571–98.
25. Oosterlaan J, Logan GD, Sergeant JA. Response inhibition in AD/HD, CD, co-morbid AD/HD + CD, anxious, and control children: a meta-analysis of studies with the stop task. J Child Psychol Psychiatry 1998; 39:411–25.
26. Muraven M, Baumeister RF. Self-regulation and depletion of limited resources: does self-control resemble a muscle? Psychol Bull 2000; 126:247–59.
27. Eisenberg N. Emotion-related regulation and its relation to quality of social functioning. Child Psychol Retrospect Prospect. Minnesota Symp Child Psychol 2002; 32:133–171.
28. Arbuthnott K, Frank J. Trail making test, part B as a measure of executive control: validation using a set-switching paradigm. J Clin Exper Neuropsychol 2000; 22:518–28.
29. Olson SL, Bates JE, Sandy JM, Schilling EM. Early developmental precursors of impulsive and inattentive behavior: from infancy to middle childhood. J Child Psychol Psychiatry 2002; 43:435–47.
30. Golden ZL, Golden CJ. Patterns of performance on the Stroop color and word test in children with learning, attentional, and psychiatric disabilities. Psychol Sch 2002; 39:489–95.
31. Schachar RJ, Tannock R, Logan G. Inhibitory control, impulsiveness, and Attention-Deficit Hyperactivity Disorder. Clin Psychol Rev 1993; 13:721–39.
32. Nakano K, Kayahara T, Tsutsumi T, Ushiro H. Neural circuits and functional organization of the striatum. J Neurol 2000; 247:1–15.
33. Robbins TW, Shallice T, Burgess PW, et al. Selective impairments in self-ordered working memory in a patient with a unilateral striatal lesion. Neurocase 1995; 1:217–30.

34. Tekin S, Cummings JL. Frontal-subcortical neuronal circuits and clinical neuropsychiatry—an update. J Psychosom Res 2002; 53:647–54.
35. Casey BJ, Durston S, Fossella JA. Evidence for a mechanistic model of cognitive control. Clin Neurosci Res 2001; 1:267–82.
36. Castellanos FX. Toward a pathophysiology of attention-deficit/hyperactivity disorder. Clin Pediat 1997; 36:381–93.
37. Castellanos FX, Lee PP, Sharp W, et al. Developmental trajectories of brain volume abnormalities in children and adolescents with attention-deficit/hyperactivity disorder. JAMA 2002; 288:1740–8.
38. Hesslinger B, Thiel T, van Elst LT, Hennig J, Ebert D. Attention-deficit disorder in adults with or without hyperactivity: where is the difference? A study in humans using short echo H-1-magnetic resonance spectroscopy. Neurosci Lett 2001; 304:117–9.
39. Rubia K, Overmeyer S, Taylor E, et al. Hypofrontality in attention deficit hyperactivity disorder during higher-order motor control: a study with functional MRI. Am J Psychiatry 1999; 156:891–6.
40. Bush G, Frazier JA, Rauch SL, et al. Anterior cingulate cortex dysfunction in attention-deficit/hyperactivity disorder revealed by fMRI and the counting Stroop. Biol Psychiatry 1999; 45:1542–52.
41. Russell VA. Hypodopaminergic and hypernoradrenergic activity in prefrontal cortex slices of an animal model for attention-deficit hyperactivity disorder—the spontaneously hypertensive rat. Behav Brain Res 2002; 130: 191–6.
42. Williams D, Tijssen M, van Bruggen G, et al. Dopamine-dependent changes in the functional connectivity between basal ganglia and cerebral cortex in humans. Brain 2002; 125:1558–69.
43. Robbins TW, Everitt BJ. Functions of dopamine in the dorsal and ventral striatum. Semin Neurosci 1992; 4:119–28.
44. Solanto MV. Dopamine dysfunction in AD/HD: integrating clinical and basic neuroscience research. Behav Brain Res 2002; 130:65–71.
45. Nigg JT, Willcutt EG, Doyle AE, Sonuga-Barke EJS. Causal heterogeneity in attention deficit/hyperactivity disorder: do we need neuro-psychologically impaired subtypes? Biol Psychiatry 2005; 57:1224–30.
46. Sagvolden T. The attention deficit disorder might be a reinforcement deficit disorder. In: Georgas J, Manthouli M, Besevegis E, Kokkevi A, eds. Contemporary Psychology in Europe: Theory, Research and Application. Goettingen: Hogrefe and Huber, 1991:131–43.
47. Sagvolden T, Aase H, Zeiner P, Berger D. Altered reinforcement mechanisms in attention-deficit/hyperactivity disorder. Behav Brain Res 1998; 94:61–71.
48. Sonuga-Barke EJS. On dysfunction and function in psychological accounts of childhood disorder. J Child Psychol Psychiatry 1994; 35:801–15.
49. Luman M, Oosterlaan J, Sergeant JA. The impact of reinforcement contingencies on AD/HD: a review and theoretical appraisal. Clin Psychol Rev 2005; 25:183–213.
50. Haelein M, Caul WF. Attention Deficit Disorder with Hyperactivity: a specific hypothesis of reward dysfunction. J Am Acad Child Adolesc Psychiatry 1987; 26:356–62.

51. Quay HC. Reward inhibition and ADHD. J Am Acad Child Adolesc Psychiatry 1988; 27:262–3.
52. van Meel CS, Oosterlaan J, Heslenfeld DJ, Sergeant JA. Telling good from bad news: ADHD differentially affects processing of positive and negative feedback during guessing. Neuropsychology 2005; 43:1946–54.
53. Kollins SH, Lane SD, Shapiro SK. Experimental analysis of childhood psychopathology: a laboratory matching analysis of the behavior of children diagnosed with Attention-Deficit Hyperactivity Disorder. Psychol Rec 1997; 47:25–44.
54. Tripp G, Alsop B. Sensitivity to reward frequency in boys with attention deficit hyperactivity disorder. J Clin Child Psychol 1999; 28:366–75.
55. Toplak ME, Jain U, Tannock R. Executive and motivational processes in adolescents with Attention-Deficit-Hyperactivity Disorder. Behav Brain Func 2005; 1:8.
56. Sonuga-Barke EJS. What role, if any, should markers of motivational dysfunction play in the diagnosis of attention deficit hyperactivity disorder? In: Rohde L, Shaffer D, Rappaport J, eds. The Future of Psychiatric Diagnosis: Externalising Childhood Disorder. US: American Psychiatric Association, 2007.
57. Sagvolden T, Johansen EB, Aase H, Russell VA. A dynamic developmental theory of attention-deficit/hyperactivity disorder (ADHD) predominantly hyperactive/impulsive and combined subtypes. Behav Brain Sci 2005; 28: 397–468.
58. Kuntsi J, Oosterlaan J, Stevenson J. Psychological mechanisms in hyperactivity. I. Response inhibition deficit, working memory impairment, delay aversion, or something else? J Child Psychol Psychiatry 2001; 42:199–210.
59. Antrop I, Stock P, Verte S, Wiersema JR, Baeyens D, Roeyers H. ADHD and delay aversion: the influence of non-temporal stimulation on choice for delayed rewards. J Child Psychol Psychiatry 2006; 47:1152–8.
60. Bitsakou P. The relationship between delay aversion and inhibitory control in ADHD. PhD thesis. University of Southampton, in preparation.
61. Marco R, Schlotz W, Melia A. Delay aversion in ADHD: a large scale assessment of the impact of pre- and post-reward delay on choice behaviour. 1st International ADHD Congress. Wurzberg, Germany, 2007.
62. Sonuga-Barke EJS, Taylor E, Sembi S, Smith J. Hyperactivity and delay aversion. The effect of delay on choice. J Child Psychol Psychiatry 1992; 33: 387–98.
63. Schweitzer JB, Sulzer-Azaroff B. Self-control in boys with attention-deficit hyperactivity disorder—effects of added stimulation and time. J Child Psychol Psychiatry 1995; 36:671–86.
64. Solanto M, Abikoff H, Sonuga-Barke EJS, et al. The ecological validity of measures related to impulsiveness in AD/HD. J Abnorm Child Psychol 2001; 29:215–28.
65. Hoerger ML, Mace FC. A computerized test of self-control predicts classroom behavior. J Applied Behav Anal 2006; 39:147–59.
66. Dalen L, Sonuga-Barke EJS, Hall M, Remington RER. Inhibitory deficits, delay aversion and preschool ADHD: implications for the dual pathway model. Neural Plast 2004; 11:1–12.

67. Antrop I, Roeyers H, Van Oost P, Buzsse A. Simulation seeking and hyperactivity in children with ADHD. J Child Psychol Psychiatry 2000; 41: 225–31.
68. Bitsakou P, Antrop I, Wiersema JR, Sonuga-Barke EJS. Probing the limits of delay intolerance: preliminary young adult data from the Delay Frustration Task (DeFT). J Neurosci Meth 2006; 151:38–44.
69. Tripp G, Alsop B. Sensitivity to reward delay in children with attention deficit hyperactivity disorder (ADHD). J Child Psychol Psychiatry 2001; 42:691–8.
70. Sonuga-Barke EJS, De Houwer J, De Ruiter K, Ajzenstzen M, Holland S. AD/HD and the capture of attention by briefly exposed delay-related cues: evidence from a conditioning paradigm. J Child Psychol Psychiatry 2004; 45:274–83.
71. Scime M, Norvilitis JM. Task performance and response to frustration in children with attention deficit hyperactivity disorder. Psychol Sch 2006; 43: 377–86.
72. Barkley RA, Edwards G, Laneri M, Fletcher K, Metevia L. Executive functioning, temporal discounting, and sense of time in adolescents with attention deficit hyperactivity disorder (ADHD) and oppositional defiant disorder (ODD). J Abnorm Child Psychol 2001; 29:541–56.
73. Scheres A, Dijkstra M, Ainslie E, et al. Temporal and probabilistic discounting of rewards in children and adolescents: effects of age and ADHD symptoms. Neuropsychologia 2006; 44:2092–103.
74. Neef NA, Marckel J, Ferreri SJ, et al. Behavioral assessment of impulsivity: a comparison of children with and without attention deficit hyperactivity disorder. J Applied Behav Anal 2005; 38:23–37.
75. Wiersema R, van der Meere J, Roeyers H, Van Coster R, Baeyens D. Event rate and event-related potentials in ADHD. J Child Psychol Psychiatry 2006; 47: 560–7.
76. Aase H, Sagvolden T. Infrequent, but not frequent, reinforcers produce more variable responding and deficient sustained attention in young children with attention-deficit/hyperactivity disorder (ADHD). J Child Psychol Psychiatry 2006; 47:457–71.
77. Robbins TW, Everitt BJ. Neurobehavioural mechanisms of reward and motivation. Curr Opin Neurobiol 1996; 6:228–36.
78. Schultz W. Predictive reward signal of dopamine neurons. J Neurophysiol 1998; 80:1–27.
79. Schultz W. Getting formal with dopamine and reward. Neuron 2002; 36: 241–63.
80. Wightman RM, Robinson DL. Transient changes in mesolimbic dopamine and their association with ‘reward’. J Neurochem 2002; 82:721–35.
81. Burk JA, Mair RG. Effects of dorsal and ventral striatal lesions on delayed matching trained with retractable levers. Behav Brain Res 2001; 122:67–78.
82. Cardinal RN, Pennicott DR, Sugathapala CL, Robbins TW, Everitt BJ. Impulsive choice induced in rats by lesions of the nucleus accumbens core. Science 2001; 292:2499–501.
83. Richardson NR, Gratton A. Changes in medial prefrontal cortical dopamine levels associated with response-contingent food reward: an electrochemical study in rat. J Neurosci 1998; 18:9130–8.

84. Wade TR, de Wit H, Richards JB. Effects of dopaminergic drugs on delayed reward as a measure of impulsive behaviour in rats. Psychopharmacology 2000; 150:90–101.
85. Max JE, Fox PT, Lancaster JL, et al. Putamen lesions and the development of attention-deficit/hyperactivity symptomatology. J Am Acad Child Adolesc Psychiatry 2002; 41:563–71.
86. Sadile AG. Multiple evidence of a segmental defect in the anterior forebrain of an animal model of hyperactivity and attention deficit. Neurosci Biobehav Rev 2000; 24:161–9.
87. Viggiano D, Grammatikopoulos G, Sadile AG. A morphometric evidence for a hyperfunctioning mesolimbic system in an animal model of AD/HD. Behav Brain Res 2002; 130:181–9.
88. Dalen, L, Sonuga-Barke EJS, Remington RE. Inhibitory deficits, delay aversion and preschool AD/HD; implications for the dual pathway model. Manuscript submitted for publication.
89. Van den Bergh F, Spronk M, Ferreira L, et al. Relationship of delay aversion and response inhibition to extinction learning, aggression, and sexual behaviour. Behav Brain Res 2006; 175:75–81.
90. Sonuga-Barke EJS. Psychological heterogeneity in AD/HD; a dual pathway model of behaviour and cognition. Behav Brain Res 2002; 130:29–36.
91. Castellanos FX, Sonuga-Barke EJS, Milham MP, Tannock R. Characterizing cognition in ADHD: beyond executive dysfunction. Trends Cogn Sci 2006; 10: 117–23.
92. Taylor EA, Sonuga-Barke EJS. Attention Deficit Hyperactivity Disorder: a developmental lifespan perspective. In: Rutter M, Taylor E, Stevenson J, et al. eds. Rutter's Child & Adolescent Psychiatry. 5th ed. In press.
93. Sergeant JA. Modeling attention-deficit/hyperactivity disorder: a critical appraisal of the cognitive-energetic model. Biol Psychiatry 2005; 57:1248–55.
94. Toplak ME, Dockstader C, Tannock R. Temporal information processing in ADHD: findings to date and new methods. J Neurosci Meth 2006; 151:15–29.

12

Cortical Excitability in ADHD as Measured by Transcranial Magnetic Stimulation

A. Rothenberger

Department of Child and Adolescent Psychiatry, University of Göttingen, Göttingen, Germany

T. Banaschewski

Department of Child and Adolescent Psychiatry, Central Institute of Mental Health, Mannheim, Germany

H. Heinrich and G.H. Moll

Department of Child and Adolescent Psychiatry, University of Göttingen, Göttingen, and Department of Child and Adolescent Psychiatry, University of Erlangen, Erlangen, Germany

J. Sergeant

Department of Clinical Neuropsychology, Vrije Universiteit Amsterdam, Amsterdam, The Netherlands

INTRODUCTION

All rating scales for attention deficit hyperactive disorder (ADHD) include items that inquire to evaluate motor hyperactivity. Although these ratings can be confounded by aggression, oppositionality, and reduced impulse control, the motor aspect of ADHD is an important one, since a general motor hyperactivity is the most apparent symptom of ADHD in young children. Further, the working group of Gillberg described as DAMP syndrome a group of children with deficits in attention, motor control, and perception (1). This combination is often found in ADHD children, particularly of the combined subtype. The motor activity in children with ADHD is not only quantitatively increased compared to healthy children but, especially in waiting situations (2), movements start earlier compared to their peers and this movement is disorganized, poorly modulated, shows problems in goal direction and cannot be inhibited properly (3). Also, some studies found that children with ADHD are not only more active during daytime than age-matched controls but even during sleep (4–6) indicating that locomotor hyperactivity is a primary symptom. Further, Rothenberger (7) and Yordanova et al. (8) demonstrated that ADHD children (registration of brain electrical activity using event-related potentials) seem to have a deficit of motor control in the primary motor cortex as well as of the frontal lobe. This view is supported by Mostofsky et al. (9) who, on the basis of MRI findings, suggested that the clinical picture of ADHD encompasses dysfunctions attributable to anomalous development of both premotor and prefrontal cortices. ADHD children do not regulate the neuronal networks responsible for voluntary motion with selective activation and sufficient precision. This possibly applies even more for spontaneous movements, which are poorly under voluntary control in ADHD children. Hence, as one example, their tendency for associative mirror movements may be better clarified by using specific experimental tasks such as transcranial magnetic stimulation (TMS). Unfortunately, in a preliminary study, Barker et al. (10) did not find a significant correlation between mirror movements and the ipsilateral silent period evoked by TMS, although they could show an abnormal transcallosal inhibition in children with ADHD.

Thus, more general neuronal processes should be investigated, since neurophysiological studies could help to determine that the disturbance in motor control processes is attributable to (1) a lack of selective neuronal ability to choose adequate motor programs, (2) to energetic deficits in the early information processing steps which translate these programs into the intended movements, and/or (3) to basic neuronal problems with excitability within the motor system. Surprisingly, such a fundamental issue remains unresolved, although nearly all attempts to produce animal models of ADHD begin with locomotor hyperactivity (11), which may be associated with both hypodopaminergic and hyperdopaminergic status in animals, which might indicate that either dopaminergic extreme can produce behavioral and cognitive dysregulation (12).

Hence, it is a great advantage that recently the noninvasive method of TMS gives us the opportunity to investigate the basic neuronal problems with excitability within the motor loops of ADHD children.

TRANSCRANIAL MAGNETIC STIMULATION

Neuroimaging techniques such as positron emission tomography (PET), single-positron emission computer tomography (SPECT), or functional magnetic resonance imaging (fMRI) offer considerable potential for studying the developing human brain; e.g., developmental changes in the efficiency of brain circuitries invoked by cognitive tasks (13). However, the activation seen in functional imaging studies probably results from excitation rather than inhibition (14). Therefore, direct conclusions concerning the significance of inhibitory neuronal processes, which are central to current theories of psychopathology (e.g., ADHD), have not been tested by using these methods. Further, the time window of these neuroimaging techniques is much broader compared to electrophysiological methods such as stimulus-evoked changes of electrical brain activity.

TMS allows investigation of activation as well as inhibition of neuronal systems. TMS uses very short (about 200 μsec), strong magnetic fields (e.g., 2 T) inducing an electric current in circumscribed brain regions (15). This method combines excellent time resolution with acceptable spatial discrimination and enables the investigation and modification of different brain functions in humans [e.g., visual system, language, memory; for review see (16–18)].[a] Stimulation of the motor cortex, and thus the cortico-striato-pallido-thalamo-cortical motor loop (19) elicits muscle twitches or suppresses ongoing voluntary movements. These effects can be assessed and quantified by measuring changes in the induced motor-evoked potentials (MEPs).

Applying single- or paired-pulse magnetic stimuli over the motor cortex, there can be derived parameters of motor system excitability such as the motor threshold (MS), the cortical silent period (CSP), and the extent of intracortical inhibition or facilitation (ICI and ICF) (20).

The MS allows determination of excitability at the level of the neuronal membrane, which is regulated by the permeability of ionic channels (21). Based on the CSP, which also depends to a limited degree on peripheral (spinal) inhibitory processes, the total magnitude of inhibitory effects on the sensorimotor system can be measured (22). By measuring ICI and ICF it is possible to draw conclusions concerning the extent of inhibitory and excitatory processes within the motor cortex itself (23).

Typically, to measure these parameters, the child sits in a comfortable chair. A magnetic coil (flat 70-mm butterfly coil) is laid on the left side of the head to evoke a muscle twitch at the (mostly) dominant right hand. By applying magnetic stimuli over the hand region of the motor cortex a transsynaptic activation of corticospinal neurons is produced. As a result of this activation, a MEP can be measured electromyographically using surface electrodes on the target muscle, in our case the abductor digiti minimi of the right hand. Three measurements can be derived:

- MS
- CSP
- ICI and ICF

---

[a] Due to ethical reason, only single- and paired-pulse TMS over the motor cortex have been applied in children so far. Because seizure elicitation is the major safety issue linked to repeated rhythmic TMS (rTMS) and little information is available about its long-term effects (19), this innovative approach should presently be restricted to adults.

For details of TMS measurement, see Ziemann et al. (24) and Moll et al. (20).

By studying the normal development of these parameters, it could be shown, that for the MS there is a significant reduction (i.e., it becomes easier to excite neuronal membranes) from 8 to 16 years (25).

A similar statistically significant age dependence was found for the duration of the CSP. This became longer with increasing age, so that an increase in the inhibitory mechanisms in the motor system may be assumed.

No age dependence could be established for the measures expressing intracortical excitability. This indicates that both inhibitory and excitatory interneurons in the motor cortex have already reached a mature functional state in prepubertal children.

DEFICITS IN MOTOR CONTROL IN CHILDREN WITH ADHD

As one of the possible neurobiological bases for ADHD, a disturbance in the control and/or regulation of motor processes has been discussed (26). The role of the sensorimotor system and its individual parts, in particular the motor cortex, which until recently has hardly been considered in proposed pathological models (in contrast to the prefrontal or parietal cortex), is still largely unclear. For this reason, it was necessary to use TMS to measure neuronal excitability in the sensorimotor system in children with ADHD in comparison with healthy children in order to test "close to the substrate" the idea of a "motor response regulation deficit" in ADHD. The hypothesis to be tested was that children with ADHD would show deficient inhibitory processes compared to healthy children. For this reason we measured and compared the neurophysiological parameters of motor system excitability of 18 children with ADHD and 18 healthy children, aged from 8 to 12 years (27).

Both for the MS and, unexpectedly, for the CSP, we could not find any differences between children with ADHD and healthy children. While there was no difference in the parameter of ICF, the children with ADHD showed a statistically significant reduction in ICI in comparison with healthy children. Because the paired stimulus paradigm used allows separate activation of inhibitory and excitatory interneurons projecting onto the motor neurons (21,23), this finding suggests a diminished expression of inhibitory processes in the region of the motor cortex in ADHD children.

Functional imaging studies can show indirect (general) differences in neuronal activity between healthy subjects and patients with ADHD, but direct conclusions concerning the significance of inhibitory neuronal processes have not been possible using these methods. Since a general deficit in behavioral inhibition is assumed to be fundamental to ADHD (28), and deficits in motor inhibition have repeatedly been described (11), the TMS method offers a means of measuring the postulated inhibitory deficit.

The normal MS found in children with ADHD gives no indication for hyperexcitability at the membrane level of cortical neurons in the motor system. Unexpectedly, children with ADHD showed normal duration of the CSP. The latter suggests in contrast to shorter CSP in children with tic disorders (20), no evidence for a generalized deficit of inhibitory processes in the sensorimotor system.

Although the deficit of ICI in ADHD was demonstrated only at the motor cortex, the TMS results could reflect a generalized inhibitory deficit in cortical areas in children with ADHD, also accounting for the attention-related abnormalities and dysfunctions in the prefrontal and parietal neuronal systems described in the literature. This explanation only partly corresponds with a model of a generally inadequate behavioral inhibition as the basis for ADHD (28), because inhibition can be found only for certain aspects (e.g., motor function) and is nonspecific for the disorder (3,20,29,30).

DEFICITS IN MOTOR CONTROL IN CHILDREN WITH COMORBID ADHD AND TIC DISORDER[b]

The two "hypermotoric syndromes" of GTS and ADHD show clinical overlap. Around 50% to 60% of children with a tic disorder show hyperkinetic signs, and about 30% of children with ADHD also have a tic disorder (31). Previous studies at several levels (e.g., morphology, neuropsychology, and neurophysiology) in children with comorbid ADHD and tic disorder compared with children with only one of these disorders have produced partly equivocal results concerning the assumption of an additive effect at all levels of investigation (7,32). For this reason the question of comorbidity, particularly concerning the excitability of the motor system (additive vs. nonadditive effects) needs to be further investigated. We wanted to test the hypothesis that in the motor system of children with comorbid ADHD and tic disorder both TMS abnormalities, i.e., shortened CSP and reduced ICI, would be present. To test this hypothesis we compared in a 2 × 2 factorial design the neurophysiological parameters of motor system excitability of a group of 16 children with comorbid ADHD and tic disorder (chronic motor tic disorder or Tourette's syndrome; ADHD + TIC) with that of 16 children with only ADHD (ADHD only), 16 children with only tic disorder (TS only), and 16 healthy children, aged 8 to 15 years (33).

In children comorbid with both disorders—ADHD plus tic disorder—both TMS abnormalities could be found in comparison with healthy children, i.e., both a significantly reduced ICI (ADHD factor) and a significantly shortened CSP (tic disorder factor) (Fig. 1).

[b] For most recent evidence based knowledge on ADHD plus TD comorbidity see Rothenberger A, Rocmner V, Banaschewstri T, Leckman J (eds., 2007) Co-existence of tic disorders and attention-deficit, hyperactivity disorder-recent advances in understanding and treatment European Child and Adolascent Psychiatry 16: Supplements.

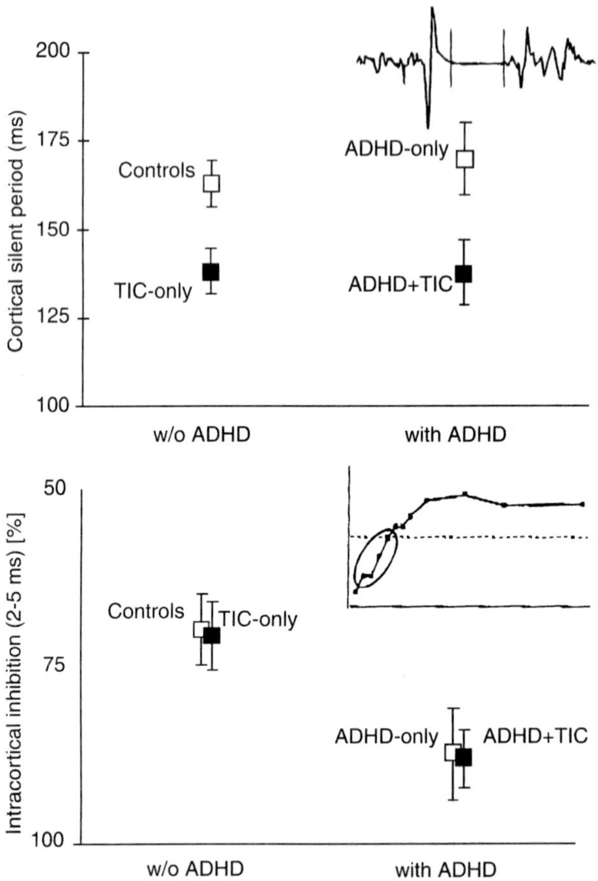

Figure 1 Additive inhibitory deficits in the sensomotor system cortical silent period (*above*) and intracortical inhibition (*below*) in children with comorbid ADHD and tic disorder. For each group mean ± mean standard error is presented. □ no tic disorer; ■: with tic disorder.

Because children with comorbid ADHD and tic disorder showed both a shortened CSP and also reduced ICI, we may assume a purely additive effect. Concerning different kinds of comorbidities in ADHD, such an additive effect could not be found in neuropathological studies of volume changes in the region of the basal ganglia (32), nor in neurophysiological studies on cognitive task-related cortical information processing (34–38). The additive effect demonstrated with TMS can therefore only be related to the excitability of the motor system.

The demonstration of both inhibitory deficits, which can be differentiated with TMS in the motor system of children with comorbid motor hyperactivity disorders—shortened CSP as evidence for inhibitory deficits probably at the level of the basal ganglia (tic disorder factor) and reduced ICI as evidence for inhibitory deficits in the region of the motor cortex (ADHD factor) corresponds phenomenologically with the simultaneous presence of both features of motor processes (pattern related in TD and general motor hyperactivity in ADHD). This finding also corresponds with the effectiveness of specific therapeutic interventions to improve the inhibitory deficits in the motor system, i.e., dopamine receptor antagonists in patients with tic disorders and methylphenidate (MPH) in patients with ADHD (39).

MPH AND INTRACORTICAL EXCITABILITY IN ADHD AND NORMALS

We know that MPH ameliorates motor problems of hyperactive children. For this reason, in children with ADHD who had not yet received any medication and where MPH treatment was indicated, we carried out a TMS study to test the acute effects of 10 mg MPH on their motor system excitability measured by TMS parameters (20). Comparison between the two TMS measurements showed (as the only statistically significant difference) an increase in ICI after MPH treatment; i.e., a tendency of normalization of their basically reduced ICI (Fig. 2).

The reported increase in inhibition in the motor system of ADHD after MPH intake shown with TMS cannot be considered as a disorder or symptom-specific phenomenon in children with ADHD, since it is not only the motor control, but the whole spectrum of ADHD symptoms—inattentiveness, impulsivity, and motor hyperactivity—that is improved. Consistent with this, the extent of motor inhibition measured using purely overt behavioral stop-signal tasks, was increased by MPH in children with ADHD (40), but attentional capacity and the overt neurophysiological parameters corresponding to information processing functions were also improved in an unspecific and more general manner (41–43).

In summary, we have a significant enhancement in ICI but no effects on ICF in children with ADHD. Since psychostimulants such as MPH lead to similar behavioral effects even in healthy children (44), and there is no developmental effect in ICI and ICF we expected a similar TMS result in healthy adults taking MPH. Hence, we investigated in healthy adults the effect of MPH on cortical excitability (29). We could demonstrate that an acute administration of a standard dose of 10 mg MPH had a pronounced effect on intracortical excitability. MPH significantly enhanced ICF. This was an unexpected observation because dopaminergic effects of MPH directly at the cortical level could explain the enhancement of the ICI but not ICF, since dopamine may act as an inhibitory agent at the level of the neocortex (45). Alternatively, MPH may also act by D2-receptor activation in the striatum via the striato-thalamo-cortical sensorimotor circuit, since the excitability of the cortical neurons is altered via the ascending synaptic input (46).

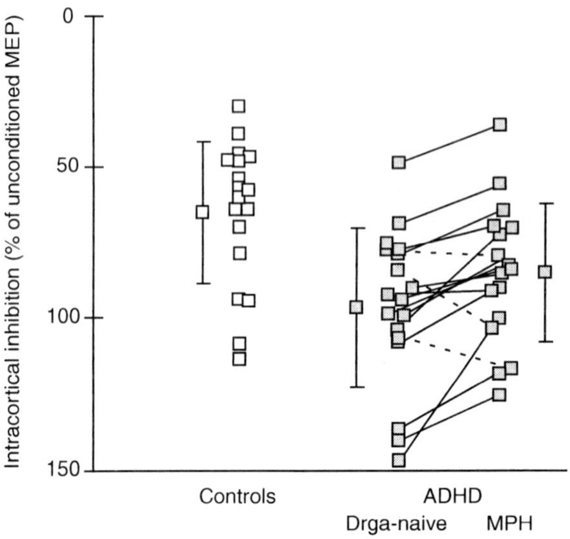

Figure 2 Intracortical inhibition [as percentage of unconditioned motor evoked potential (MEP) mean value over interstimulus intervals (ISI) 2–5 ms] in 18 drug-naive children with attention-deficit hyperactivity disorder (ADHD) aged 8–12 years compared to 18 age-matched healthy children. For each ADHD child, the effect of 10 mg methylphenidate (MP) on intracortical inhibition is also depicted. The group's mean values and standard deviations are plotted beside each group and condition, respectively. The insert shows MEPs of a representative ADHD patient (drug-naive, thick line; MP, thin line) to the test stimulus alone (upper trace) and conditioned by a subthreshold stimulus at ISI 13 ms ($\hat{=}$ inhibitory interval, lower traces).

In contrast to ICI the enhancement of ICF by MPH in healthy adults cannot readily be explained by the activation of D2-like receptors, because other D2-agonists such as bromocriptine do not significantly enhance the ICF (24). On the other hand, noradrenergic projections (such as those from locus coeruleus) are widely distributed in the neocortex, and studies from other authors indicate that norepinephrine modulates excitatory neuronal transmission (47). Further, intake of 40 but not 20 mg yohimbine, a central norepinephrine enhancing drug has been shown to increase ICF (48). Hence, it may be speculated whether MPH enhances ICF by increasing the excitatory neurotransmission via indirect noradrenergic neurons, similar to-amphetamine (49).

It is unclear, whether the acute effects of MPH in ADHD treatment results from drug-induced catecholamine changes at presynaptic and/or postsynaptic sites (50). Nevertheless, an increased striatal dopamine transporter availability was reported in adult patients with ADHD compared with healthy controls using SPECT (51,52). Therefore, a different status of dopaminergic innervation (the different level in ADHD may be "functionally normalized" by MPH) might contribute to opposite effects of MPH on intracortical excitability in ADHD compared to healthy subjects (29). In this context, it should be noted that changes in ICI and ICF may also be due to other reasons which are not related to intracortical effects (33). Therefore, not only different dosage effects, but also input–output curves of MEP with and without MPH as well as direct measures of spinal motor neuron excitability are required to substantiate these findings. Moreover, also adult patients with ADHD need to be examined, although it seems unlikely that the observed opposite effects of MPH depend on a developmental process, since no age-dependent changes could be found in intracortical excitability during adolescence (25).

CONCLUSION

With these TMS studies on motor system excitability in children and adolescents with ADHD we have been able to obtain substantial new information to further support the notion that motor excitability plays an important role in ADHD. Further insight into the pathophysiological background of child psychiatric disorders may be expected by combining TMS with brain electrical methods and neuroimaging techniques, especially fMRI.

REFERENCES

1. Pereira HS, Landgren M, Gillberg C, Forssberg H. Parametric control of fingertip forces during precision grip lifts in children with DCD (developmental coordination disorder) and DAMP (deficits in attention, motor control and perception). Neuropsychologia 2001; 39:478–88.
2. Kalverboer AF. A Neurobehavioural Study in Pre-school Children. Lavenham, England: Spastics International Medical Publications, 1975.
3. Oosterlaan J, Logan GD, Sergeant JA. Response inhibition in AD/HD, CD, comorbid AD/HD+CD, anxious and control children: a meta-analysis of studies with the stop task. J Child Psychol Psychiatry 1998; 39:411–26.
4. Porrino JL, Rapoport JL, Behar D, Sceery W, Ismond DR, Bunney WE Jr. A naturalistic assessment of the motor activity of hyperactive boys. I. Comparison with normal controls. Arch Gen Psychiatry 1983; 40:681–7.
5. Porrino JL, Rapoport JL, Behar D, Sceery W, Ismond DR, Bunney WE Jr. A naturalistic assessment of the motor activity of hyperactive boys. II. Stimulant drug effects. Arch Gen Psychiatry 1983; 40:688–93.
6. Konofal E, Lecendreux M, Bouvard MP, Mouren-Simeoni MC. High levels of nocturnal activity in children with attention-deficit hyperactivity disorder: a video analysis. Psychiatr Clin Neurosci 2001; 55:97–103.
7. Rothenberger A. In: Garreau B, ed. Neuroimaging In Child Neuropsychiatric Disorders. Chapter: Electrical Brain Activity and Motor Control In Tourette's Syndrome and Attention Deficit Hyperactivity Disorder. Heidelberg, Berlin: Springer, 1998:141–51.

8. Yordanova J, Kolev V, Heinrich H, Woerner W, Banaschewski T, Rothenberger A. Developmental event-related gamma oscillations: effects of auditory selective attention. Eur J Neurosci 2002; 16:2214–24.
9. Mostofsky SH, Cooper KL, Kates WR, Denckla MB, Kaufmann WE. Smaller prefrontal and premotor volumes in boys with attention-deficit/hyperactivity disorder. Biol Psychiatry 2002; 52:785–94.
10. Barker CA, Garvey MA, Bartko JJ, et al. The ipsilateral silent period (iSP) in children with attention deficit hyperactivity disorder (ADHS). Neurology 2001; 56(Suppl. 3):A321.
11. Sagvolden T, Sergeant JA. Attention deficit/hyperactivity disorder—from brain dysfunctions to behaviour. Behav Brain Res 1998; 94:1–10.
12. Castellanos FX, Tannock R. Neuroscience of attention-deficit/hyperactivity disorder: the search for endophenotypes. Nat Rev Neurosci 2002; 3:617–28.
13. Casey BJ, Giedd JN, Thomas KM. Structural and functional brain development and its relation to cognitive development. Biol Psychol 2000; 54:241–57.
14. Waldvogel D, van Gelderen P, Muellbacher W, Ziemann U, Immisch I, Hallett M. The relative metabolic demand of inhibition and excitation. Nature 2000; 406:995–8.
15. Barker AT, Jalinous R, Freeston IL. Non-invasive magnetic stimulation of the human motor cortex. Lancet 1985; 1:1106–7.
16. George MS, Lisanby SH, Sackein HA. Transcranial magnetic stimulation. Arch Gen Psychiatry 1999; 56:300–11.
17. Boylan LS, Sackheim HA. Magnetoelectric brain stimulation in the assessment of brain physiology and pathophysiology. Clin Neurophysiol 2000; 111:504–12.
18. Fitzgerald PB, Brown TL, Daskalakis ZJ. The application of transcranial magnetic stimulation in psychiatry and neurosciences research. Acta Psychiatry Scan 2002; 105:324–40.
19. Parent A, Hazrati LN. Functional anatomy of the basal ganglia. I. The cortico-basal ganglia-thalamo cortical loop. Brain Res Brain Res Rev 1995; 20:91–127.
20. Moll GH, Heinrich H, Rothenberger R. Transcranial magnetic stimulation in child psychiatry—disturbed motor system excitability in hypermotoric syndromes. Dev Sci 2002; 5:381–91.
21. Ziemann U, Rothwell JC, Ridding MC. Interaction between intracortical inhibition and facilitation in human motor cortex. J Physiol (Lond) 1996; 496: 873–81.
22. Inghillerie M, Berardelli A, Cruccu G, Manfredi M. Silent period evoked by transcranial stimulation of the human cortex and cervicomedullary junction. J Physiol 1993; 466:521–34.
23. Kujirai T, Caramia MD, Rothwell JC, et al. Corticocortical inhibition in human motor cortex. J Physiol (Lond) 1993; 471:501–19.
24. Ziemann U, Paulus W, Rothenberger A. Decreased motor inhibition in Tourette's disorder: evidence from transcranial magnetic stimulation. Am J Psychiatry 1997; 154:1277–84
25. Moll GH, Heinrich H, Wischer S, Tergau F, Paulus W, Rothenberger A. Motor system excitability in healthy children: developmental aspects from transcranial magnetic stimulation. Electroenc Clin Neurophysiol 1999; 51(Suppl 51):243–9.

26. Meere van der JJ, Vreeling HJ, Sergeant JA. A motor pre-setting study in hyperactives, learning disabled and control children. J Child Psychol Psychiatry 1992; 34:1347–54.
27. Moll GH, Heinrich H, Trott G-E, Wirth S, Rothenberger A. Deficient intracortical inhibition in drug-naive children with attention-deficit hyperactivity disorder is enhanced by methylphenidate. Neurosci Lett 2000; 284:121–5.
28. Barkley RA. Behavioral inhibition, sustained attention, and executive functions: constructing a unifying theory of ADHD. Psychol Bull 1997; 121: 65–94.
29. Moll GH, Heinrich H, Rothenberger A. Methylphenidate and intracortical excitability: opposite effects in healthy subjects and attention-deficit hyperactivity disorder. Acta Psychiatr Scand 2003; 107:1–4.
30. Banaschewski T, Brandeis D, Heinrich H, Albrecht B, Brunner E, Rothenberger A. Questioning inhibitory control as a specific deficit of ADHD—evidence from brain electrical activity. J Neurol Transmission 111: 841–64.
31. Spencer T, Biederman J, Wilens T. Attention-deficit/hyperactivity disorder and comorbidity. Pediatr Clin N Am 1999; 46:915–27.
32. Castellanos FX, Giedd JN, Hamburger SD, March WL, Rapoport JL. Brain morphometry in Tourette's syndrome: the influence of comorbid attention-deficit/hyperactivity disorder. Neurology 1996; 47:1581–3.
33. Moll GH, Heinrich H, Trott GE, Wirth S, Bock N, Rothenberger A. Children with comorbid attention-deficit hyperactivity disorder and tic disorder: evidence for additive inhibitory deficits within the motor system. Ann Neurol 2001; 49:393–6.
34. Rothenberger A, Banaschewski T, Heinrich H, Moll GH, Schmidt MH, van't Klooster B. Comorbidity in ADHD children: effects of coexisting conduct disorder or tic disorder on event-related potentials in an auditory selective attention task. Eur Arch Psychiatr Clin Neurosci 2000; 250:101–10.
35. Schuerholz LJ, Baumgardner TL, Singer HS, Reiss AL, Denckla MG. Neuropsychological status of children with Tourette's syndrome with and without attention deficit hyperactivity disorder. Neurology 1996; 46:958–65.
36. Yordanova J, Dumais-Huber C, Rothenberger A. Coexistence of tics and hyperactivity in children: no additive effect at the psychophysiological level. Int J Psychophysiol 1996; 21:121–33.
37. Yordanova J, Dumais-Huber C, Rothenberger A, Woerner W. Frontocortical activity in children with comorbidity of tic disorder and attention deficit hyperactivity disorder. Biol Psychiatry 1997; 41:585–94.
38. Banaschewski T, Brandeis D, Heinrich H, Albrecht B, Brunner E, Rothenberger A. Association of ADHD and conduct disorder—brain electrical evidence for the existence of a distinct subtype. J Child Psychol Psychiatry 2003; 4:356–76.
39. Gadow KD, Sverd J, Sprafkin J, Nolan EE, Grossman S. Long-term methylphenidate therapy in children with comorbid attention-deficit hyperactivity disorder and chronic multiple tic disorder. Arch Gen Psychiatry 1999; 56:330–6.

40. Tannock R, Purvis KL, Schachar RJ. Narrative abilities in children with attention deficit hyperactivity disorder and normal peers. J Abnorm Child Psychol 1992; 21:103–17.
41. Klorman R, Brumaghim JT, Fitzpatrick PA, Borgstedt AD. Methylphenidate reduces abnormalities of stimulus classification in adolescents with attention deficit disorder. J Abnorm Psychol 1992; 101:130–8.
42. Jonkman LM, Kemmer C, Verbaten MN, et al. Effects of methylphenidate on event-related potentials and performance of attention-deficit-hyperactivity disorder in children in auditory and visual selective attention tasks. Biol Psychiatr 1997; 41:690–702.
43. Vaidya CJ, Austin G, Kirkorian G, et al. Selective effects of methylphenidate in attention deficit hyperactivity disorder: a functional magnetic resonance study. Proc Am Acad Sci 1998; 95:14494–9.
44. Rapoport JL, Buchsbaum MS, Weingarten H, Zahn TP, Ludlow C, Mikkelsen EJ. Dextroamphetamine—its cognitive and behavioral effects in normal and hyperactive boys and normal men. Arch Gen Psychiatry 1980; 37:933–43.
45. Cepeda C, Radisavljevic Z, Peacock W, Levine MS, Buchwald NA. Differential modulation by dopamine of responses evoked by excitatory amino acids in human cortex. Synapse 1992; 11:330–41.
46. DeLong MR. Primate models of movement disorders of basal ganglia origin. Trend Neurosci 1990; 13:281–5.
47. Radisavljevic Z, Cepeda C, Peacock W, Buchwald NA, Levine MS. Norepinephrine modulates excitatory amino-acid responses in developing human and adult rat cerebral cortex. Int J Dev Neurosci 1994; 12:353–61.
48. Plewnia C, Bartels M, Cohen L, Gerloff C. Noradrenergic modulation of human cortex excitability by the presynaptic alpha (2)-antagonist yohimbine. Neurosci Lett 2001; 307:41–4.
49. Boroojerdi B, Battaglia F, Muellbacher W, Cohen LG. Mechanisms influencing stimulus-response properties of the human corticospinal system. Clin Neurophysiol 2001; 112:931–7.
50. Ziemann U, Tergau F, Bruns D, Baudewig J, Paulus W. Changes in human motor cortex excitability induced by dopaminergic and anti-dopaminergic drugs. Electroenc Clin Neurophysiol 1997; 105:430–73.
51. Dougherty DD, Bonab AA, Spencer TC, Rauch SL, Madras BK, Fischman AJ. Dopamine transporter density in patients with attention deficit hyperactivity disorder Lancet 1999; 354:2132–3.
52. Krause KH, Dresel SH, Krause J, Kung HF, Tatsch K. Increased striatal dopamine transporter in adult patients with attention deficit hyperactivity disorder: effects of methylphenidate as measured by single photon emission computed tomography. Neurosci Lett 2000; 28:107–10.

Section IV: Management

13

Assessment and Remediation of Organizational Skills Deficits in Children with ADHD

Howard Abikoff and Richard Gallagher

Department of Child and Adolescent Psychiatry, New York University School of Medicine, New York, New York, U.S.A.

INTRODUCTION

Attention deficit hyperactivity disorder (ADHD) affects about 6% of the school age population, and is the most prevalent disorder in child psychiatric clinics. It is characterized by age inappropriate inattention, motor activity, and impulsivity, to the point of causing meaningful impairment in the child's function. In addition to the cardinal signs of ADHD, it is generally recognized that other clinical features affect children's function. Among these other features are problems in organizing tasks and activities, with disorganized work habits, and a tendency to scatter, lose, or carelessly mishandle materials necessary for tasks (1). These characteristics have been conceptualized as reflecting deficits in executive function (EF). A prominent model of ADHD (2,3) posits that deficits in EF represent the underlying pathological process in ADHD. Although this view has been influential, it has not been translated into therapeutic action. Multiple psychosocial strategies have been developed for the management of children with ADHD (4,5), but none has incorporated the reversal of organizational deficits as a key component. The relative lack of attention paid to the organizational, time management, and planning (OTMP) skills in ADHD is noteworthy, given that ineffective OTMP skills compromise school success, and also result in family conflict, and decreased work performance.

We have attempted to address this neglected clinical issue through the development of a treatment approach specifically designed to ameliorate deficits in time management, organizational, and planning skills in elementary school-aged children with ADHD. This chapter provides an overview of an intervention we developed and evaluated with the support of an NIMH R21 Treatment Development grant.

BACKGROUND

There is converging theoretical, clinical, and empirical consensus that an essential element of ADHD is poor organization of materials, time, and actions, and that these deficits play a critical role in the adjustment and functioning of individuals with ADHD. Recent models of the core cognitive and behavioral characteristics of ADHD (2,3), and findings on the adult adjustment of ADHD children highlight the impact that poor skills in organization of time, activity and materials, have on ultimate functioning (6–8). Barkley's theoretical model suggests that EF, including deficits in the capacity to plan actions into the future and organize actions for current situations is at the core of the disorder (2,3). Although this model is perhaps best formulated by Barkley, others as well have discussed the importance of EF deficits in ADHD (9,10). These formulations imply that weak executive functioning accounts not only for overt behavioral problems of impulsivity and unfocused restlessness, but also for poor attention to details, for poor time management, and for deficient planning of future actions, all characteristics of ADHD. These OTMP deficits have negative repercussions on multiple aspects of youngsters' function, including academic performance. For example, poor organizational skills result in misplacing or losing materials at school and home, forgetting to bring home materials needed for school assignments, losing or forgetting to bring completed homework to school, etc. Further, a poor sense of time (11,12) and deficiencies in time management, coupled with procrastination and inefficient planning add to the difficulty ADHD children have in starting and completing daily, as well as long-term academic assignments. Not surprisingly, these related difficulties lead not only to suboptimal academic work, which impacts negatively on the children's scholastic performance and grades, but also frequent conflicts with parents and teachers. Moreover, children's OTMP deficits affect social functioning. Lateness, and losing or misplacing materials needed for games and sports, impact negatively on peer relationships.

Of note, OTMP difficulties typically continue into adolescence and adulthood, and adversely affect work performance and occupational status. Follow-up studies of ADHD children grown-up indicate significant problems with fulfilling work expectations, working independently, and completing tasks (13). Moreover, in a norms adult ADHD rating scale (14,15), the factor that best distinguishes ADHD and nonimpaired adults is "inattention/memory problems," which consists almost entirely of items that reflect OTMP behaviors (e.g., "disorganized," "lose things I need," "don't plan ahead," "absent-minded," "misjudge time," etc.). These findings are consistent with the clinical description of ADHD in the DSM-IV.

Despite recognition of the salience of organizational skills in ADHD, there are neither comprehensive assessment measures of OTMP skills in children nor have there been efforts to develop and test interventions that specifically target OTMP deficits in ADHD. The Adolescent Subcommittee of Children and Adults with Attention-Deficit/Hyperactivity Disorder (CHADD) Public and Professional Education Committee developed the classroom performance survey in 1995 (16). However, the instrument evaluates only a handful of OTMP relevant behaviors, and lacks normative data. Relatedly, the revised Conners scales, among the most widely used ADHD assessment and outcome measures, have a limited item pool for OTMP behaviors (two items on the teacher scale, and four on the parent scale). The Child Organization Hyperactivity Index (17), a 26-item parent scale includes items about organization of materials and time, but the 8-item subscale that has shown discriminative utility assesses a restricted range of OTMP behaviors. The Behavior Rating Inventory of Executive Function (BRIEF) (18), a measure for teachers and parents with representative norms for children and adolescents, has two clusters that assess aspects of organization of materials and planning and organization and appears useful in screening children for disturbances in some OTMP behaviors. Children with ADHD, learning disorders, and brain injury were more impaired than nondisordered children on these item clusters and on a general factor (Metacognitive Index) (18–20). However, the scale has numerous repetitions and non-specific items. Items overlap considerably with core symptoms of ADHD. As a result, the BRIEF does not provide a profile specific to deficits in organization, or details of OTMP behaviors necessary to develop interventions and monitor progress.

There is a similar dearth of validated OTMP skills intervention programs. In lieu of empirically based programs, there are published guides for teachers that highlight the need to instruct ADHD students in management of materials and schedules (21–23). Levine (23) has provided several guidelines for helping children with "persistent organizational failure." Remediation recommendations include strategies to: (1) provide children with assistance in managing their notebooks, (2) monitor their study areas to be free from distractions and clutter, and (3) develop awareness of time demands. These recommendations, though creative in addressing the needs of students with deficient OTMP skills, have not been put to the test.

Cognitive remediation for individuals with acquired brain damage has focused on the facilitation of OTMP skills. Many patients with brain injuries experience deficits in executive skills, including disturbances in planning and organization (24,25). Although some remedial training has focused on these deficits (26), efforts have primarily emphasized assistance to adults with loss of function. There are efforts underway in youngsters with sequelae from injury, or CNS radiation or chemotherapy treatments, but their application to children with developmental disorders is unclear and effectiveness has not been established to date (27).

Classroom interventions in ADHD typically focus on improving on-task and related behaviors (28–30). Treatment studies rarely evaluate students' responses to the organizational demands in school settings, even though "persistent organizational failure" is recognized as a major problem (23). To our knowledge, no empirical studies have assessed the impact of OTMP interventions, which, if they exist at all, are small components of a larger treatment program (30,31). For example, a brief organizational skills treatment module was developed for the multimodal treatment of attention deficit hyperactivity disorder (MTA) school-based psychosocial treatment component (32). The behavioral strategies in this module integrated a variety of procedures, including prompting, external reinforcement (including contingency management and token economies), self-monitoring and self-reinforcement, all of which were intended to modify and improve organizational skills. Targeted behaviors included general organization of the child's desk and materials, organization of homework-related behaviors, and planning of long-term assignments. Additionally, in consultation with the children's teachers, MTA therapist–consultants reviewed the teachers' organizational skills and how they impacted on classroom functioning. The program allowed for flexibility in teachers' presentation of assignments and management of classroom materials in response to individual children's needs. However the organizational skills module was only a minor component of the MTA psychosocial intervention package. Moreover, because the MTA was not designed for component analyses, determination of the clinical efficacy of the organizational skills module was not possible.

Although there is an extensive literature regarding the effects of stimulant medication on the core symptoms of ADHD, there is a dearth of controlled studies that have evaluated medication's impact on children's organizational skills. A recent placebo (PL) controlled crossover study evaluated methylphenidate (MPH) effects on OTMP behaviors in nineteen 8–13 year old stimulant naïve youngsters with ADHD and organizational skills deficits. These deficits were ascertained via the Children's Organizational Skills Scale (COSS), a measure developed in conjunction with our training program (described in the following sections). Although children's OTMP scores were significantly improved with MPH compared to PL, 61% of children had COSS scores that were not normalized with MPH, and these youngsters continued to meet the study entry criteria for impaired OTMP skills (33).

In summary, although there has been increasing awareness of the deficits in EF among children with ADHD, there has been little systematic assessment of "real-world" functionally relevant organizational, time management, and planning skills of children with ADHD. There have been even fewer efforts to develop treatments specifically designed to target these skills and to ascertain the utility of the intervention to ameliorate OTMP deficits, maintain improvements, and enable children to generalize treatment gains to new functional domains. In recognition of the dearth of OTMP assessment measures and interventions, our research efforts have focused on three interrelated activities: (1) instrument development, (2) treatment development, and (3) pilot intervention testing. These efforts are described in the following sections.

ASSESSMENT OF OTMP BEHAVIORS

In light of the paucity of OTMP behavioral measures, we considered the development of such measures an essential component of treatment development and evaluation. Thus, the first goal was to develop "real-life" measures of OTMP skills to (1) inform the development of the training program, including the content and focus of treatment; (2) identify each child's specific areas of impairment, and (3) assess treatment outcome. To this end, we developed parent, teacher, and child self-rating scales to determine children's OTMP skills, and to identify specific problem areas in these domains.

Children's Organizational Skills Scales

Development of the scales was conducted through consultation with clinicians, teachers, and parents to obtain behaviors that reflected the day-to-day organizational difficulties that children with ADHD demonstrate. Lists were composed, critically evaluated by parents and teachers, revised to alter reading level, and compiled into versions that were used to gather data on a normal sample of children in the New York Metropolitan Region. Ratings of children by teachers, parents, and children were obtained. A sample of over 900 third to eighth grade children was rated by teachers and a separate sample of 137 children was rated by parents and themselves. Analysis of the teacher ratings (using principal components factor analysis with varimax rotation) yielded a three-factor solution: "organized behaviors" consists of 11 items that describe actions that facilitate school efforts, the effective use of organizational tools such as folders and calendars, and neat results (e.g., "This student is organized"; "This student makes lists, schedules, and reminders to keep him/herself organized"); "lapses in memory and materials management" consists of 11 items reflecting problems in forgetting assignments, forgetting the materials needed for those assignments, and losing, misplacing, or poorly organizing materials for assignments (e.g., "This student has trouble finding school supplies when they are needed"; "This student loses things at school"); and "task planning," which consists of 6 items that reflect actions related to time management and steps needed to complete a plan (e.g., "This student seems to run out of time before assignments are finished"; "When this student has a big project to do, he/she doesn't know where to begin"). In addition, a "cross-factor cluster" consisting of 7 items that load on more than one factor was retained because the items reflect important functional concerns that have implications for day-to-day functioning (e.g. "The child's backpack is messy"). A 41-item version of the measure, which includes 6 items that assess the degree of impairment associated with these skills deficits, is used to provide the clinical profile for intervention and ranking on the factors. The measure has been found effective in distinguishing children who receive supplemental special educational services from those that do not and in distinguishing girls from boys in the normative sample. Children who obtain special educational services and boys were rated as less effective on all factors. An independent sample of clinically diagnosed children with ADHD has been found to be significantly more impaired on all factors and the cross-cluster items (34).

Smaller sample sizes have prevented the completion of a factor analysis of the parent and child versions. Thus far, only a Total summary score has been utilized with the parent version. Significantly, a sample of children with ADHD has a lower total score on the parent COSS, reflecting less effective organization. Arrangements to obtain a nationally representative sample are under way. All three versions of the COSS will be used to obtain multiple-rater information on each child in the sample. Analytic strategies for this sample include reliability studies, validity studies, confirmatory factor analysis on the teacher version, and initial factor analysis on the parent and child versions of the scale.

OTMP INTERVENTION PROGRAM

Rationale

The intervention program was developed for 8- to 11-year-old children with ADHD, in grades 3–5. This age group was selected to reflect the elementary school grades in which demands for independent function become salient. The program attempts to ameliorate OTMP deficits through the use of child-focused behaviorally based skills training facilitated via the involvement of parents and teachers. Skills training that incorporates important adults in the child's environment has been shown to be an appropriate behavioral treatment strategy for ADHD children (30,35). It is not assumed that the intervention directly affects the putative deficits in EF theorized to underlie ADHD symptomatology. Rather, our position is that children can be taught to minimize their functional consequences. If proven effective, the treatment is intended to serve as an important adjunct to other validated treatments such as pharmacotherapy and parent management training, and not as a stand-alone intervention for the treatment of ADHD.

Overview of Treatment Principles and Features

The 10-week, 20-session manualized, flexible individual intervention program consists of a number of integrated procedures that are intended to maximize the development and appropriate use of OTMP skills in children with ADHD. There are several key principles and assumptions upon which the intervention is based. These are described in the following sections.

Treatment Tailoring

There has been increasing recognition of the need to incorporate tailored treatment strategies in ADHD interventions (36–38). The training program consists of modules that focus on specific OTMP skills (e.g., management of materials, planning for short and long-term projects, use of organizational aids, and time management). Although all children are exposed to all training modules, the emphasis placed on each module is individualized for each child. A needs assessment approach is used to identify each child's relative OTMP strengths and deficits so that tailoring procedures can target OTMP skills that have been determined to be especially salient for each child.

Needs assessment is ascertained via consideration of information from several sources. Each child's OTMP domain scores on the teacher, parent, and child versions of the COSS are compared to each other and to normative levels to determine the child's relative deficits in the OTMP skills domains targeted in the training program. Additionally, discussions with the teacher, parent and child are used to confirm the initial interpretation of the child's OTMP scores and to better clarify the specific nature of each child's difficulties.

As per procedures implemented in the MTA school consultation program (32), teacher interventions are individualized as well. Careful attention is paid to establishing a relationship with the teacher and assessing his/her current classroom behavioral and environmental procedures relevant to OTMP behaviors (e.g., use of homework assignment sheets, side-of-desk folders for each academic subject, etc.). Rather than foisting an inflexible protocol on teachers, clinicians assist teachers to use whatever strategies from the OTMP intervention protocol are feasible. In addition, teachers are involved in decision-making processes to assure that behaviors selected for intervention are socially valid (i.e., important to the teacher, and therefore likely to be reinforced by the teacher).

Skills Acquisition

The intervention program is based on the assumption that children with ADHD are more likely to use skills appropriately if they have demonstrated a high level of skills acquisition. Thus, shaping and successive approximation procedures are used early on in each training module to facilitate the initial stages of skills acquisition. This is followed by multiple opportunities to practice and master target skills during and in-between clinic-based sessions. The behavioral skills training approach integrates a number of behavior therapy strategies, including verbal instruction, modeling, behavioral rehearsal with feedback, cueing and use of lists, behavior prompting and reward, self-monitoring, as well as guided and rewarded practice between sessions.

Generalization

To be successful, ADHD intervention programs that target broad functional domains, such as social skills, require that the children learn and/or hone these skills in training and use them appropriately in a host of complex, multidimensional interpersonal situations and contexts. Unfortunately, these programs have been relatively unsuccessful. We considered possible reasons for their limited effectiveness. By their very nature, such training programs, whether they occur in the clinic or in specialized treatment settings, restrict the opportunities to provide training and practice in the exact interpersonal situations that a youngster confronts in daily life. Consequently, to use these broad functional skills appropriately, a child must demonstrate generalization skills in an extremely wide-range of heterogeneous social situations. That is, the child must recognize that the situation (s)he is confronting is a variant of the situation encountered in training (stimulus generalization), and then engage in social behaviors that are often a variant of the specific social behaviors focused on during training (response generalization). The disappointing results of social skills training programs (39) attest to the difficulty in achieving generalization effects.

In contrast, the OTMP skills targeted for intervention in this program focus on a somewhat circumscribed set of behaviors and recurring situations (e.g., getting ready for school, leaving school, initiating and completing homework). As such, there is an opportunity to target a relatively delimited number of skills and settings. Because these specific skills are typically required in real-world settings that do not vary much from day-to-day, the child has the opportunity to practice and refine these specific skills on a regular basis.

Notwithstanding the relatively limited range of situations requiring the use of OTMP skills, the intervention program incorporates systematic approaches throughout training to facilitate and evaluate generalization effects. Included here are efforts to involve parents and teachers via training in prompting, cueing and reinforcement procedures to be used with the child throughout the training program. Between-session practice and homework assignments are also included as generalization aids. Numerous exemplars are used in training to facilitate generalization, including the use of the child's own school-related assignments and materials.

Reinforcement

To facilitate learning of new OTMP skills and increase the children's motivation to use these skills outside of training, reinforcement procedures are used throughout the training program. During clinic-based sessions as well as between training sessions, a variety of contingency-based reward procedures are implemented. For example, to facilitate tracking and monitoring of assignments, tests and managing materials, children are taught to use a daily assignment record (DAR). By using step-wise training procedures, children learn to use the DAR to write down homework assignments for each subject, their due dates, and the exact materials that are needed to complete this assignment. The teachers provide feedback (by signing the DAR) in accord with the specific step(s) focused on in training. Teacher feedback is backed up with reinforcements provided by parents at home. Eventually, with the inclusion of cues (e.g., a small "reminder" card attached to the child's book bag zipper), at the end of each school day the youngster self-monitors whether all the necessary homework-related materials are in the book bag. Similar procedures regarding materials management are used at home.

Maintenance

A primary intervention goal is to facilitate OTMP skills maintenance after the completion of training. To this end, maintenance probes are conducted throughout the program. These probes, which rely on parent, teacher and child ratings and reports, are intended to evaluate whether learned skills, no longer targeted directly in clinic sessions, continue to be used appropriately outside of training. Problems regarding maintenance of specific skills are followed-up by reexposure to and reinforcement of these skills in and outside the clinic. Additionally, at the end of treatment parents are provided with an owner's guide, which provides a summary of training procedures and copies of key forms used in treatment. Therapists discuss with parents how they can make use of the guide once treatment has ended.

Engagement

Children function as collaborators in the treatment process. The tone of treatment emphasizes the mutual efforts that the child, therapists, parents, and teachers are making to overcome the impact of ADHD on the child's life. In the process, training exercises, although understood as having a serious intent, are playful and interactions with the child are informal. Also, to foster an alliance with the child and to facilitate engagement in the goal, children are presented with a rationale for overcoming the effects of ADHD so that the disorder does not interfere with their success. Similar to successful efforts used to help children overcome anxiety disorders utilized by Kendall in his Coping Cat procedure (40) and March and Mülle (41) in their method to "Run OCD Off My Land," we describe the child's and helpers' goal as "Controlling the glitches" that interfere with: keeping track of materials, remembering items and events, managing time, and planning steps. We use drawings to convert the "glitches" into characters that reside in the minds of people. We also provide children with workbooks that help them keep another aspect of their mind, the "mastermind," as active as possible in controlling the glitches. Our methods are intended to enhance success by objectifying the disorder's impact, by making the treatment "child-friendly" (42), by creating a collaborative team, and by converting the conflicts often encountered by the child when he or she fails to remain organized into fun exercises that can be incorporated into new habits.

Overview of OTMP Program

Treatment consists of 20 sessions, which occur twice weekly for 10 weeks. The content of the sessions includes: (1) parent and child Orientation; (2) parent guidance in building new skills through behavior modification; (3) module for keeping track of assignments; (4) module for organizing materials and papers; (5) module for time management; (6) module for planning tasks; (7) module on transfer of skills to other typical activities; (8) maintenance module; (9) phone contact and coaching; (10) graduation ceremony and a child's video-taped summary of skills learned and skills to be kept.

Parents and children are oriented to the program to help them understand the model of training utilized so that they are invested in the process. Participants are informed that evidence suggests that persons with ADHD learn new behaviors (even those that seem easy to carry out) most effectively when those responses are prompted in detail, when the responses are monitored carefully, and when the responses are praised and rewarded. Repetitive practice of small behavior chains is described as a necessary step for building skills, leading to skills mastery. This strategy is considered a viable means of increasing the likelihood that the behaviors will become embedded in the child's habitual response to situations that call for OTMP skills. Each training session integrates behavior therapy procedures to build skills through psychoeducation, modeling, guided practice, prompting and practice with reward in several situations, and use of home exercises to utilize the skill in the child's usual routine. Teachers as well receive training in the use of prompting and labeled praise. Teachers are asked to monitor the results of the child's efforts on the DAR, to be sent home each day. Graduated privileges are provided to the child based on the success indicated by the DAR. Thus, prompting, reinforcement with rewards in several settings, and repetitive practices are used to facilitate skill development.

Generalization Procedures

Overview: We adhere to a specific model to monitor and train for generalization in the main training modules (i.e., materials management, time management, and planning). First, training is conducted in the clinic setting for a specific task, and ratings of how well the child completes that task at home and at school are gathered. The task is practiced in the clinic session with a number of trials. The trials involve situations that are similar to the child's day-to-day circumstances. However, to facilitate generalization and recognition of the steps involved, a "fantasy" situation is also presented. Next, children explain the skill steps to parents and parents are educated to prompt and praise the use of those skills at home on a daily basis. Third, prompting and praise for use of the steps in school is fostered through the use of teacher consultation procedures used in previous clinical trials (32,43). Fourth, other situations that require the same skills are monitored and rated by parents and teachers to determine generalization across tasks.

Training Example: For example, when working on space and materials management as applied to a desk work area, children are presented with steps to review as they prepare to complete work. They are trained to determine what materials are needed for the task, what materials are present on the desk, what materials need to be added to the supplies present, and what materials need to be put away because they are unnecessary and may be distracting. They are presented with a task involving writing, a task involving taking notes from a book, a task to construct a 3D model, and a task to complete math problems using a ruler and calculator. As a generalization "fantasy" task, they may be asked to use the steps to prepare a work area for mapping a rocket ship course to Mars. Additionally, parents are trained to prompt and monitor the steps as the child completes daily homework. Teachers as well are asked to monitor the child's material and space management for select times during the school day. Parents and teachers rate the child's use of skills and the end result in-between training sessions. If the child has a low rating at home, the clinic setting is used to simulate home situations and practice continues until parents report an effective transfer of skills to the home setting. Meanwhile, teachers report on the school desk. The DAR provides information for monitoring by the treating clinician. Training in the clinic setting that simulates the school desk is or is not conducted depending on the teacher's report. Thus, application of the skills in several settings is monitored and addressed as needed to facilitate generalization across situations.

For task generalization, parents monitor the child's organization of his/her school book bag or backpack. How well the child puts in necessary items and keeps out unnecessary items are tracked. This information is used to determine how effectively skills are applied to similar tasks. Specific training is utilized in this task if transfer is not documented. For further extension, children's use of other bags for sports equipment, for example, is reviewed and trained if necessary.

Recognizing Where and When to Use OTMP Skills: In addition to using multiple exemplars, a procedure recommended to facilitate generalization, other key generalization training procedures are implemented to help children learn to recognize when and in what situations OTMP skills can be used in their day-to-day activities. The recognition procedures include the use of between-session diaries where children list situations in which they believe that OTMP skills would be useful. Children are also asked to develop a label for each skill and are asked to list when they used the varied skills. Relatedly, parents are asked to keep a separate diary of episodes in which they observe their children using OTMP skills. Finally, children are directed to review their upcoming schedule and anticipate when OTMP skills could be used in those activities.

Maintenance Procedures

A systematic sequence to fade prompts and rewards is followed to facilitate maintenance in the natural environment. As a first step, the number of steps prompted to complete a task is decreased in a planned way. For example, when space management for the work area is the task, prompts to place materials into groups and to leave a clear area for writing may be faded to the single prompt: "Please straighten out your work area." Rewards are provided for the end goal. Eventually, all prompts are faded and children are monitored and rewarded. Rewards are eventually faded to an intermittent schedule. Initially, praise and rewards are available as the task is ongoing; subsequently, they are faded to task completion, and then to daily, weekly, and longer time periods. Following fading, subsequent "maintenance probes" are used to determine if behavior has become embedded in the child's repertoire. Behaviors that are not demonstrated appropriately receive additional training.

Treatment Adherence and Fidelity

Measures of treatment adherence are implemented throughout the training program to ascertain the degree to which children, parents, and teachers carry out requisite treatment activities. Tracking adherence includes monitoring children's between-session "home exercises," including completion of calendars and school-assignment planners, parents' record sheets of behavioral procedures implemented at home, and teachers' completion of the DAR. Similarly, in-clinic sessions are monitored to track treatment fidelity and integrity.

Manuals Features

The treatment manual ("Organizational Skills Training"; OST) consists of specific instructions for each session.

Session Guidelines: Each session contains descriptions of the session goal and target skills, an overview, rationale, tasks, and the materials required. Detailed descriptions of the content of each session are presented, including the behavioral procedures to be implemented in the session tasks. Specific guidelines for in-clinic, home, and school activities are provided. Between-session "home exercises" are specified for the child, parent, and teacher.

Treatment Monitoring Forms: Each session contains treatment adherence, treatment fidelity, and performance forms. Treatment adherence forms track the degree to which the previous session's assignments were carried out; treatment fidelity forms track how much and which components of the session were completed during the session; session performance forms assess how well the child performed the session tasks.

Pilot Study of Intervention

The OST program was evaluated for feasibility and effectiveness in an open pilot study in 20 children with ADHD and organizational skills deficits. The youngsters were in grades 3–5; 60% had a diagnosis of ADHD Inattentive type and 40% Combined type; 50% were receiving stimulant treatment in the community and the remainder was medication free. Treatment was delivered by behaviorally trained Ph.D. clinical psychologists. The findings were positive and provided a signal of the intervention's effectiveness. Significant pre-post improvements were found on: teacher and parent ratings on the COSS ($p<0.01$); parent ratings of homework problems ($p<0.05$); and children's performance on an academic planning task ($p<0.001$). Improvements were not related to children's medication status or type of ADHD. No children dropped out of the program, and there was a high level of attendance, with all youngsters completing at least 17 sessions. Further, both parents' and teachers' ratings indicated satisfaction with the program.

Future Directions

We are currently evaluating the efficacy of the OST intervention in the context of a dual-site randomized controlled trial. The study design includes a wait-list group to control for the effects of repeated assessments and time, and an active treatment comparator. The latter, entitled "Parents and Teachers Helping Kids get Organized" (PATHKO), excludes any skills training with the child. Rather, it utilizes contingency management procedures, implemented by parents and to a lesser extent teachers, to target the end results of behavior chains that are likely to require effective OTMP behaviors (e.g., bringing home school assignments, handing in work on time), and reinforces children for engaging in relevant OTMP identified "end behaviors."

In addition to comparing the impact of skills versus performance-based interventions on children's organizational and academic functioning, the study is designed to evaluate maintenance and moderator effects. To this end, children's functioning is evaluated during the school year following their participation in treatment, and the moderating effects of parental ADHD on outcome are assessed as well.

Finally, the study includes children with OTMP deficits, regardless of their medication status. This sample will enable us to explore whether medicated children, whose OTMP deficits presumably reflect a skills rather than performance deficit, show greater improvement with OST than PATHKO, Such findings would have important implications for tailoring treatment interventions based on the nature of children's OTMP impairments.

REFERENCES

1. American Psychiatric Association. Diagnostic and Statistical Manual of Mental Disorders. 4th ed. Washington, DC: Author, 1994.
2. Barkley RA. ADHD and the Nature of Self-control. New York: Guilford Press, 1997.
3. Barkley RA. Attention-deficit Hyperactivity Disorder: A Handbook for Diagnosis and Treatment. 2nd ed. New York: Guilford, 1999.
4. Hinshaw SP, Klein RG, Abikoff H. Childhood Attention-Deficit Hyperactivity Disorder: Nonpharmacologic and Combination Treatments. In: PE Nathan, JM Gorman, eds. A Guide to Treatments That Work. Oxford: Oxford University Press, 1998:26–41.
5. Hinshaw SP, Klein RG, Abikoff H. Childhood Attention-Deficit/Hyperactivity Disorder: Nonpharmacologic Treatments and their combination with medication. In: Nathan PE, Gorman JM, eds. A Guide to Treatments That Work. 2nd ed. Oxford: Oxford University Press, 2002:1–23.
6. Mannuzza S, Klein RG, Bessler A, Malloy P, LaPadula M. Adult outcomes of hyperactive boys: Educational achievement, occupational rank, and psychiatric status. Arch Gen Psychiatry 1993; 50:565–76.
7. Mannuzza S, Klein RG, Bessler A, Malloy P, Hynes ME. Educational and occupational outcome of hyperactive boys grown up. J Am Acad Child Adol Psychiatry 1997; 36:1222–27.
8. Weiss G, Hechtman L, Milroy T, Perlman T. Psychiatric status of hyperactives as adults: a controlled prospective 15-year follow-up of 63 hyperactive children. J Am Acad Child Adol Psychiatry 1985; 24:211–20.
9. Brown TE. Emerging understandings of attention-deficit disorders and comorbidities. In: TE Brown, ed. Attention-Deficit Disorders and Comorbidities in Children, Adolescents, and Adults. Washington, DC: American Psychiatric Press, 2000.

10. Pennington BF, Ozonoff S. Executive functions and developmental psychopathology. J Child Psychol Psychiatry 1996; 37:51–87.
11. Barkley RA, Koplowitz S, Anderson T, McMurray MB. Sense of time in children with ADHD: Effects of duration, distraction, and stimulant medication. J Intl Neuropsychol Soc 1997; 3:359–69.
12. Grskovic JA, Zentall SS, Stormont-Spurgin M. Time estimation and planning abilities: Students with and without mild disabilities. Behav Disord 1995; 20: 197–203.
13. Weiss G, Hechtman L. Hyperactive Children Grown Up. 2nd ed. New York: Guilford, 1993.
14. Conners CK, Erhardt D, Epstein JN, Parker JDA, Sitarenios R, Sparrow E. Self-ratings of ADHD symptoms in adults I: Factor structure and normative data. J Atten Disord 1999; 3:141–51.
15. Erhartdt D, Epstein JN, Conners CK, Parker JDA, Sitarenios G. Self-ratings of ADHD symptoms in adults II: Reliability, validity, and diagnostic sensitivity. J Atten Disord 1999; 3:153–8.
16. Robin AL. ADHD in Adolescents. New York: Guilford Press, 1998.
17. Zentall SS, Harper GW, Stormont-Spurgin M. Children with hyperactivity and their organizational skills. J Educ Res 1993; 87:112–7.
18. Gioia GA, Isquith PK, Guy SC, Kenworthy L. BRIEF: Behavior Rating Inventory of Executive Function: Professional manual. Lutz, FL: Psychological Assessment Resources, Inc., 1996.
19. Denckla MB. The Brief Rating Inventory of Executive Function: Commentary. Child Neuropsychol 2002; 4:304–6.
20. Mahone EM, Cirino PT, Cutting LE, Cerrone PM, Hagelthorn KM, Hiemenz JR, Singer HS, Denckla MB. Validity of the behavior rating inventory of executive function in children with ADHD and/or Tourette syndrome. Arch Clin Neuropsychol 2002; 17:643–62.
21. Braswell L, August GJ, Bloomquist ML, Realmuto GM, Skare SS, Crosby RD. School-based secondary prevention for children with disruptive behavior: Initial outcomes. J Abnorm Child Psychol 1997; 25:197–208.
22. Braswell L, Bloomquist ML. Cognitive-Behavioral Therapy with ADHD Children. New York: Guilford, 1991.
23. Levine M. Educational Care: A System of Understanding and Helping Children with Learning Problems at Home and in School. Cambridge, MA: Educators Publishing Service, 1994.
24. Mattson AJ, Levin HS. Frontal lobe dysfunction following closed head injury. J Nerv Ment Dis 1990; 178:282–91.
25. Stuss DT, Gow CA. "Frontal dysfunction" after traumatic brain injury. Neuropsychiatry Neuropsychol Behav Neurol 1992; 5:272–82.
26. Matteer CA. The rehabilitation of executive disorders. In: DT Stuss, G Winocur, IH Robertson, eds. Cognitive Neurorehabilitation. Cambridge, England: Cambridge University Press, 1999:314–32.
27. Butler RW, Copeland DR. Attentional processes and their remediation in children treated for cancer: a literature review and the development of a therapeutic approach. J Intl Neuropsych Soc 2002; 8:115–24.

28. DuPaul GJ, Eckert TL. The effects of school-based interventions for attention deficit hyperactivity disorder: A meta-analysis. School Psychol Rev 1997; 26:5–27.
29. Klein RG, Abikoff H. Behavior therapy and methylphenidate in the treatment of children with ADHD. J Attn Disord 1997; 2:89–114.
30. MTA Cooperative Group. A 14-month randomized clinical trial of treatment strategies for attention-deficit/hyperactivity disorder. Arch Gen Psychiatry 1999; 56:1073–86.
31. Hechtman L, Abikoff H, Klein R, Weiss G, Respitz C, Kouri J, Blum C, Greenfield B, Etcovitch J, Fleiss K, Pollack S. Academic achievement and emotional status of children with ADHD treated with long-term methylphenidate and multimodal psychosocial treatment. J Amer Acad Child Adol Psych 2004; 43:820–9.
32. Wells KC, Pelham WE, Kotkin R Et al. Psychosocial treatment strategies in the MTA study: Rationale, methods, and critical issues in design and implementation. J Abnorm Child Psychol 2000; 28:483–505.
33. Abikoff H, Gallagher R, Nissley-Tsiopinis J, Stotter R, Zambenedetti M, Seyffert M, Boorady R, McCarthy J. Stimulant treatment of ADHD-related organizational, time management and planning deficits. Poster presented at the Annual Meeting of the American Academy of Child and Adolescent Psychiatry, San Diego, CA, 2006, October.
34. Abikoff, H, Gallagher R, Alvir J. A teacher rating scale of children's organizational, time management and planning skills: The COSS-T. Poster presented at the Annual Meeting of the International Society for Research in Child and Adolescent Psychopathology, Sydney, Australia, 2003, June.
35. Pfiffner LJ, McBurnett K. Social skills training with parent generalization: treatment effects for children with attention deficit disorder. J Consult Clin Psychol 1997; 65:749–57.
36. Abikoff H. Tailored psychosocial treatments for ADHD: the search for a good fit. J Clin Child Psychol 2001; 30:122–5.
37. Greene R, Ablon SJ. What does the MTA study tell us about effective psychosocial treatment for ADHD? J Clin Child Psychol 2001; 30:114–21.
38. Jensen PS, Abikoff HA. Tailoring treatment for individuals with attention-deficit/hyperactivity disorder: clinical and research perspectives. In: TE Brown, ed. Attention-Deficit Disorders and Comorbidities in Children, Adolescents, and Adults. Washington, DC: American Psychiatric Press, 2000:637–52.
39. Gresham FM. Social skills training: should we raze, remodel, or rebuild? Behav Disord 1998; 24:19–25.
40. Kendall PC. Coping Cat Workbook. Ardmore, PA: Workbook Publishing, 1992.
41. March J, Mulle K. OCD in Children and Adolescents: A Cognitive-Behavioral Treatment Manual. New York: Guilford Press, 1998.
42. Stern MB. Child friendly Therapy: Biopsychosocial Innovations for Children and Families. New York: WW Norton & Company, Inc., 2002.
43. Gittelman-Klein R, Abikoff H, Pollack E, Klein DF, Katz S, Mattes J. A controlled trial of behavior modification and methylphenidate in hyperactive children. In: C Whalen, B Henker, eds. Hyperactive Children: The Social Ecology of Identification and Treatment. New York: Academic Press, 1980: 221–43.

14

School Consultation for the Mental Health Professional Working with ADHD

Ann Abramowitz

Department of Psychology, Emory University, Atlanta, Georgia, U.S.A.

RATIONALE FOR SCHOOL CONSULTATION BY THE MENTAL HEALTH PROFESSIONAL

For a mental health professional trained in traditional approaches to therapy with children and adolescents, it may be tempting to follow a practice of primarily conducting individual therapy with the youngster, additionally conferring with the parents. However, therapists with current knowledge of attention deficit hyperactivity disorder (ADHD) treatment will be far more likely to conduct behaviorally oriented family therapy to address the primary and secondary behavioral concerns often associated with ADHD. This includes creating structure within the home that facilitates follow-through with instructions, reducing oppositional behavior, alleviating "homework hassles," and establishing rules and contingencies to prevent and deal with problems. While these strategies will address difficulties occurring within the family, they will not be sufficient to address the youngster's difficulties at school. Improvements at home likely will not generalize to the school setting, and similar approaches will need to be employed there (1). Ideally, the school personnel will be well-trained in working with youngsters with ADHD, and perhaps school-wide interventions, or at least strategies to assist the particular youngster, are already in place. Often, however, this is not the case. The main point of this chapter is that mental health professionals treating youngsters with ADHD need to be proficient in school consultation skills. Such consultations typically involve visits to the school to develop strategies and to assist with their implementation. When assessing problems or requesting that particular strategies be implemented, mental health professionals should not rely exclusively on written contact with the school, telephone calls, or using the parents or the youngster him/herself as a conduit.

For several reasons, the mental health professional is the ideal person to assist the school with interventions for ADHD. First, he or she knows the youngster and family. Youngsters with ADHD may have depression, anxiety, troubled families, poverty, and any of the other mental health problems and psychosocial stressors endured by those without ADHD. The youngster's ADHD or that of another family member also may predispose the youngster to any of these conditions (2). The mental health professional often is the individual most aware of these issues in a child's life, and is in an ideal position to interpret these issues to school personnel. Second, the mental health professional usually has expertise with medications for ADHD and is in the best position to facilitate treatment that maximizes the effects of both medication and classroom interventions, possibly even making it possible to reduce medication doses (3). Third, he or she can facilitate communication between the school and home, and reduce the tendency for these interactions to become adversarial.

CONSIDERATION OF RESEARCH IN SELECTING INTERVENTIONS

Interventions selected should be supported by research. They should be feasible for the setting and acceptable to those who will be involved in implementing them, as well as to the youngster him/herself. Mental health professionals who are abreast of the literature pertaining to the treatment of ADHD may have concerns about the recently published MTA results suggesting that psychosocial interventions, including school consultation and school-based behavioral strategies, do not offer an incremental benefit over stimulant medication in the treatment of ADHD (4). While this interpretation of the MTA results is accurate when interpreting the effects of the treatments on ADHD symptoms in the overall study sample, mental health professionals should be cautioned that the issue is far more complicated, and any implications of the MTA for community practice are unclear. First, not all youngsters with ADHD receive stimulant medication, for reasons that include parent and/or student preference and adverse side effects. Second, the abundant literature on the management of disruptive behavior in the school setting informs the practice of ADHD intervention in the school setting. Medicated or not, a youngster's disruptive behavior must be dealt with. Third, youngsters with ADHD, medicated or not, typically exhibit disorganization and inattention, both of which can be fatal to school success. While research targeting these behaviors is less extensive than research targeting disruptive behavior, well-documented strategies do exist, and work is continually being done to expand this area. Fourth, the medication protocol followed in the MTA was far more meticulous than that typically employed in community practice, and it is logical to infer that benefits accruing from medication will be more variable than those attained in the MTA (5). Fifth, the MTA children who had both comorbid conduct problems and anxiety responded best to the condition that combined psychosocial intervention and medication (6).

STEPS IN PROVIDING SCHOOL CONSULTATION

Prior to conducting a school consultation, it is important to gather relevant information. Comparable to the information gathered in the process of assessing for ADHD, this should include an in-depth history of the child, including family, school and home behavior, health, social, and academic. It is helpful to know what school interventions have been particularly helpful for this youngster in the past. In addition to checklists that assess for the presence of ADHD-related behaviors, behavior rating scales that assess for social or emotional difficulties and atypical behavior should be obtained from all teachers presently involved with the youngster. Having this information in advance of the school visit enables the mental health specialist to consider the teachers' concerns while observing.

The next step should be a planned observation of the youngster in the school setting. There are published methodologies for conducting the observation (7), or the observation may be informal, but it is important to observe the youngster in as many as possible of the settings where he or she reported to be experiencing difficulties. The key here is that the manifestation of ADHD-related behaviors in any particular setting should be viewed as a function not only of the ADHD, but also of the characteristics. Ultimately, it may prove easier to modify aspects of the setting than to change the ADHD itself. For the observation, relevant characteristics include, but certainly are not limited to:

- teaching style (enthusiasm, clarity, warmth, confidence, etc.),
- teacher's typical responses to off-task or disruptive behavior exhibited by any student,
- degree to which distractions are present,
- aspects of the classroom organization such as seat arrangement and placement of shared materials,
- extent to which a clear time limit is imposed for completion of individual tasks,
- interest level of instruction and other tasks, and
- degree to which youngster possesses the academic and organizational skills needed to comply with teacher's expectations.

The next step is to meet with the teacher(s) and any other relevant personnel. To facilitate communication and cooperation among all those helping the youngster, it is most helpful to invite the parents to this meeting, and often the youngster as well, particularly at the high school level. Involvement by members of the student support team (SST) can be very helpful in the process of generating ideas, as SST members ultimately will be involved in the implementation of interventions and in the process of maintaining those interventions as the youngster moves to the next grade. Interventions should be designed collaboratively, along with a plan for ongoing evaluation of their success. They should target specific behaviors of concern and strategies should be specific, along with procedures to monitor their effectiveness. The roles of the mental health professional, teachers, and others should be spelled out.

Finally, follow-up should be systematic. Subsequent visits to the school may be necessary, or phone contacts with key personnel may suffice. Behavior rating scales should be used at regular intervals to assess the extent of remaining problems, just as they are used for medication monitoring. Often, follow-up can be accomplished through office visits to the mental health professional and phone calls to the school, but when school difficulties persist, or when issues change, successive visits may be needed.

TECHNIQUES THAT CAN BE APPROPRIATE OUTCOMES FOLLOWING CONSULTATION

Techniques based on contingency management—systematic positive reinforcement of appropriate behavior and systematic ignoring and punishment of inappropriate behaviors—can be highly effective. Systematic verbal feedback by the teacher has been demonstrated to be a powerful consequence in classroom management. In particular, reprimands that are firm, delivered in a neutral as opposed to emotional manner, brief, and as immediate as possible following the onset of off-task behavior have been shown to be a key component of successful management of off-task and disruptive classroom behavior (8). To initially establish their maximum effectiveness, the teacher should pair reprimands with back-up consequences, generally loss of a privilege, as needed. Besides teacher feedback, one of the best supported interventions is home-based contingencies, also referred to as a daily report card, or DRC for short. With this procedure, the teacher rates several specific behaviors on a checklist that the child brings home daily. Parents can provide praise and other positive consequences contingent on a positive report; sometimes loss of points or a privilege are made contingent on a negative report or failure to bring the DRC home (9). Other strategies include systematic use by the teacher of positive reinforcement, including points toward tangible rewards and privileges; response cost, involving loss of points or direct loss of privileges; and extinction (ignoring) of minor inappropriate behaviors. Relatively simple yet sophisticated systems utilizing these approaches can be tailored using individualized checklists for particular youngsters or implemented as classroom-wide strategies (8). Peer-mediated interventions, where the teacher enlists peers to withhold attention from the youngster's inappropriate behavior and where the whole group benefits from supporting his or her appropriate behavior, can also be very useful. Peer-mediated strategies have an advantage over exclusive use of direct contingent reinforcement administered by the teacher, in that they can dramatically reduce the amount of peer reinforcement of inappropriate behavior that is competing with teacher-administered reinforcers, thereby decreasing not only the amount of teacher effort expended on counteracting peer attention, but also lessening the need for punishment (8).

In addition to strategies based on principles of contingency management, and particularly to address behaviors primarily reflecting inattention and disorganization, the mental health professional may suggest modifications of the classroom environment, the way tasks or instructions are provided, or the nature of the tasks themselves. Excellent resources are available that list suggest modifications along these lines (10,11). Some commonly recommended strategies include shortening the length of tasks, providing more frequent feedback to youngsters as they work independently, varying the type of activity to reduce boredom, and providing the youngster with a quiet area shielded from classroom stimulation. However, in the author's experience, such recommendations are best offered, and tailored to the youngster, following an observation that focuses on the specifics of a particular classroom and teaching style.

SPECIAL CONSIDERATIONS FOR SECONDARY STUDENTS

Managing ADHD within middle schools and high schools is challenging. These settings demand a high level of organization with respect to assignments and materials, and youngsters with ADHD often need ongoing assistance. Securing consistency between teachers in applying systems involving contingency management or organizational strategies is challenging. Finding relevant reinforcers and negative consequences becomes far more complicated for older students. Several consultation techniques can be useful in addressing these challenges. First, the mental health professional should try to involve a central person through such as the team leader (middle school) or guidance counselor (high school) for obtaining rating scales from teachers, scheduling the visit, and coordinating the meeting that follows. This is more effective than the mental health professional's trying to communicate individually with teachers. Second, secondary teachers may be reluctant to provide accommodations, particularly because ADHD is an "invisible" disability whose symptoms they may attribute to poor motivation or disinterest. This issue must be addressed forthrightly, and the follow-up meeting is an ideal forum in which to do that. Often, some members of the school team are quite enlightened regarding ADHD and the need for accommodations, while other members are not. The consultation meeting can provide an ideal forum for less enlightened teachers to hear from their peers about strategies they use to assist youngsters with ADHD, and considerable attitude change may result from this discussion. Third, the youngster him/herself often can be included in meetings whose goal it is to establish accommodations. With the support of the mental health professional, the student can become skilled in communicating with his/her teachers about his/her needs. This can have the added benefit of helping the youngster be seen by his/her teachers as positively involved, rather than unmotivated or oppositional.

When working with teens with ADHD, the mental health professional often is addressing issues of depression, struggles with peer relationships, academic failure, planning for the future, and temptations regarding substance use, among others. As compared with school personnel, the mental health professional often is better positioned to integrate information from all available sources including school, parents, and the youngster, as well as knowledge about educational and vocational choices that can capitalize on the youngster's strengths and avoid pitfalls. The information gleaned through therapy with the teen and his/her parents should be shared as needed (and as requested by the family) with the school, in support of a genuine team effort to address the ADHD and the related concerns.

FORMALIZED SPECIAL SERVICES

Many youngsters with ADHD exhibit considerable residual symptomatology despite good efforts at treatment. In such cases it is often advisable to formalize the intervention plan via an individualized educational program (IEP). This plan serves as a guarantee that the necessary services will be provided, specifies personnel and amount of service, and indicates goals and objectives for academic and behavioral targets. For ADHD, the two primary avenues to obtaining an IEP are special education eligibility under the 2004 revision of the Individuals with Disabilities Education Act (IDEA) and Section 504 of the Americans with Disabilities Act. Any mental health professional working with youngsters with ADHD who wants to conduct meaningful school consultation should be familiar with the provisions of both, including the circumstances under which it is advisable to request that the youngster's eligibility for either be considered by the school. Depending on the presentation of the youngster's issues, one or the other may be the more appropriate avenue to pursue. In general, it is more difficult for a youngster to qualify for an IEP under IDEA than 504.

Within IDEA, ADHD falls in the category other health impairment (OHI). When other difficulties besides ADHD are present, such as significant behavioral or learning problems, the OHI eligibility can be preferable, as the IEP process includes a broader range of services and guarantees than is involved with 504 plans, which involve only accommodations. For example, under IDEA the IEP specifies any additional "related services" for which the youngster is eligible, such as speech and language therapy or occupational therapy. There is also a section that specifies a behavior intervention plan for the youngster. Further, the IDEA IEP provides for any academic support for which the youngster qualifies, such as the services of a learning disabilities specialist.

In contrast to IDEA, IEPs written under 504 are designed only to specify accommodations made necessary by the youngster's condition, in this case ADHD. Typical accommodations include additional time or a quiet place in which to take tests, a reminder system for homework assignments, class notes supplied to the student, extra time for completion of work, and notification to parents of both due and uncompleted assignments. Accommodations such as these are commonly included in IEPs written as part of OHI eligibility as well.

An important provision of IDEA is that it mandates a SST, sometimes known by other names such as "child study team," at each school. This team evolves into the eligibility committee that considers the question of special services, and then into the committee that designs the IEP. Membership changes as appropriate, but includes both regular and special education teachers, an individual qualified to supervise special education services, the school psychologist, others such as the guidance counselor, and the parents. This team meets regularly to discuss all youngsters who are experiencing difficulties at school, provide teachers with strategies to address these, and evaluate the success of these strategies. The SST manages the process of determining whether a youngster should be evaluated for special education support under IDEA, or for accommodations under Section 504. Mental health professionals should become comfortable attending SST meetings when their input is needed, and likely will find that communicating with SST members as needed can facilitate the consistent provision of services to the youngster. Often the mental health professional must play an advocacy role in order to facilitate the process of having the youngster found eligible for services, seeing that the necessary services are written into the IEP, and ensuring that the school follows through with the provision of the services.

CONCLUSION

School psychologists and other school personnel, including teachers, guidance counselors, and administrators, have increasingly taken up the challenge of providing the necessary services to youngsters with ADHD. It has been the author's experience that school personnel are increasingly aware of empirically supported interventions. With this trend, the primary responsibility of the mental health professional in the school consultation process can shift from that of educating school personnel about ADHD to one of collaborating with the school to provide smart, sophisticated interventions that hone in on the youngster's difficulties without being excessively burdensome to teachers. No matter how great a youngster's need may be for school intervention, the mental health professional should remain keenly aware of the amount of responsibility teachers carry for large numbers of students. Interventions should not overburden teachers. Just as the mental health professional must advocate for services for youngsters, they should also urge support for the teachers who must implement those services. Mental health professionals involved in school consultation should look for opportunities to influence policies—Federal, state and local—that impact services provided to youngsters with ADHD.

REFERENCES

1. Breiner JB, Forehand R. An assessment of the effects of parent training on clinic-referred children's school behavior. Behav Assess 1981; 3:31–42.
2. Barkley RA. Attention-deficit Hyperactivity Disorder: A Handbook for Diagnosis and Treatment. New York: Guilford Press, 1998.
3. Pelham WE. The NIMH multimodal treatment study for attention-deficit hyperactivity disorder: just say no to drugs alone? Can J Psychiatry 1999; 44: 981–90.
4. The MTA Cooperative Group. A 14-month randomized clinical trial of treatment strategies for attention-deficit/hyperactivity disorder. Arch Gen Psychiatry 1999; 56:1073–86.
5. Greenhill LL, Abikoff HB, Arnold LE, et al. Medication treatment strategies in the MTA study: relevance to clinicians and researchers. J Am Acad Child Adolesc Psychiatry 1996; 35:1304–13.
6. Jensen PS, Hinshaw SP, Kraemer HC, et al. ADHD comorbidity findings from the MTA study: comparing comorbid subgroups. J Am Acad Child Adolesc Psychiatry 2001; 40:147–58.
7. Reynolds DR, Kamphaus RW. BASC: Behavior Assessment System for Children Manual. Circle Pines, MN: American Guidance, 1992.
8. Abramowitz AJ, O'Leary SG. Behavioral interventions for the classroom: implications for students with ADHD. School Psychol Rev 1991; 2:220–34.
9. Kelley ML. School-home Notes: Promoting Children's Classroom Success. New York: Guilford Press, 1990.
10. DuPaul GJ, Stoner G. ADHD in the Schools: Assessment and Intervention Strategies. New York: Guilford Press, 2003.
11. Dendy CAZ. Teaching Teens with ADD and ADHD: A Quick Reference Guide for Teachers and Parents. Bethesda, MD: Woodbine House, 2000.

15

Daily Report Cards

Nichole Jurbergs and Mary Lou Kelley
Department of Psychology, Louisiana State University, Baton Rouge, Louisiana, U.S.A.

HOME-BASED TREATMENT FOR ACADEMIC AND BEHAVIOR PROBLEMS IN THE CLASSROOM

Barkley (1) stresses the importance of parent involvement in the management of the academic performance of attention deficit hyperactivity disorder (ADHD) in children. Home-based behavioral interventions include teaching parents how to deliver time-out, the use of token economies, and contingent attention (2). Academic interventions in the home include homework routines, goal setting and contingency contracting for homework (3), and response cost and positive reinforcement contingent on academic performance (4,5). Grolnick and colleagues (6) note that parents' involvement in their children's academic career is associated with children's success in school. Parents have an important role in their children's education, and home–school communication has been shown to lead to better educational outcomes (7). One way to facilitate such a relationship is to involve both parent and teacher in home-based interventions for classroom problems.

ADVANTAGES OF DAILY REPORT CARDS

A daily report card is a home-based classroom intervention that allows parents to receive frequent feedback about their child's classroom behavior. The reports are completed and sent home daily by the teacher. The notes contain information rating the student's performance on that day. Parents are responsible for providing rewards for the child's appropriate behavior. Home-based intervention has many advantages over school-based intervention.

Daily report cards, also known as school-home notes, provide increased communication between parent and teacher and encourage greater parent involvement. This is a vast improvement over the more common practice of parents receiving intermittent, negative feedback from the school when children misbehave. School-home notes allow parents to offer powerful reinforcers that may not be available to teachers at school. Also, daily report cards are a quick and simple intervention, making them more likely to be utilized by teachers. The use of the note relieves teachers of the duties to discover effective reinforcers for the students and to spend time providing consequences. The note puts these responsibilities on the parents of each individual student. The simplicity, ease, and non-time-consuming nature of daily report cards are valuable advantages of this home-based intervention (8).

DECIDING TO UTILIZE A DAILY REPORT CARD AND DEFINING TARGET BEHAVIORS

Daily report cards may be individually tailored to suit a wide variety of students with a range of classroom problems. Children as young as preschool and as old as high school may receive treatment benefits from school-home notes. They have proven effective in reducing behaviors such as talking in class, leaving the desk without permission, and other disruptive behaviors. Daily report cards also have been used to increase positive behaviors such as paying attention, completing positive social behaviors, and following teacher instructions. Although positive changes in classroom behavior are often accompanied by improved grades, specific academic behaviors may also be targeted, including completing and properly turning in classwork and homework. School-home notes have also been utilized as a treatment component for strengthening appropriate behaviors that are inhibited by anxiety. Targets may include working without crying for school-phobic children and talking in a loud voice for shy or selectively mute children. However, much of the literature on the efficacy of daily report cards has focused on externalizing behavior problems and students with ADHD.

Another consideration in the design of the note itself is its comprehensiveness. Students may be evaluated during multiple intervals throughout the day, such as every class period or before and after lunch, or at one specific time of day, such as lunchtime or math class.

Essential to the success of daily report cards are parents' willingness and commitment to review the note daily and provide contracted consequences consistently. It is also necessary for teachers to consistently and fairly complete the report card. It is important that the child is able to perform the behaviors defined by the note. For example, a student with a learning disability may not be capable of completing class assignments without additional help. Such a case may be better treated with an academic intervention plan.

After deciding to implement a school-home note, parents and teachers, as well as a consultant if available, should collaborate in determining the behaviors to be targeted by the note. They should include socially valid behaviors important to the child's academic success, such as "completed classwork" and "followed directions." Conduct behaviors including "kept hands to self" and "talked only with permission" may also be included. It is essential to define each behavior as operationally as possible in order to decrease the subjectivity of its ratings. Also, the target behaviors should be stated positively, as behaviors to increase rather to decrease. For instance, if a student is perpetually leaving his seat in the classroom, the behavior to be rated by his teacher on his school-home note should read "stayed in seat" rather than "left seat without permission."

HOW TO IMPLEMENT A DAILY REPORT CARD

Kelley (8) offers general guidelines for the use of school-home notes. Parents and teachers should be trained in the use of basic contingency management procedures. The note should evaluate the target behaviors during several different time intervals throughout the day, giving frequent, time-specific feedback about student performance. Parents, students, and teachers should collaborate when developing performance goals and appropriate reinforcement. They should all be involved in constructing a "contract" outlining what constitutes appropriate behavior and, in turn, a "good note" worthy of positive consequences.

The majority of daily report card interventions require parents to positively reinforce any acceptable notes brought home with either tangibles or activities that the child may enjoy that day after school. Praise alone does not appear to be adequate. Typically, parents are not instructed which specific reinforcers to utilize, but common suggestions in the literature include: special snacks, TV time, late bedtime, verbal praise, and freedom from chores (9–11). The daily behavioral criteria for earning rewards are spelled out in the contract. For example, one child's criteria for an acceptable note may be 8 of 10 behaviors rated by the teacher as good or fair and only 2 or less rated as bad. The school-home note contract should also include specific rewards that may be earned based on the performance ratings. Many home-based reward programs include more valuable weekly rewards in addition to smaller daily rewards.

The daily report card should be reviewed by the parent with the child each day. Parents should attempt to focus equal time on the positive and negative ratings received by the child. After proceeding through the entire note from the beginning of the child's day to the end, parents are encouraged to provide the contracted consequences as soon as possible. The reward given should be recorded in order to document treatment integrity.

RESEARCH ON TREATMENT OUTCOME

Ayllon et al. (12) used a "good behavior" daily report card targeting disruptive behaviors including out-of-seat, vocalizations, and any motor activity that interfered with the other students' studying in a third-grade classroom of 23 children. Parents provided appropriate rewards on days the child's behavior warranted a "good behavior" letter. The average level of disruption decreased from 90% during baseline to zero during the treatment phase. In another study, Blechman et al. (13) used a "good news note" to decrease inconsistency of math classwork in a group of elementary students with inconsistent math performance. Teachers sent a note home on days the student's math performance equaled or exceeded performance during baseline. Parents delivered positive reinforcement on days the child received a "good news note." The note significantly increased consistency in math performance.

ADDING NEGATIVE CONSEQUENCES

Research has consistently shown, however, that positive consequences alone are not sufficient to maintain the desired behavior of ADHD children (14–17). These studies suggest that both positive and negative consequences are necessary to achieve optimal levels of appropriate classroom behavior. Response cost is a behavior modification technique that may be incorporated into a daily report card so that a child's classroom behavior may earn positive or negative consequences. Response cost has been defined as a punishment procedure which involves the loss of positive reinforcement (privileges, points, rewards) contingent on misbehavior or failure to meet specified behavioral or academic criteria (18). In the case of a school-home note, a child may be instructed by the teacher to cross off a smiley face from his note contingent upon inappropriate behavior. The loss of the smiley face decreases the child's chance of bringing home a "good note" for the day and earning a reward.

McCain and Kelley (19) compared the effectiveness of a school-home note with and without response cost in improving the classroom performance of three fourth-grade boys in a public school. A multiple-baseline design with alternating treatments was used. On-task (oriented toward work), off-task (not oriented toward work), and disruptive behaviors (out of seat, making noise, other teacher disapproved behaviors) were recorded. Parents were instructed to reward good notes with positive reinforcement according to a contract that outlined contingencies for reinforcement. In addition, the school-home notes with response cost required parents to provide consequences contingent on satisfactory on-task behavior and minimal loss of response cost points. The addition of response cost increased the effectiveness of the intervention beyond the traditional school-home note without response cost. That is, all three students showed decreases in off-task behavior and exhibited low, stabilized levels of disruptive behavior during the response cost intervention as compared to the traditional school-home note.

Kelley and McCain (20) found similar results in a study that compared the effectiveness of a school-home note with and without response cost for increasing academic productivity and appropriate classroom behavior in five elementary-aged children. Both notes included the target behaviors "completed classwork satisfactorily" and "used classtime well." Teachers rated each behavior as "yes," "so-so," or "no." Notes were taken home and parents provided rewards contingent upon satisfactory behavior. The note used during the response cost condition had the addition of five smiley faces on the page. Teachers instructed students to mark off a smiley face every time they were off-task or behaved disruptively. Notes were taken home and rewards were provided contingent upon satisfactory behavior ratings as well as minimal loss of smiley faces. Both appropriate classroom behavior and academic productivity increased in all five children with the use of school-home notes. In three of the subjects, the inclusion of the response cost component lead to significantly greater improvement over the traditional school-home note.

More recently, Jurbergs (21) compared the effectiveness of similar school-home notes with and without response cost in improving the classroom performance of six, minority, first- and second-grade students with ADHD. A reversal design with alternating treatments was utilized. On- and off-task behavior was measured using direct observation. Academic productivity was measured in percentage complete and percentage correct during each phase. Again, both on-task classroom behavior and academic productivity increased in all participants during treatment phases. Also, accurate classwork completion increased substantially. However, no consistent added benefits of the response cost component were found. The school-home note with response cost was more effective in increasing on-task behavior for two of the subjects, while the no response cost note was more effective for one of the subjects. The other three subjects, however, showed no difference in levels of on-task behavior between the two notes.

TREATMENT ACCEPTABILITY

The same study also examined treatment acceptability of daily report cards. The interview data collected after the conclusion of the study indicated that both notes were highly acceptable to all teachers, parents, and students involved.

Although no differences in treatment efficacy were demonstrated, all participants reported finding the response cost note more acceptable.

In summary, school-home notes have been shown to be effective in the classroom management of children with ADHD (5,10,12,13,19–21). Various aspects of school-home notes such as target behaviors, consequences, and age of subjects have been varied in the literature without diminishing effectiveness. Home-based contingency interventions have been effective in increasing both academic performance and appropriate classroom behavior. Such techniques have also been described as very highly acceptable by parents, teachers, and students. These findings as well as the advantages of parent involvement in their children's classroom behavior make daily report cards an important behavior modification intervention for use in educational settings.

REFERENCES

1. Barkley RA. Taking Charge of ADHD: The Complete, Authoritative Guide for Parents. New York: Guilford Press, 2000.
2. Pelham WE, Hinshaw SP. Behavioral intervention for attention-deficit/hyperactivity disorder. In: Turner SS, Calhoun KS, Adams HE, eds. Handbook for Clinical Behavior Therapy. New York: John Wiley & Sons, 1992.
3. Miller DL, Kelley ML. The use of goal setting and contingency contracting for improving children's homework performance. J Appl Behav Anal 1994; 27: 73–84.
4. Karraker RJ. Increasing academic performance through home-managed contingency programs. J School Psychol 1972; 10:173–9.
5. Rosen LA, Gabardi L, Miller CD, Miller L. Home-based treatment of disruptive junior high school students: an analysis of the differential effects of positive and negative consequences. Behavior Disord 1990; 15:227–32.
6. Grolnick WS, Benjet C, Kurowski CO, Apostoleris NH. Predictors of parent involvement in children's schooling. J Educ Psychol 1997; 89:538–48.
7. Christenson SL, Conoley JC. Home-school Collaboration: Enhancing Children's Academic and Social Competence. Silver Springs, MD: National Association of School Psychologists, 1992.
8. Kelley ML. School-home Notes: Promoting Children's Classroom Success. New York: Guilford Press, 1990.
9. Heaton RC, Safer DJ, Allen RP, Spinnato NC, Prumo FM. A motivational environment for behaviorally deviant junior high school students. J Abnorm Child Psychol 1976; 4:263–75.
10. Schumaker JB, Hovel MF, Sherman JA. An analysis of daily report cards and parent-managed privileges in the improvement of adolescents' classroom performance. J Appl Behav Anal 1977; 10:449–64.
11. Taylor VL, Cornwell DD, Riley MT. Home-based contingency management programs that teachers can use. Psychol Schools 1984; 21:368–74.

12. Ayllon T, Garber S, Pisor K. The elimination of discipline problems through a combined school-home motivational system. Behav Ther 1975; 6:616–26.
13. Blechman EA, Taylor CJ, Schrader SM. Family problem solving versus home notes as early intervention with high-risk children. J Consult Clin Psychol 1981; 49:919–26.
14. Forehand R. Parental positive reinforcement with deviant children: does it make a difference? Child Fam Behav Ther 1987; 8:19–25.
15. Acker MM, O'Leary SG. Effects of reprimands and praise on appropriate behavior in the classroom. J Abnorm Child Psychol 1987; 15:549–57.
16. Pfiffner LJ, O'Leary SG. The efficacy of all-positive management as a function of the prior use of negative consequences. J Appl Behav Anal 1987; 20:265–71.
17. Rosen LA, O'Leary SG, Joyce SA, Conway G, Pfiffner LJ. The importance of prudent negative consequences for maintaining the appropriate behavior of hyperactive students. J Abnorm Child Psychol 1984; 12:581–604.
18. Abramowitz AJ, O'Leary SG. Behavioral interventions for the classroom: implications for students with ADHD. School Psychol Rev 1991; 20:220–34.
19. McCain AP, Kelley ML. Improving classroom performance in underachieving preadolescents: the additive effects of response cost to a school-home note system. Child Fam Behav Ther 1994; 16:27–41.
20. Kelley ML, McCain AP. Promoting academic performance in inattentive children: The relative efficacy of school-home notes with and without response cost. Behav Modif 1995; 19:357–75.
21. Jurbergs N, Palcic J, Kelley ML. School-home notes with and without response cost: Increasing attention and academic performance in low-income with attention-deficit/hyperactivity disorder. School Psychol Quarterly, 2007; 22: 358–79.

16

Tailoring Psychosocial Treatment for ADHD-Inattentive Type

Linda J. Pfiffner

Department of Psychiatry, University of California San Francisco, San Francisco, California, U.S.A.

Despite the prevalence and significant impairment associated with attention deficit hyperactivity disorder-predominantly inattentive type (ADHD-I), treatment studies of this subtype are lacking, partially because the field has focused on the combined type of ADHD (ADHD-C), and also because the specification of ADHD-I as a distinct condition only occurred in 1994 (1). The critical lack of any treatment studies of ADHD-I was noted in the NIH Consensus Development Conference on ADHD (2) with the recommendation that more systematized treatment strategies be developed and evaluated for ADHD-I.

Stimulant treatment (ST) and behavioral interventions are both evidence-based treatments for the combined type of ADHD and it stands to reason that these interventions also would be helpful for ADHD-I. Findings from recent studies (6) show that many children with ADHD-I can benefit from ST. However, psychosocial interventions (PST) may be especially important for those with ADHD-I based on reports that medication may be somewhat less helpful for this subtype (3,4), that the social impairment in ADHD-I (e.g., social passivity, withdrawal, lack of social knowledge) may be more amenable to PST than ST (5), and that even in cases showing a positive response to ST, normalized functioning is often not achieved and the inclusion of PST may be necessary to produce "excellent" treatment response. Also, acceptability of treatments is an important factor to be considered in the selection of treatments. Parents show a significant preference for behavioral treatments over pharmacological treatment alone (7), and there is growing concern among the public and government over the proliferation of ST with children. This chapter will describe the characteristics of ADHD-I important for targeting in psychosocial intervention and a new multicomponent psychosocial intervention for this subtype of ADHD.

TAILORING PSYCHOSOCIAL TREATMENT TO ADHD-I

The evidence-based psychosocial interventions developed for ADHD-C appear to be appropriate for addressing the needs of ADHD-I. These include training parents in behavioral strategies and classroom accommodations and consulting with teachers to implement behavioral strategies at school (including daily report cards) (8). In addition, social-interaction training provided in the context of a behavior modification program and parent involvement may be helpful for improving social skill deficits (9,10).

Unique characteristics of ADHD-I, however, suggest the need to tailor these interventions. Evidence is emerging that the cognitive/attentional deficits of ADHD-I overlap only partially with those of ADHD-C. Several studies suggest that children with ADHD-I show more severe alertness/orientation problems or sluggish cognitive tempo than those with ADHD-C (11–13). Both ADHD-I and ADHD-C share deficits on tests of frontal lobe functions, but slowness in perceptual motor speed and automatic information processing may be specific to the attention-deficit disorder (ADD) without H group (14–17). It is also worth noting that the "sluggish cognitive tempo" and excessive passivity aspects of ADHD-I bear similarities to impairments seen in patients with mild traumatic brain injury (TBI). Adults with mild TBI often exhibit a reduced level of alertness and a reduced ability to initiate behavioral sequences (18,19). Rehabilitation psychologists and psychiatrists use a broad array of techniques to help these patients, ranging from behavior modification, cognitive rehabilitation and other neuropsychological approaches, mnemonics, and ecological supports. Psychosocial treatment for ADHD-I would likewise do well to emphasize adaptive skills, functional competence, and compensatory strategies. Specific teaching strategies used with TBI also are likely to be helpful with ADHD-I. These include use of cues and prompts, routinization of recurring problem situations, increased rehearsal of information used in daily life, and metacognitive strategies such as self-identification of off-task cognitive states and self-redirection to task. On the other hand, there is no evidence that cognitive remediation emphasizing computer-based practice/learning of deficient cognitive skills, often used with TBI, would be helpful for ADHD-I. Even for TBI, the efficacy of these approaches is less recognized than that of compensatory-substitutive approaches (20), and task-specific training appears to provide greater benefit than more generalized training (21).

Academic impairment appears to be especially pronounced, relative to other problems, in children with ADHD-I. They show considerable impairment in academic functioning including underachievement, underproductivity, and learning disabilities (22–24). Homework problems are ubiquitous (25). These serious academic concerns necessitate close involvement with the school and direct intervention for homework.

Recent findings suggest that ADHD-I is associated with a pattern of low motivation for learning, less interest in challenging tasks, less persistence and being more easily discouraged (26). Although children with ADHD-C also have motivational deficits (particularly during low interest activities without external reinforcement), Booth et al. (26) report differences between the two subtypes. Children with ADHD-I were found to prefer a cooperative work setting relative to those with ADHD-C who tended to prefer a more competitive environment. Also, children with ADHD-I seemed to be more motivated to perform well to please the teacher and make good grades rather than for their own curiosity, interest, or internal drive. Perhaps, as the authors speculated, this is due to a more passive approach to academic work. In contrast, those with ADHD-C were significantly more likely to value being perceived as high performing and successful than those with ADHD-I. Recently Huang-Pollock et al. (27) reported subtype differences in motivation on a reward-based variation of the stop-signal paradigm, whereby children with ADHD-I tended to give up more easily than those with ADHD-C when rewards were not as available.

The findings of relatively slow cognitive processing, low levels of curiosity, interest, and enjoyment of learning, preference for less challenging tasks, preference for cooperative work environments, and greater reliance on external criteria for determining success all need to be considered in planning optimal learning environments at school and at home. Those that emphasize noncompetitive external rewards for meeting specific goals and accommodations to tasks and assignments to address slow work style appear indicated.

Social impairment is also marked in ADHD-I, but is distinct from ADHD-C. Those with ADHD-I tend to be unpopular and socially withdrawn (23) and have social skill deficits rather than only performance problems (28,29). Children with ADHD-I receive more peer nominations of being very shy and being teased and left out than those with ADHD-C (who receive nominations for fighting and arguing). Teachers and parents report that those with ADHD-I are more socially passive (28) and they have been observed to be more socially withdrawn during play groups—engaging in solitary play to a greater degree and having less sustained interaction (30). Their attentional problems may lead to poor tracking and processing of social cues and faulty timing during interpersonal interactions (31). Recently, Mikami et al. (27) reported further evidence for unique social deficits in ADHD-I on a computer-based chat room task: those with

ADHD-I were more disengaged and had poorer memory for social conversation than those with ADHD-C. The social difficulties of ADHD-I youth including passivity, withdrawal, lack of skill, and inaccurate processing of social cues point to the need to carefully teach and practice specific skills, and provide opportunities and reinforcement for approaching and interacting with peers. Interventions to help parents with programming social activities in cases where a child's proclivity is to select passive, nonsocial activities would seem important. Likewise, daily living skills are also deficient, pointing to the need to increase levels of independence in completing daily tasks, most efficiently done with parent monitoring and reinforcement.

In addition, children with ADHD-I are known to have fewer disruptive behavior problems. Children with ADHD-I exhibit less aggression, fewer oppositional problems, and are less likely to meet criteria for oppositional-defiant disorder or conduct disorder than children with ADHD-C (32,33). As a result, limit setting strategies, such as time-out, are likely to be less useful with these children than they are for ADHD-C where behavioral control is so important. Instead, positive reinforcement targeting specific goals and routines may be especially helpful as noted above.

THE CHILD LIFE AND ATTENTION SKILLS PROGRAM FOR ADHD-I

We have developed a multicomponent package of integrated behavioral and cognitive-behavioral interventions to address the unique impairments of ADHD-I, described above. The package includes three components: teacher consultation, parenting skills, and child life skills training. The teacher and parent components are designed to facilitate generalization and maintenance of strategies taught directly to children during the child training. The teacher and parent components are expected to exert effects on core ADHD-I problems (e.g., disorganization, failure to sustain attention to task, forgetfulness) and related impairments (e.g., academic underproductivity, social withdrawal, homework problems, lack of independence in self-care and daily activities) by structuring school and home environments to enhance functioning in these areas. To accomplish this, the parent and teacher interventions specifically target these areas in contingency management programs and by altering environmental "antecedents" (e.g., by establishing routines, using organizational lists and plans, using assignment books, simplifying tasks, using strategic reminders). The child skills component provides children with instruction and practice in strategies for improving attention to task, work productivity and organization at school and home, and for improving interpersonal relationships (with adults and peers). The child groups provide direct instruction in strategies to remediate skill deficits (e.g., how to enter peer groups, complete work, keep work space organized, track homework) and provide practice (behavioral rehearsal) to remediate skill performance deficits. The program also integrates cognitive-behavioral components (e.g., problem solving, self-monitoring/self-evaluation) with the behavioral approaches based on published work suggesting this combination is beneficial (10,34).

The program includes 8 to 10 concurrent group sessions of 90 min (one for the parents and one for the children), up to 5 individual family sessions and up to 5 meetings between the teacher, therapist, parent, and child over a 12-week period. It is important to note that these interventions, although manualized, are individualized for each family. For example, target behaviors, rewards, and negative consequences are based on the specific needs and proclivities of the child and family and strategies are tailored to the child's cognitive functioning. This individualization occurs during each group session and is a specific focus of the individual family sessions and teacher consultation meetings. Thus, this plan begins with group-based interventions that target needs that virtually all ADHD-I cases have, followed by distribution of intensive problem-focused treatment where and when it is needed.

Teacher Consultation Component

This component is intended to provide the teacher with consultation in behavioral interventions and classroom accommodations, with a focus on development and implementation of an individualized daily home–school report card and classroom accommodations specific to concerns of each child. Interventions for this component are based on numerous studies documenting efficacy of classroom behavior modification and teacher consultation for children having ADHD (8,35). Consultation consists of an orientation meeting providing an overview of behavioral interventions and classroom-based accommodations for working with children having ADHD-I (1 hr), followed by up to four meetings of teacher, parent, child, and therapist. In the first two of these meetings, a school-home daily report card (classroom challenge, CC) is designed and implemented. The CC is intended to provide the needed structure and reinforcement to support improvement on school-based tasks. Target behaviors are individualized based on the needs of the child and typically include common problem areas for ADHD-I including: academic work (e.g., completion of assigned work, completion and return of homework, accuracy of completed work), work behavior/study skills (e.g., following directions, having necessary materials to begin work, getting started on work, staying on-task), and social interactions (e.g., entering peer groups, accepting consequences, being a good sport, using assertive behavior). Skills taught in the child group are shared with teachers so that the child's use of these skills can be reinforced (often by including as a target on the CC) in the naturalistic environment of the school. During the remaining two meetings, the program is reviewed using the "Challenge Review" script to ensure that all critical points are covered and to help parents develop a set of transferable skills for working with their child's teachers. The therapist may model use of the script, but the parent is shaped into taking the lead role in the teacher meetings. In addition to the daily report card, the therapist may also suggest environmental or academic accommodations (e.g., additional time or "time challenges" to complete work, preferential seating, reduction in workload, use of assignment book, use of completed work folder, time limits) depending on the needs of the child and the teacher's overall teaching style.

Parent Skills Component

Our approach to teaching parenting skills is similar to the approaches used in a number of studies of parent training (36–39), but adapted to more fully address the concerns facing ADHD-I. These include an increased emphasis on improving homework routines (bringing home materials, completing assignment, returning it back to class), improving independence, self-care skills, and follow through to parent requests, increasing organizational and time-management skills, and facilitating peer interactions. The program begins with an overview of ADHD-I and the social learning model. Thereafter, a set of strategies is presented over the course of the 8–10 group sessions. Strategies covered include: use of attending, rewards, and other positive consequences; establishing effective routines for the morning, for homework, and for the evening; planning activities, giving directions and commands, and using prudent negative consequences, to promote attention and adaptive functioning. Parents also are taught communication skills for interacting effectively with teachers and are introduced to the school-home note (CC, the primary school-based intervention described in the teacher consultation component above). Additionally, the modules covered in the children's groups (see below) are reviewed each week and parents are taught methods to promote and reinforce their child's use of skills taught during these sessions (e.g., independence skills, positive social interactions).

Child Skills Component

The child program is divided into modules that teach children skills to be independent at school and home (academic, study and organization skills, self-care and daily living skills), and modules to improve social interactions and increase social competence. These modules address both skill knowledge deficits and performance problems through didactic instruction, behavior rehearsal and in vivo practice in the context of a dense, reward-based contingency management program. Self-management of alertness is supported by group-reinforced "attention checks" (40) during which time children are prompted to repeat back the last comment made or activity that occurred. In addition to the behavioral interventions, children are taught cognitive-behavioral strategies (e.g., problem-solving steps, how to use cues/verbal mediation strategies to stay on-task and focused, use of reminder lists of activities to be completed) including skills for self-monitoring and self-evaluation (e.g., "Match Game") in light of studies supporting their use with ADHD youth (10,34). The social skills modules are based on a previous treatment study for ADHD (10) and include the following: being a good sport, accepting consequences, assertion, ignoring provocation, problem-solving, friendship-making skills, and emotion management. Additional focus on friendship-making skills and planning playdates is included due to the specific deficits in these areas associated with ADHD-I. Modules focused on independence include the following: homework/study skills, self-care skills (e.g., getting ready for school) and getting chores done independently. Role-plays of common problem scenarios for ADHD-I are covered as a part of each module (e.g., joining a game, being teased, being left out of an activity, "spaciness" during a game, staying on-task during homework, staying focused when getting ready in the morning) and solutions are practiced until success is achieved. Children also practice new skills during play activities and mock school/home routines with high doses of positive reinforcement. The module focused on homework/academic skills is reinforced by having children and parents participate in "mock" homework sessions during which time they are coached in strategies to improve homework success. During the last 15 minutes of group, parents and children meet together to go over the "skill of the week" and plan homework for the upcoming week.

RESULTS OF RANDOMIZED-CONTROLLED TRIAL OF THE CHILD LIFE AND ATTENTION SKILLS PROGRAM

With funding from the National Institute of Mental Health, we completed a randomized-controlled trial of this intervention with children between 7 and 11 years of age (41,42). Sixty-nine children were randomized to the intervention (Child Life and Attention Skills Program) or to a control group which did not receive the intervention. Our findings reveal significant treatment-related improvement on the number and severity of DSM-IV inattention symptoms and symptoms of sluggish cognitive tempo as well as on functional impairment associated with ADHD-I including organizational skills, homework problems, and social skills. These findings were maintained into the next school year. Our program was well-received by parents, teachers, and children. Feedback from the teachers suggests that the school component is suitable for implementation in general education classrooms (where most students with ADHD-I are taught). The fact that gains were sustained after treatment was completed (which is often not the case in treatment studies with ADHD-C), is consistent with theories (29) that ADHD-I may be more associated with remediable skills deficits and less associated with disinhibition compared to ADHD-C. We attribute the efficacy of our program to the focus on specific areas of impairment for this subtype and the integrated approach that puts parents, teachers, and the children themselves on the same game plan. This integrated approach appears to improve functioning for children with ADHD-I to a greater extent, and for longer period of time, than the sum of the individual treatment effects would suggest.

NEXT STEPS

Continued development and evaluation of psychosocial treatments for ADHD-I are in order. Our results suggest behavioral approaches integrated between home and school can have a significant impact, but more needs to be known about the moderating and mediating mechanisms underlying treatment response to allow for more refined tailoring of intervention. Future studies should also evaluate when and how psychosocial interventions may best be combined with medication for optimal response. Equally important will be studies on how best to disseminate these treatments in the community.

REFERENCES

1. American Psychological Association. Diagnostic and Statistical Manual for Mental Disorders. 4th ed. Washington, D.C.: APA, 1994.
2. NIH. Diagnosis and Treatment of Attention Deficit Hyperactivity Disorder. Washington, D.C.: NIH, 1998.
3. Barkley RA, DuPaul GJ, McMurray MB. Attention deficit disorder with and without hyperactivity: clinical response to three dose levels of methylphenidate. Pediatrics 1991; 87:519–31.
4. Greenhill LL, McDaniel D, CoChien C. Subtypes of ADHD: differentiated by response to methylphenidate? 47th Annual conference for the American Academy of Child and Adolescent Psychiatry New York, NY, 2000.
5. Pfiffner LJ, Calzada E, McBurnett K. Interventions to enhance social competence. In: Stubbe D, ed. Child and Adolescent Psychiatric Clinics. Philadelphia, PA: W.B. Saunders, 2000:689–709.
6. Stein M, Sarampote CS, Waldman ID, et al. A dose-response study of OROS methylphenidate in children with attention-deficit/hyperactivity disorder. Pediatrics 2003; 112:e404.
7. Pelham WE. The NIMH multimodal treatment study for ADHD: just say yes to drugs alone? Can J Psychiatry 1999; 44:981–90.
8. Pelham WE Jr, Wheeler T, Chronis A. Empirically supported psychosocial treatments for attention deficit hyperactivity disorder. J Clin Child Psychol 1998; 27:190–205.
9. Frankel F, Myatt R, Cantwell DP, Feinberg DT. Parent-assisted transfer of children's social skills training: effects on children with and without attention-deficit hyperactivity disorder. J Am Acad Child Adolesc Psychiatry 1997; 36: 1056–64.

10. Pfiffner LJ, McBurnett K. Social skills training with parent generalization: treatment effects for children with attention deficit disorder. J Consult Clin Psychol 1997; 65:749–57.
11. Carlson CL, Mann M. Attention-deficit/hyperactivity disorder, predominantly inattentive subtype. Child Adolesc Psychiatric Clin North Am 2000; 9:499–510.
12. Carlson CL, Mann M. Sluggish cognitive tempo predicts a different pattern of impairment in the attention deficit hyperactivity disorder, predominantly inattentive type. J Clin Child Adolesc Psychol 2002; 31:123–9.
13. McBurnett K, Pfiffner LJ, Frick PJ. Symptom properties as a function of ADHD type: an argument for continued study of sluggish cognitive tempo. J Abnorm Child Psychol 2001; 29:207–13.
14. Barkley RA, Grodzinsky G, DuPaul GJ. Frontal lobe functions in attention deficit disorder with and without hyperactivity: a review and research report. J Abnorm Child Psychol 1992; 20:163–88.
15. Goodyear P, Hynd GW. Attention-deficit disorder with (ADD/H) and without (ADD/WO) hyperactivity: behavioral and neuropsychological differentiation. J Clin Child Psychol 1992; 21:273–305.
16. Lockwood KA, Marcotte AC, Stern C. Differentiation of attention deficit hyperactivity disorder subtypes: application of a neuropsychological model of attention. J Clin Exp Neuropsychol 2001; 23:317–30.
17. Weiler MD, Bernstein JH, Bellinger DC, Waber DP. Processing speed in children with attention deficit hyperactivity disorder, inattentive type. Child Neuropsychol 2000; 6:218–34.
18. Trexler LE, Zappala G. Neuropathological determinants of acquired attention disorders in traumatic brain injury. Brain Cogn 1998; 8:291–302.
19. Wilson BA. Case Studies in Neuropsychological Rehabilitation. New York: Oxford University Press, 1999.
20. Ben-Yishay Y, Diller L. Cognitive remediation in traumatic brain injury: update and issues. Arch Phys Med Rehabil 1993; 74:204–13.
21. Ben-Yishay Y, Piasetsky E, Rattok J. A systematic method for ameliorating disorders in basic attention. In: Meier MJ, Diller L, Benton AL, eds. Neuropsychological Rehabilitation. London: Churchill-Livingstone, 1987: 165–81.
22. Faraone SV, Biederman J, Weber W, Russell RL. Psychiatric, neuropsychological, and psychosocial features of DSM-IV subtypes of attention-deficit/hyperactivity disorder: results from a clinically referred sample. J Am Acad Child Adolesc Psychiatry 1998; 37:185–93.
23. McBurnett K, Pfiffner LJ, Willcutt E, et al. Experimental cross-validation of DSM-IV types of attention-deficit/hyperactivity disorder. J Am Acad Child Adolesc Psychiatry 1999; 38:1–8.
24. Willcutt E, Chhabildas N, Pennington BF. Validity of the DSM-IV subtypes of ADHD. ADHD Rep 2001; 9:2–5.
25. Lahey BB, Applegate B, McBurnett K, et al. DSM-IV field trials for attention deficit/hyperactivity disorder in children and adolescents. Am J Psychiatry 1994; 151:1673–85.
26. Booth J, Carlson C, Shin M, Canu W. Parent, teacher, and self-rated motivational styles in the ADHD subtypes. ADHD Rep 2001; 9:8–11.

27. Mikami A, Huang-Pollock C, Pfiffner L, McBurnett K, Hangai D. Social skills differences among attention deficit/hyperactivity disorder types in a chat room assessment task. J Abnorm Child Psychol 2007; 35:509–21.
28. Maedgen JW, Carlson CL. Social functioning and emotional regulation in the attention deficit hyperactivity disorder subtypes. J Clin Child Psychol 2000; 29: 30–42.
29. Wheeler J, Carlson CL. The social functioning of children with ADD with and without hyperactivity: a comparison of their peer relations and social deficits. Emot Behav Disord 2000; 2:2–12.
30. Hodgens JB, Cole J, Boldizar J. Peer-based differences among boys with ADHD. J Clin Child Psychol 2000; 29:443–52.
31. Bellanti CJ, Bierman KL, Group CPPR. Disentangling the impact of low cognitive ability and inattention on social behavior and peer relationships. J Clin Child Psychol 2000; 29:66–75.
32. Eiraldi RB, Power TJ, Nezu CM. Patterns of comorbidity associated with subtypes of attention-deficit hyperactivity disorder among 6- to 12-year-old children. J Am Acad Child Adolesc Psychiatry 1997; 36:503–14.
33. Hinshaw SP. Attention-deficit hyperactivity disorder: the search for viable treatments. In: Kendall PC, ed. Child and Adolescent Therapy: Cognitive-Behavioral Procedures. 2nd ed. New York: Guilford Press, 2000.
34. Morgan AE, Hynd GW, Riccio CA, Hall J. Validity of DSM-IV ADHD predominantly inattentive and combined types: relationship to previous DSM diagnoses/subtype differences. J Am Acad Child Adolesc Psychiatry 1996; 35: 325–33.
35. Pfiffner LJ, Barkley RA. Treatment of ADHD in school settings. In: Barkley RA, ed. ADHD in Children and Adults: A Handbook for Diagnosis, Assessment, and Treatment. New York: Guilford Press, 1998.
36. Anastopoulos AD, Shelton TL, DuPaul GJ, Guevremont DC. Parent training for attention-deficit hyperactivity disorder: its impact on parent functioning. J Abnorm Child Psychol 1993; 21:581–96.
37. Barkley RA. Defiant Children: A Clinician's Manual for Parent Training. New York: Guilford Press, 1987.
38. Forehand R, McMahon R. Helping the Noncompliant Child: A Clinician's Guide to Parent Training New York: Guilford Press, 1981.
39. Patterson GR, Reid JB, Dishion TJ. Antisocial Boys. Eugene, OR: Castalia Publishing Company, 1992.
40. Pelham WE, Hoza B. Intensive treatment: a summer treatment program for children with ADHD. In: Hibbs E, Jensen P, eds. Psychosocial Treatments for Child and Adolescent Disorders: Empirically Based Strategies for Clinical Practice. New York: APA Press, 1996:311–40.
41. Pfiffner L. Psychosocial treatment for ADHD-inattentive type. ADHD Rep 2003; 11:1–8.
42. Pfiffner LJ, Mikami A, Huang-Pollock C, Zalecki C, Easterlin B, McBurnett K. A randomized controlled trial of integrated home-school behavioral treatment for ADHD, predominantly inattentive type. J Am Acad Child Adolesc Psychiatry 2007; 46:1041–6.

17

Social Skills Training

Linda J. Pfiffner
Department of Psychiatry, University of California San Francisco, San Francisco, California, U.S.A.

Difficulties in peer relations plague many, if not most, youth with attention deficit hyperactivity disorder (ADHD). These problems can be extremely debilitating and can cascade into a variety of serious outcomes, including academic failure, school dropout, substance abuse, other mental health issues, and legal problems (1,2). Not only are social problems enduring, among the most impairing issues for those with ADHD and often the reason for referral to mental health clinics, they are difficult to treat (3). This chapter summarizes the social profile of youth with ADHD and social skills training programs that have been developed to address the problems.

SOCIAL PROFILES OF ADHD YOUTH

While most youth with ADHD exhibit considerable impairment in the social arena, these problems are not uniform across subtypes and also seem to be influenced by the presence of comorbid disorders. The literature on peer relations in ADHD is based on studies of children with the "classic" triad of symptoms of ADHD: inattention, hyperactivity, and impulsivity, now referred to as ADHD-Combined Type. In some ways, the behavior of those with ADHD-Combined Type is not different from their non-ADHD counterparts. They tend to exhibit similar rates of positive behaviors and neutral verbal interchanges (3). However, negative behaviors, often a result of high activity levels and impulsivity, are excessive. Parent and teacher reports and observations of children in classrooms and on the playground, indicate that youth with ADHD are more dominating, controlling, and aggressive (3,4). They issue more commands, grab desired objects from others, cut in line, and quickly change the rules of a game (or cheat) when the rules do not suit them (5). Their tendency to blurt out comments is often disruptive in a classroom and annoys other children who are trying to concentrate on their work. Often the comments are insensitive or insulting, and even though unintentional, can be hurtful to peers. Recently, Mikami et al. (6) also reported this pattern on a computer chat room task: children with ADHD-C were far more likely to be off-task and hostile in their responses to computerized peers compared to comparison children. Children with ADHD-C also have a pattern of emotional dysregulation characterized by intense emotional reactions, which they have difficulty adjusting to the changing demands of social situations (7). They frequently do not recognize the physical boundaries of others, touching or poking them or otherwise "getting in their space." Excessive physical activity, over-exuberance, and talkativeness are often bothersome to peers. To add to their problems, they are often unaware of the negative impact of their behavior on others (8).

Although much less is known about social functioning in ADHD-I, existing data suggest that these children are less disruptive than those with ADHD-C but still exhibit social problems. In several studies, both boys and girls with ADHD-I were rated as being passive and socially withdrawn relative to those with ADHD-C and to comparison children (7,9–11). In a recent observational study, those with ADHD-I, relative to ADHD-C and nonclinical controls, engaged in more solitary play and spent more time as onlookers of their peer's activities (10). When they did play with other children, it was for shorter periods of time relative to those with ADHD-C and nonclinical controls. Similarly, Mikami et al. (6) found that while children with ADHD-I were equally off-topic as those with ADHD-C during a computerized chat room interaction, they were far less engaged and had poorer memory of the chat room conversation relative to children with ADHD-C.

The peer status of youth with ADHD is, not surprisingly, compromised. Peer status, like peer interactions, appears to differ by type of ADHD. Boys and girls with hyperactivity and impulsivity (both the combined and hyperactive-impulsive types) are more often openly rejected by their peer group and rarely receive positive nominations from their peers. Children with only attentional problems also have low popularity, but they tend to have less extreme ratings of rejection (although still elevated), and seem to show more evidence of being neglected (12). The more withdrawn disposition of youth with ADHD-I may make them less visible to peers. However, they are not completely overlooked since they are often rated as being very shy, teased, and left out. Hodgens et al. (10) posit that their withdrawn behavior may be what leads to the low levels of peer acceptance.

Recent research has also begun to evaluate friendships in youth with ADHD. Dyadic friendships, being characterized by reciprocity and mutual affection, are distinct from general acceptance by peer groups and appear to contribute independently to mental health (13). Few studies have investigated friendships among children with ADHD, but those that have show that ADHD children have fewer friends than others and are seen as less desirable friends (13). Lack of friendships may be particularly deleterious in girls. During a summer camp experience, girls with ADHD were found to have fewer friendships than comparison girls—due to having either fewer multiple friends or no friends at all. The stability and quality of the friendships were compromised for girls of both subtypes (9).

Comorbid aggression, oppositional or antisocial behavior exacerbates the social problems of children with ADHD to the extent that this combination of problems leads to the worst social outcomes. Boys with ADHD and these comorbidities exhibit more aggressive verbal (e.g., yelling, teasing) and nonverbal (e.g., pushing, hitting) behavior than boys with only ADHD and they are least preferred by peers (4). While girls, in general, exhibit less physical aggression than boys, girls with ADHD-C show more overt aggression than those without and such aggression is linked to fewer nominations from peers as being "liked most" and more nominations of being "liked least" (14). A more common form of aggression for girls has been termed "relational aggression." This type of aggression includes a range of behaviors (e.g., social exclusion, spreading rumors, teasing) intended to hurt another child's friendships or peer status (15). Similar to physical aggression, high levels of relational aggression have been shown to adversely affect the quality of friendships and overall social acceptance (9,14). These studies found that girls with ADHD (especially the combined type) exhibited greater conflict and relational aggression than those without ADHD and that those with high levels of relational aggression also had the most compromised peer status and friendships.

MECHANISMS UNDERLYING SOCIAL PROBLEMS

These behavioral descriptions provide important information about what children with ADHD might be doing that contributes to their peer problems. Theories regarding why these problems occur are also important for development of effective intervention programs. A number of studies suggest underlying problems of affect regulation, behavioral intensity, cognitive distortions, and lack of skills (4). Barkley's theory of self-control of ADHD implicates the lack of behavioral inhibition as a key mechanism underlying social impairment (16). Based on this theory, difficulties with the executive functions of nonverbal working memory, internalized self-speech, affective and motivational self-regulation and reconstitution occur and markedly affect the ability to self-regulate social interactions. These factors might account for the excessive behavioral intensity, affect dysregulation, and aberrant social information processing often seen in these children.

They seem to take insufficient time to process and evaluate social information, fail to attend to important information, not talk themselves through potential responses, overreact to emotional factors, and/or fail to evaluate the appropriateness of their behaviors.

Social information processing deficits may also underlie the peer relationship problems among youth with ADHD. Encoding deficits have been found such that children with ADHD tend to form decisions about a situation utilizing less information than those without ADHD (17). Furthermore, they are less able to utilize the social cues they do observe to appropriately modulate their behavior in different situations. Social problem-solving skills also are deficient in that they generate less friendly, more assertive and impulsive, and less effective solutions (5). Other social information processing abnormalities appear to underlie the aggressive behavior of youth with ADHD. These include: overattributions of hostile intent in the behavior of peers, social agendas that prioritize troublemaking and having fun at the expense of breaking rules and teasing kids, and greater confidence in one's ability to succeed with aggression (4).

Recent theorizing by Wheeler and Carlson (7) suggests that the extent to which skill knowledge or performance problems account for social problems may differ by subtype of ADHD. Those with the hyperactive-impulsive component may be more likely to exhibit performance problems rather than skill deficits. That is, when asked, they know what they should be doing, but in actual practice they do not exhibit those behaviors. Performance problems may be due to excessive negative behaviors (e.g., grabbing, interrupting, breaking rules) or too few prosocial behaviors (attending to another child, initiating an interaction). In either case, motivational factors or lack of behavioral inhibition is thought to underlie the performance problems. Skill deficits may be a relatively stronger mechanism in ADHD-I. Children with this subtype may simply not know what to do in various social situations. In addition, their attentional problems may lead to poor tracking and processing of social cues from other people, apparent disinterest in carrying on a conversation, and faulty timing during interpersonal interactions. These problems may be particularly impairing for girls with ADHD due to their greater focus on verbal communication. Based on findings of Blachman and Hinshaw (9), they may have specific difficulty balancing multiple friendships, perhaps due to their lack of active engagement and focus.

Given the complexity of the problem, it is likely that differences in subtype are relative rather than absolute, and that children with ADHD will vary in the degree to which skill remediation or performance motivation is beneficial. The challenge of modifying these problems is complicated by data showing youth with ADHD lack awareness of their social ineptitude and tend not to take responsibility for their transgressions (8). The lack of accurate self-appraisal limits their ability to learn how to modulate their behavior to different circumstances (13).

SOCIAL SKILLS TRAINING TO REMEDIATE PEER PROBLEMS IN ADHD

Historically, social skills training has been used to treat children identified as being rejected or neglected by peers and also to treat children with aggression and conduct problems (18–20). A number of studies report improvement in social behaviors as a result of the training, however, the involvement of parents and teachers was necessary to support their use of the social skills outside of the therapy setting (21). Social skills training programs were first systematically investigated with youth having ADHD in the early 1980s. In one of the first studies of social skills training (SST) with ADHD, Pelham and Bender (22) applied a variant of the program developed for socially isolated youth. The concepts of cooperation, communication, participation, and validation-support were taught in small groups via direct instruction, modeling, role-playing, and coaching. SST alone did not lead to improvement, although when positive reinforcement was added for prosocial behavior, improvement was observed. Over the next decade or so, several other studies attempted to improve social interactions via self-instruction training in which children were taught to modify their self-talk in order to self-regulate their behavior. Short-term beneficial effects were found for impulsive children (23), but this approach has not been shown to be effective for ADHD. During this time, commercially available social skills training programs proliferated and became quite popular (24).

Clearly, there is intuitive appeal for the idea of training children in skills to improve their social relations. However, reviews of the SST literature provided little evidence that such training changed the way children behaved or were received in the natural environments of home and school (24,25). The typical approach to training referred to as "train and hope," wherein children are taught skills in an office (or other contrived) setting via didactics and modeling and without explicit programming for generalization outside of the training setting, showed little effect.

Since then, several well-controlled studies of SST tailored to the needs of ADHD and incorporating strategies to address the generalization problems have shown beneficial effects. Pfiffner and McBurnett (26) evaluated a broad-based SST program for ADHD children with the goals of teaching skills of social significance, using motivational systems to reduce performance problems, increasing awareness and understanding of verbal and nonverbal social cues, and promoting generalization and maintenance by incorporating significant others (parent and teachers) in treatment. The SST program included eight 90-min group sessions covering the following modules: good sportsmanship, accepting consequences, assertiveness, ignoring mild provocation, problem-solving, and recognizing and dealing with feelings. Didactic instruction, modeling, role-plays, and a variety of games were used to teach the skills. Children were taught to evaluate their own performance each week. A token reinforcement system was implemented to reinforce skill use during sessions. Children were randomly assigned to three groups: SST only, SST plus parent generalization training, or a wait-list control group. Parents in the parent generalization group were taught methods for supporting their child's use of the skills at home and also worked with their child's teacher to set up systems for reinforcing their child's use of the skills at school. The token system used in the group was also used at home by parents and at school by the teachers. At the end of treatment both the SST groups resulted in gains in child social skill knowledge and in parent report of improvement in social interactions and home behavior problems with the gains maintaining for 3–4 months following treatment. Some generalization to the school setting was also found for the parent generalization group only.

Frankel et al. (27) also found positive effects of their 12-week SST program focused on training in conversational skills, group entry, handling teasing and rejection, negotiation skills for changing activities and praising others. At posttreatment, parents rated significant reductions in social skills deficits relative to a wait-list control group. Children without oppositional defiant disorder (ODD) showed significant drops in teacher-rated aggression and withdrawal. In a subsequent study in which they added modules for addressing disruptive classroom behavior and aggression and also trained parents in homework compliance, methods for working with teachers to decrease disruptive behavior at school and methods for coaching their child in peer interactions significant gains also were made for children with ODD (28). In another study, concurrent parent and child behavioral skills groups resulted in reductions in ADHD symptoms and improvement in parenting at home for medicated children in an outpatient primary care clinic (29). The efficacy of SST with young (age 4–8 year olds) children having conduct problems has been demonstrated recently with equivalent benefit for the subgroup with ADHD. Here too, treatment included direct involvement of parents and teachers for facilitating generalization of skills to home and school (30). While the greatest improvement seems to occur from programs that actively include parents and/or teachers in the treatment, SST has shown some effect with minimal parent involvement. Antshel and Remer (31) implemented an 8-week SST program with medicated youth having ADHD (ages 8–12) focused on training in a variety of social skills (e.g., cooperation, problem-solving, recognizing and controlling anger, assertiveness, conversations, and accepting consequences) and included several informational sessions for parents. Both parents and children reported significant improvement in assertiveness at posttreatment relative to a wait-list control group.

As these studies indicate, there is accumulating evidence to support use of SST with ADHD youth. The positive effects are seen on parent and teacher ratings of social behaviors; whether training effects extend to observations of the children's actual interactions with peers or peer acceptance requires further study. To maximize positive effects of SST, the following factors are important:

1. The curriculum should be based on problems exhibited by ADHD. For ADHD-C this means addressing problems such as intrusiveness, impulsivity, and emotional dysregulation. For ADHD-I this means addressing problems such as disengagement, social withdrawal, and passivity (32). For both subtypes, it means learning to adjust their behavior to the nuances of the social environment. It follows then that treatment should be tailored to the specific social-cognitive deficits associated with ADHD. For example, to address attentional problems, children can be taught how to be better observers of other children; to address lack of social problem-solving skills, children can be supplied with a range of effective solutions for a variety of problems; to address the lack of self-appraisal or insight into their own behavior and consequences, treatments may incorporate strategies such as Match Game (33) wherein children are taught and reinforced for accurate self-appraisals. Another approach may involve having children view and evaluate videotaped samples of their own interactions with peers. Attributional problems may also be remedied by using specific cognitive strategies and behavioral rehearsal (34).
2. Strategies to decrease aggressive behavior, be it physical or relational, need to be in place. This should include contingency management and other behavioral interventions to manage aggression as well as methods for altering the aggressive social agendas, distorted cognitive appraisals, and poor social problem-solving skills characteristic of those with comorbid aggression. Programs such as those developed by Lochman and Lenhart (19) for aggressive children may be useful models.
3. SST is best implemented in the context of a group in order to facilitate peer modeling and practice of skills. However, if a group is not available, individual training may be effective if adequate opportunity for peer interaction is provided. For example, Colton and Sheridan (35) successfully trained several individual children via individualized coaching, role-plays, prompts for skill use ("friendship cards"), self-monitoring of recess behaviors, and a home–school communication system with positive reinforcement at home for school success. Importantly, parents and teachers also were encouraged to provide ample monitoring and feedback of the children's social behavior.
4. A behavior management component is necessary to handle behavior excesses in group, particularly for ADHD-Combined Type (28).

Without this component, the attention and focus needed from children to learn new skills will be limited.

5. A generalization component needs to be in place since children do not usually transfer the skills they learn in SST on their own to their interactions with peers (26,28). The greatest gains result from programs where parents and teachers are actively involved in reinforcing the social skills taught during SST. In classrooms, playgrounds or families where negative, coercive behaviors are prominent, this may require altering the environmental milieu so that prosocial behavior becomes desirable and the norm among all individuals.
6. Even after children learn new skills and modify their behavior, peers may not alter their negative assessment of them. Reputational biases may be addressed by making treatment class-wide, incorporating cooperative play activities, and making sure the skills taught are of value to peers (13). In some cases, reputations may be virtually impossible to change; switching classes or schools may be the best solution for these children.
7. SST should not be considered a sole treatment for the social problems accompanying ADHD. Parent training and classroom-based interventions, the primary evidence-based psychosocial treatments for ADHD, are necessary to help supervising adults develop needed skills for monitoring, prompting and reinforcing prosocial behaviors, and decreasing aggressive behaviors. Stimulant medication also has been shown to improve peer interactions and in conjunction with SST and other psychosocial interventions leads to optimal effects, especially in moderate to severe cases of ADHD. The combination of medication and behavioral interventions is recommended due to their effects on different underlying processes of social impairment with medication affecting inhibitory processes and SST affecting skill, social cognition, and judgment (4).

IMPROVING PEER INTERVENTIONS

Although SST shows benefit, the intensive environmental support needed for optimal maintenance and generalization of treatment gains is often difficult to accomplish, making the need for further development of peer interventions a priority. One area usually not addressed in SST is the development of dyadic friendships. Based on a number of studies indicating that good friendships may compensate for the negative impact of peer rejection and seem to predict better adjustment later in life, greater focus on developing dyadic friendships is important. One promising approach has been developed by Hoza et al. (36). The focus of this intervention is on developing a positive relationship with one specific peer rather than improving peer relations in general. The program was implemented in the context of an intensive, camp-like behavioral treatment program which included SST. It involved pairing children with one buddy based on interests, competencies, and practical considerations (how close the families lived to one another). Buddy pairs were scheduled to spend more time together, received special privileges as a pair, and were evaluated and rewarded for good friendships. The children's parents were encouraged to have the children get together during playdates outside of the program to promote the friendship. Buddy coaches helped work out problems between the buddies while at the treatment program. Initial results show that frequent playdates significantly contributed to the quality of the friendships. Also, children paired with less disruptive/antisocial children showed the most benefit. The positive effects of the playdates appear dependent on control of disruptive and aggressive behavior of the buddies by supervising adults. The actual efficacy of the intervention requires further study due to the lack of a comparison group not receiving the intervention. However, strategies focused on developing dyadic friendships appear readily integrated into traditional SST programs via prescribed playdates and training for parents to support these interactions and friendships (32,37,38). They also may be integrated into classrooms (13). The focus on dyadic friendships may be especially helpful to address the social withdrawal often seen in the inattentive type.

Environmental accommodations to improve the fit between the child and the demands of the environment are an additional method for augmenting social skills or friendship interventions. In the classroom, accommodations to assignments, seating, instructional format, etc., are routinely implemented to improve classroom behavior and academic functioning. However, accommodations to the environment are less often emphasized for improving peer relations, but may be effective for reducing unfocused, impulsive, or disruptive behavior. For example, during playdates this may include having a structured play activity planned in advance, keeping the activity brief and relatively fast-paced, having play activities in the child's areas of interest and rotating these activities to maintain motivation. For after-school activities, small peer groups with close adult supervision are advisable and activities should allow the child to be active and involved most of the time.

Peer tutoring in social interaction skills also may be of benefit as it has been for academic skills (39). Such tutoring may involve pairing children and having them work together on cooperative tasks for successful outcomes during recess and lunch. A variant of this concept is the student-mediated conflict resolution program developed by Cunningham and Cunningham (40). This program involves teams of older children, trained as mediators, helping peers solve interpersonal conflicts when they occur such as during recess or lunch. The mediators help negotiate resolutions and plan strategies for preventing future problems. Initial outcomes of this program have been quite positive with evidence for reduced conflicts of the type often experienced by children with ADHD. Although not specifically evaluated for effects with ADHD, training in mediation skills and serving as a mediator could offer significant benefits for the child with ADHD including improvements in one's reputation among peers, and acquisition of skills in perspective-taking, self-awareness, and resolving conflicts.

CONCLUSION

Recent advances in SST suggest that this form of treatment shows promise for treating the social difficulties of youth with ADHD. However, positive effects are limited to programs that address the specific social problems of children with ADHD and those that actively program generalization via involvement of parents and/or teachers. Further development of SST should incorporate greater focus on development of dyadic friendships and environmental accommodations to promote successful peer interactions. Additionally, peer-mediated conflict resolution programs show promise for addressing conflict in the natural environment.

REFERENCES

1. Greene RW, Biederman J, Faraone SV, Sienna M, Garcia-Jetton J. Adolescent outcome of boys with attention-deficit/hyperactivity disorder and social disability: results from a 4-year longitudinal follow-up study. J Consult Clin Psychol 1997; 65:758–67.
2. Greene RW, Biederman J, Faraone SV, Wilens TE, Mick E, Blier HK. Further validation of social impairment as a predictor of substance use disorders: findings from a sample of siblings of boys with and without ADHD. J Clin Child Psychol 1999; 28:349–54.
3. Hinshaw SP. Intervention for social competence and social skill. Child Adolesc Psychiatr Clin N Am 1992; 1:539–52.
4. Pfiffner LJ, Calzada E, McBurnett K. Interventions to enhance social competence. In: Stubbe D, ed. Child and Adolescent Psychiatric Clinics. Philadelphia: W.B. Saunders, 2000:689–709.
5. Grenell MM, Glass CR, Katz KS. Hyperactive children and peer interaction: knowledge and performance of social skills. J Abnorm Child Psychol 1987; 15: 1–13.
6. Mikami A, Huang-Pollock C, Pfiffner L, McBurnett K, Hangai D. Social skills differences among Attention Deficit/Hyperactivity Disorder types in a chat room assessment task. J Abnorm Child Psychol, 2007; 35:509–21.
7. Wheeler J, Carlson CL. The social functioning of children with ADD with hyperactivity and ADD without hyperactivity: a comparison of their peer relations and social deficits. J Emotional Behav Disord 1994; 2:2–12.

8. Hoza B. Attention-Deficit/Hyperactivity Disordered and control boys responses to social success and failure. Child Dev 2000; 71:432–46.
9. Blachman DR, Hinshaw SP. Patterns of friendship among girls with and without attention-deficit/hyperactivity disorder. J Abnorm Child Psychol 2002; 30:625–40.
10. Hodgens J, Cole J, Boldizar J. Peer-based differences among boys with ADHD. J Clin Child Psychol 2000; 29:443–52.
11. Milich RM, Balentine AC, Lynam DR. ADHD combined type and ADHD predominantly inattentive type are distinct and unrelated disorders. Clin Psychol: Sci Pract 2001; 8:463–88.
12. McBurnett K, Pfiffner LJ, Willcutt E, et al. Experimental cross-validation of DSM-IV types of Attention-Deficit/Hyperactivity Disorder. J Acad Child Adolesc Psychiatry 1999; 38:17–24.
13. Mrug S, Hoza B, Gertdes AC. Children with attention-deficit/hyperactivity disorder: peer relationships and peer-oriented interventions. In: Nangle DW, Erdley CA, ed. The Role of Friendship in Psychological Adjustment. New Directions for Child and Adolescent Development, Vol 91. San Francisco, CA: Jossey-Bass, 2001:51–77.
14. Zalecki CA, Hinshaw S. Overt and relational aggression in girls with Attention Deficit Hyperactivity Disorder. J Clin Child Adolesc Psychol 2004; 33:131–43.
15. Crick NR, Grotpeter JK. Relational aggression, gender, and social-psychological adjustment. Child Dev 1995; 66:710–22.
16. Barkley RA. ADHD and the Nature of Self-Control. New York: Guilford Press, 1997.
17. Matthys W, Cuperus JM, Van Engeland H. Deficient social problem-solving in boys with ODD/CD, with ADHD, and with both disorders. J Am Acad Child Adolesc Psychiatry 1999; 38:311–21.
18. Bierman KL. Peer Rejection: Developmental Processes and Intervention Strategies. New York: Guilford Publications, 2003.
19. Lochman JE, Lenhart L. Cognitive behavioral therapy of aggressive children: effects of schemas, In: van Bilsen HPJG, Kendall PC, Slavenburg JH, eds. Behavioral Approaches for Children and Adolescents: Challenges for the next century. New York: Plenum Press, 1995 pp. 145–66.
20. Oden S, Asher SR. Coaching children in social skills for friendship making. Child Dev 1977; 48:495–506.
21. Kolko DJ, Loar LL, Sturnick D. Inpatient social-cognitive skills training groups with conduct disordered and attention deficit disordered children. J Child Psychol Psychiatry 1990; 31:737–48.
22. Pelham WE, Bender ME. Peer relationships in hyperactive children: description and treatment. Adv Learn Behav Disabil 1982; 1:365–436.
23. Kendall PC, Braswell L. Cognitive-behavioral self-control therapy for children: a components analysis. J Consult Clin Psychol 1982; 50:672–89.
24. DuPaul GJ, Eckert TL. The effects of social skills curricula: now you see them, now you don't. Sch Psychol Quarterly 1994; 9:113–32.
25. Landau S, Moore LA. Social skill deficits in children with Attention-Deficit Hyperactivity Disorder. Sch Psychol Rev 1991; 20:235–51.

26. Pfiffner LJ, McBurnett K. Social skills training with parent generalization: treatment effects for children with attention deficit disorder. J Consult Clin Psychol 1997; 65:749–57.
27. Frankel F, Myatt R, Cantwell DP. Training outpatient boys to conform with the social ecology of popular peers: effects on parent and teacher ratings. J Clin Child Psychol 1995; 24:300–10.
28. Frankel F, Myatt R, Cantwell DP, Feinberg DT. Parent-assisted transfer of children's social skills training: effects on children with and without Attention-Deficit Hyperactivity Disorder. J Am Acad Child Adolesc Psychiatry 1997; 36: 1056–64.
29. Tutty S, Gephart H, Wurzbacher K. Enhancing behavioral and social skill functioning in children newly diagnosed with attention-deficit hyperactivity disorder in a pediatric setting. J Dev Behav Pediatr 2003; 24:51–7.
30. Webster-Stratton C, Reid J, Hammond M. Social skills and problem-solving training for children with early-onset conduct problems: who benefits? J Child Psychol Psychiatry 2001; 42:943–53.
31. Antshel KM, Remer R. Social skills training in children with attention deficit hyperactivity disorder: a randomized-controlled clinical trial. J Clin Child Adolesc Psychol 2003; 32:153–65.
32. Pfiffner LJ, Mikami A, Huang-Pollock C, Zalecki C, Easterlin B, McBurnett K. A randomized controlled trial of integrated home-school behavioral treatment for ADHD, Predominantly Inattentive Type. J Am Acad Child Adolesc Psychiatry 2007; 46: 1041–6.
33. Hinshaw SP, Melnick S. Self-management therapies and attention-deficit hyperactivity disorder. Reinforced self-evaluation and anger control interventions. Behav Modif 1992; 16:253–73.
34. Hinshaw SP, Henker B, Whalen CK. Self-control in hyperactive boys in anger-inducing situations: effects of cognitive-behavioral training and of methylphenidate. J Abnorm Child Psychol 1984; 12:55–77.
35. Colton DL, Sheridan SM. Conjoint behavioral consultation and social skills training: Enhancing the play behaviors of boys with Attention Deficit Hyperactivity Disorder. J Educ Psychol Consultat 1998; 9:3–28.
36. Hoza B, Mrug S, Pelham WEJ, Greiner AR, Gnagy EM. A friendship intervention for children with attention-deficit/hyperactivity disorder: preliminary findings. J Atten Disord 2003; 6:87–98.
37. Frankel F, Myatt R. Children's Friendship Training. New York: Brunner-Routledge, 2003.
38. Pfiffner LJ. Training Manual for Child Life Skills Program. San Francisco, CA: UCSF, 2003.
39. DuPaul GJ, Henningson PN. Peer tutoring effects on the classroom performance of children with attention deficit hyperactivity disorder. Sch Psychol Rev 1993; 22:134–43.
40. Cunningham CE, Cunningham LJ. Student-mediated conflict resolution problems. In: Barkley RA, ed. Attention-Deficit Hyperactivity Disorder: A Handbook for Diagnosis and Treatment. 2nd ed. New York: The Guilford Press, 1998:491–509.

18

Parent Training in the Treatment of ADHD

Karen C. Wells
Department of Psychiatry, Duke University Medical Center, Durham, North Carolina, U.S.A.

Attention deficit hyperactivity disorder (ADHD) is a chronic and impairing disorder of childhood, adolescence, and adulthood and is characterized by primary symptoms of inattention, impulsivity, and overactivity (1). In addition, ADHD is usually associated with one or more comorbid conditions, associated features, and functional deficits, or combination of these, which add to the impairment picture and complicate treatment planning. Oppositional defiant disorder (ODD) is the most common comorbid condition with 35% to 60% of ADHD children also meeting criteria for an ODD diagnosis (2,3). Conduct disorder (CD), another significant comorbid condition occurs in 30% to 50% of ADHD cases. Among the functional impairments, difficulties within the family and parenting domains are prominent.

The primary difficulties with inattention, impulsivity, and overactivity present parenting challenges to the mothers and fathers of ADHD children. Inattentive children have a difficult time sustaining attention and completing tasks as they move through the structured activities of the day. The impulsivity of these children often results in verbal or even physical aggression directed toward siblings or other family members as well as other social disruptions that require parent intervention (e.g., grabbing toys away from siblings; inability to wait to take one's turn; loud verbal outbursts that are annoying to others; etc.). Overactivity can produce behaviors that are very disruptive or require constant intervention by parents (e.g., running around the table at mealtime; inability to sit still and play quietly while parents are occupied).

Within the parenting and family domain, the parent–child interactions of ADHD children and adolescents with their mothers and fathers are frequently disturbed and conflictual. Parents of ADHD children display more negative reactivity, more commanding, directive behavior, and less positive responsivity to ADHD children than do parents of normal children (4–6). While disrupted parent–child interaction is probably not etiologic in ADHD, it may have a primary causal role in the development, escalation and maintenance of the oppositional and aggressive behavior that is characteristic of ODD and CD.

These comorbid conditions (ODD and CD) also carry implications for parent training interventions. Research has documented that the presence of ODD is associated with much of the parent–child interactional conflicts in ADHD families (7,8). Nevertheless, parental intrusiveness and overstimulation in the infant–child relationship are significant early antecedents of later hyperactivity in kindergarten (9) and parents and children with ADHD alone still display interactions that deviate from normal (6,8). This suggests that intervening in parent–child interactions may be important not just with ADHD comorbid with ODD and CD but with pure ADHD.

For all of these reasons, parent training interventions have developed and been utilized as one of the primary psychosocial treatment strategies in the armamentarium of clinicians working with ADHD children. Parent training may be used as a frontline treatment but is often used in conjunction with stimulant medication therapy and school interventions for those children who have significant difficulties in the school environment.

Although a number of clinical researchers have employed Parent Training programs with families of children with behavior problems, the investigators most associated with this approach for use with ADHD populations are Barkley (10) and Wells and colleagues (11,12). Barkley adapted an 8–10 session intervention for use with ADHD children from the Parent Training program first developed by Constance Hanf. Wells and colleagues developed an extended Parent Training program that incorporated many of Barkley's adaptations, but embellished and extended the basic program to include attention to school and other parent factors that are often issues in ADHD families. Each of these will be described briefly.

In Barkley's version of parent training for ADHD, treatment begins with a review of information on ADHD as well as causes of oppositional and defiant behavior, including diagnosis, theories of etiology, and principles of social learning theory that are relevant to parent–child interactions. Once this background has been discussed with parents, presentation of parent management skills begins, starting first with increasing positive parental attention to children during a 10–20 min "special time" every day. Once parent attention has been established as a reinforcer, parents are next taught how to apply their positive attention to two critical target behaviors for ADHD children; compliance to parent instructions and independent play. Parents are taught to "catch the child being good" (i.e., compliant) and also to attend and praise the child when the child is playing independently while the parent is engaged in some other activity (such as working or cooking).

Compliance to parental instructions is felt to be a critical target behavior to increase in ADHD children. Noncompliance is the keystone characteristic of ODD and decreasing this comorbidity is important in the clinical management of these children. However, even in children with pure ADHD, improving compliance to parental instructions is often the key if parents are to assist the child with managing his/her inattentive, impulsive, and overactive behaviors. That is, management of these behaviors can only be accomplished via parental instructions to the child (e.g., "sit down at the table and don't get up again until dinner is finished") and establishment of house rules (e.g., "grabbing your sister's toys without asking is not permitted"). If the child cannot or will not follow these instructions and house rules, then the parent will be unsuccessful in assisting the child with his overactive and impulsive behaviors. Likewise, independent play is felt to be a critical target behavior in these children since staying "on task" for an age-appropriate amount of time is a frequent, primary problem behavior.

For young children improving parent positive attention may be sufficient. For older children, the next step is establishing a home token economy which sets up a reward system for compliance as well as an expanded array of target behaviors, such as social behaviors related to impulsivity (e.g., hitting, swearing, etc.), age-appropriate chores and other responsibilities. Later, parents are taught a "time-out" procedure to use as a mild punishment procedure for decreasing noncompliance and later, other disruptive behaviors that may still be occurring (violations of house rules, etc.).

In the final stage of the basic Parent Training program, attention is paid to establishing generalization of treatment effects across settings and time. Parents are taught procedures for managing disruptive behavior in public places and at school [using the home-school daily report card (DRC) system]; as well as strategies for managing future behavior problems. A booster session is then held 1 month after the final intensive phase session, to review treatment goals and consolidate treatment gains.

The Parent Training program developed by Wells and colleagues (11,12) was used in the MTA study of multimodal treatment of ADHD. This program is a 27-session treatment program that incorporates adaptations of the 8–12 session program described above, but extends well beyond the basic program. It provides more discussion of clinical nuances that arise in treatment of ADHD families, and more step-by-step instructions of basic procedures. However, beyond embellishments to the basic program, the Parent Training program of Wells et al. (11) was designed more intensively and comprehensively to address multiple settings and domains of child and family functioning in ADHD. First, great emphasis is placed on intervention in the school setting, since most ADHD children display considerable difficulties related to primary ADHD symptoms in school. Many sessions are devoted to discussing, modeling, and role-playing with parents, both in therapy sessions as well as in visits to the school, parent advocacy, and teacher consultation skills. Other innovations include training parents in cognitive strategies for changing their own maladaptive cognitions and attributions related to parenting a child with ADHD (e.g., "my child is bad; I must be a very bad parent"), as well as stress management strategies, including calming "self-talk" and relaxation skills, to use in disciplinary encounters with the child. These innovations were added to address findings from empirical research that have shown that parents of ADHD children experience more parenting stress, anger, and irritability and a decreased sense of parenting self-competence compared to other parents (13–15).

Since 1980, there have been several controlled studies in the published literature that have examined Parent Training as a single treatment or as a component of a clinical behavior therapy package for youth with ADHD. These studies have shown that parent training produces reductions in inattention and overactivity (16–18) in child noncompliance and conduct problems (18–20) and in child aggression (16). As would be expected, improvements in parenting skills (19,21) also have been found. Some studies also have reported reductions in parent stress, and improvements in parent self-esteem with parent training (16,18,21). Effect sizes for parent training for ADHD of 1.2 have been reported on ADHD symptoms. Anastopoulos et al. reported that 64% of their sample demonstrated clinically significant changes in terms of percentage of children no longer in the clinical range on ADHD Rating Scale with Parent Training compared with 27% for a waitlist control group.

Other studies have examined multicomponent behavior therapy programs of which Parent Training is one component. The most typical combination involves Parent Training plus Teacher Consultation. In Teacher Consultation, the therapist works with the teacher to set up a DRC focusing on classroom behavior and academic performance and may also consult with the teacher on classroom-wide behavior management strategies as well. Several studies have combined Parent Training and Teacher Consultation (22–24) and compared them to medication, with results generally showing that the combination of Parent Training plus Teacher Consultation results in significant improvement in children's home and school behavior. Even greater improvements are noted when Parent Training and Teacher Consultation are combined with stimulant medications (24).

The two large-scale randomized clinical trials in the published literature each included Parent Training as one component of comprehensive behavior therapy programs, and compared behavior therapy to medication alone and their combination (25–27). While the effects of Parent Training alone can not be elucidated from these studies, they are instructive when considering the best multimodal treatment for ADHD children. In both studies, medication outperformed behavior therapy alone on several measures of ADHD children's functioning. However, on some measures, the combination of medication and behavior therapy resulted in greater improvement than medication alone (25), or than community-treated controls whereas medication alone did not result in greater improvement than community-treated controls (26). Full normalization on objective classroom measures was only achieved with combination treatment (25) and parents were more satisfied with behavior therapy alone and with combination treatment than with medication alone (26). These results suggest that a comprehensive behavior therapy approach that includes Parent Training will be most effective (on some but not all symptoms) and result in greater normalization of ADHD children. All of these studies confirm that Parent Training is and will remain an important component of the treatment armamentarium for the families of children with ADHD and should be considered to be an essential "leg" in the three-legged stool comprising treatment of these children (i.e., stimulant medication, Parent Training, and School Intervention).

REFERENCES

1. American Psychiatric Association. Diagnostic and Statistical Manual of Mental Disorders. 4th ed. Washington, D.C.: Author, 1994.
2. Barkley RA. Attention-deficit/hyperactivity disorder. In: Mash EJ, Barkley RA, eds. Child Psychopathology. New York: Guilford Press, 1996:63–112.
3. Biederman J, Faraone SV, Lapey K. Comorbidity of diagnosis in attention-deficit hyperactivity disorder. In: Weiss G, ed. Child and Adolescent Psychiatric Clinics of North America: Attention-Deficit Hyperactivity Disorder. Philadelphia: Saunders, 1992:335–60.
4. Anderson CA, Hinshaw SP, Simmel C. Mother–child interactions in ADHD and comparison boys: relationships with overt and covert externalizing behavior. J Abnorm Child Psychol 1994; 22:247–65.
5. Danforth JS, Barkley RA, Stokes TF. Observations of parent–child interactions with hyperactive children: research and clinical implications. Clin Psychol Rev 1991; 11:703–27.
6. Johnston C. Parent characteristics and parent–child interactions in families of nonproblem children and ADHD children with higher and lower levels of oppositional-defiant behavior. J Abnorm Child Psychol 1996; 24:85–104.
7. Barkley RA, Anastopoulos AD, Guevremont DG, Fletcher KF. Adolescents with attention deficit hyperactivity disorder: mother-adolescent interactions, family beliefs and conflicts, and maternal psychopathology. J Abnorm Child Psychol 1992; 20:263–88.

8. Fletcher KE, Fisher M, Barkley RA, Smallish L. A sequential analysis of the mother-adolescent interactions of ADHD, ADHD/ODD, and normal teenagers during neutral and conflict discussions. J Abnorm Child Psychol 1996; 24: 271–97.
9. Jacobvitz D, Sroufe LA. The early caregiver–child relationship and attention-deficit disorder with hyperactivity in kindergarten: a prospective study. Child Dev 1987; 58:1488–95.
10. Barkley RA. Attention-Deficit Hyperactivity Disorder: A Handbook for Diagnosis and Treatment. 2nd ed. New York: Guilford Press, 1998.
11. Wells KC, Abikoff H, Abramowitz A, et al. Parent Training for Attention Deficit Hyperactivity Disorder: MTA Study Manual. Duke University Medical Center, Durham, NC, 1996.
12. Wells KC, Pelham WE Jr, Kotkin RA, et al. Psychosocial treatment strategies in the MTA Study: rationale, methods, and critical issues in design and implementation. J Abnorm Child Psychol 2000; 28:483–505.
13. Fischer M. Parenting stress and the child with attention deficit hyperactivity disorder. J Clin Child Psychol 1990; 19:337–46.
14. Mash EJ, Johnston C. Determinants of parenting stress: illustrations from families of hyperactive children and families of physically abused children. J Clin Child Psychol 1990; 19:313–28.
15. Podolski CL, Nigg JT. Parent stress and coping in relation to child ADHD severity and associated child disruptive behavior problems. J Clin Child Psychol 2001; 30:503–13.
16. Anastopoulos AD, Shelton T, DuPaul GJ, Guevremont DC. Parent training for attention deficit hyperactivity disorder: its impact on parent functioning. J Abnorm Child Psychol 1993; 21:581–95.
17. Dubey DR, O'Leary SG, Kaufman KF. Training parents of hyperactive children in childmanagement: a comparative outcome study. J Abnorm Child Psychol 1983; 11:229–46.
18. Sonuga-Barke EJS, Daley D, Thompson M, Laver-Bradbury C, Weeks A. Parent-based therapies for preschool attention-deficit/hyperactivity disorder: a randomized, controlled trial with a community sample. J Am Acad Child Adolesc Psychiatry 2001; 40:402–8.
19. Pisterman S, McGrath P, Firestone P, Goodman JT, Webster I, Mallory R. Outcome of parent-mediated treatment of preschoolers with attention deficit disorder with hyperactivity. J Consult Clin Psychol 1989; 57:628–35.
20. Pollard S, Ward E, Barkley RA. The effects of parent training and Ritalin on the parent-child interactions of hyperactive boys. Child Fam Ther 1983; 5:51–69.
21. Pisterman S, Firestone P, McGrath P, et al. The role of parent training in treatment of preschoolers with ADDH. Am J Orthopsychiatry 1992; 62: 397–408.
22. Horn WF, Ialongo N, Greenberg G, Packard T, Smith-Winberry C. Additive effects of behavioral parent training and self-control therapy with attention deficit hyperactivity disordered children. J Clin Child Psychol 1990; 19:98–110.
23. Horn WF, Ialongo NS, Pascoe JM, et al. Additive effects of psychostimulants, parent training, and self-control therapy with ADHD children. J Am Acad Child Adolesc Psychiatry 1991; 30:233–40.

24. Pelham WE, Schnedler RW, Bender M, et al. The combination of behavior therapy and methylphenidate in the treatment of attention deficit disorder: a therapy outcome study. In: Bloomingdale LM, ed. Attention Deficit Disorder, Vol. 3. Oxford, UK: Pergamon, 1988:29–48.
25. Klein RG, Abikoff H. Behavior therapy and methylphenidate in the treatment of children with ADHD. J Attent Disord 1997; 2:89–114.
26. Multimodal Treatment Study of Children with Attention Deficit Hyperactivity Disorder (MTA) Cooperative Group. A 14-month randomized clinical trial of treatment strategies for Attention Deficit Hyperactivity Disorder (ADHD). Arch Gen Psychiatry 1999a; 56:1073–86.
27. Multimodal Treatment Study of Children with Attention Deficit Hyperactivity Disorder (MTA) Cooperative Group. Effects of co-morbid anxiety disorder, family poverty, session attendance, and community medication on treatment outcome for Attention-Deficit Hyperactivity Disorder. Arch Gen Psychiatry 1999b; 56:1088–96.

19

Summer Treatment Programs for Children with ADHD

Daniel A. Waschbusch, William E. Pelham Jr., Elizabeth M. Gnagy, Andrew R. Greiner, and Greg A. Fabiano

Center for Children and Families, State University of New York at Buffalo, Buffalo, New York, U.S.A.

OVERVIEW AND DESCRIPTION

For more than 20 years, the summer treatment program (STP) has been used to treat children with attention deficit hyperactivity disorder (ADHD). The STP was first implemented by the senior author (WEP) at Florida State University in 1980. The program has been continually developed and expanded since that time and has been used in over 20 locations throughout North America. The STP was included as a key component of psychosocial treatment in the Multimodal Treatment Study of Children with ADHD, which was the largest study ever conducted to evaluate treatment of ADHD or any other child mental health problem (1).

The STP takes place in the summer, typically for 8 weeks. Children attend weekdays for approximately 9 hr/day (8 a.m. to 5 p.m.). Children spend 3 hr each day in education settings (art classroom, academic classroom), which are conducted by a teacher (usually a special education teacher) and an aide. The remainder of the day is spent in recreational activities. The STP provides treatment to children with ADHD in a summer camp-like setting. From the children's point of view, they are participating in a summer camp; they play soccer, softball, and basketball; go swimming; do arts and crafts; work on computers; and have free time. They participate in these activities in groups that consist of 12 age-matched children and five counselors (undergraduate and graduate students). The same children and counselors stay together all summer so that children have a chance to make new friends and keep them for a number of weeks (a novel experience for some campers) and so that counselors gain detailed knowledge of the nature and extent of the children's psychosocial difficulties. Each group of children and counselors is under the supervision of senior level staff, typically psychiatrists and/or psychologists, who monitor and evaluate the children's treatment response, as well the counselors' delivery of treatment, throughout the summer (2).

In the context of these activities, numerous empirically supported treatments are delivered, including: a comprehensive token economy (i.e., a point system), sports skills training and practice, group problem-solving training and practice, social skills training and practice, group and individualized parent education, ubiquitous positive reinforcement, time-out, daily report cards (DRCs), and academic training and practice. These interventions are adapted or supplemented with other, individualized treatments when necessary, and individualized medication assessments are also employed when appropriate. In addition, all staff members are taught to use positive reinforcement to encourage adaptive behavior and to avoid positive reinforcement following maladaptive behavior. Commands are issued in a manner that maximizes the likelihood of compliance. Consistency is emphasized by having children follow the same schedule each day, with rules for each activity repeatedly rehearsed, to help ensure that children know where they are supposed to be and what they are supposed to be doing. All of these interventions are implemented at a developmentally appropriate level for each child. They are also integrated into the context of the ongoing activities such that for both the children and the counselors these treatments become an integral part of the child's day at summer camp.

These interventions are the means through which the STP attempts to achieve six treatment goals: (1) developing children's problem-solving skills, social skills, and the social awareness necessary to enable them to get along better with other children; (2) improving the children's learning skills and academic achievement; (3) developing the children's abilities to follow through with instructions, to complete tasks that they commonly fail to finish, and to comply with adults' requests; (4) improving children's self-esteem by developing competencies in areas necessary for daily life functioning (e.g., interpersonal, recreational, academic) and other task-related areas; (5) teaching the children's parents how to develop, reinforce, and maintain these positive changes; and (6) evaluating the effects of medication on the child's academic and social functioning in a natural setting. These treatment goals represent the areas that research and clinical experience suggests are typical among most impaired in children with ADHD. They are also the areas that are of most concern to their parents and teachers.

THEORETICAL RATIONALE

The pervasive impairment experienced by a child with ADHD across important functional domains (e.g., academic functioning, peer and adult relationships, self-esteem, parenting) cannot be treated in an office setting, and it is impractical to think such profound impairments could be treated through periodic counseling visits. The STP is notable in that it explicitly targets the maladaptive behaviors (e.g., aggression, noncompliance), functional impairments (e.g., peer relationship problems, academic problems), and weak competencies (e.g., poor knowledge of sports rules and skills) that are hypothesized to be important predictors of long-term outcome. For example, because children receive treatment in the context of peer group activities, peer relationship problems are direct targets of interventions in the STP. There is considerable evidence that children with ADHD often have seriously impaired relationships with their peers (3,4). In fact, a number of recent studies suggest that peer problems may be more highly associated with the features of ADHD than with the features of other disruptive behavior problems, such as aggression (5–9). This is noteworthy in light of evidence that problems with peer relationships tend to be stable over time (10), and strongly predictive of poor developmental outcome (11), and may thus mediate the poor long-term outcome experienced by many children with ADHD (12). Typically used treatments, including outpatient behavior therapy and psychostimulant medication, have been largely unsuccessful in ameliorating problems with peers (4,13–15). One explanation for this lack of success is that typical treatments are not able to directly target peer relationships. The STP overcomes this weakness by providing treatment in the context of ongoing peer relationships in real-world situations (sports, classroom activities).

Second, the treatment approach in the STP is intensive. The STP takes place during the summer, when children are able to attend full time without interfering with their participation in school. By providing full-time treatment, children receive at least 360 hr of intensive treatment in a very short period of time—more intervention time than a child would receive in 6 years of typical outpatient treatment. This fact is especially compelling when one considers that alternative summer activities (often unsupervised, unstructured activities) may result in a decline in behavior. By offering intensive treatment over a considerable period of time, the STP is able to overcome some of the most common problems of implementing behavior therapy. For example, it is sometimes the case that children will show an initial negative reaction to behavioral interventions, exhibiting higher rates or degrees of the undesired behavior after introducing treatment. This is a well-known, widely studied phenomenon known as an extinction burst (16) and it is usually followed by a dramatic reduction in undesired behavior. Unfortunately, parents and teachers will often stop the new treatment in response to an extinction burst, thereby reinforcing the child's higher rate of negative behavior. The STP helps avoid this problem by providing treatment that is of sufficient duration and intensity to overcome an extinction burst, allowing for subsequent improvements that parents and teachers can then maintain.

Third, the treatment in the STP is multimodal and multicomponent. The STP uses numerous specific interventions (behavior, cognitive-behavioral, social skills, recreation therapy, and medication) to assist the children with ADHD, as well as their parents and schools. The parenting components include daily meetings between the child's counselors and parents to discuss the child's daily progress, weekly parent education and support meetings, and individualized meetings between parents and a clinician. The school components include not only the classroom interventions in the STP, but also the development and implementation of a daily home-school note. By developing a home-school note in the STP, the family can easily adapt the goals and reward procedures when the child returns to the normal school setting. Finally, we provide recommendations and consultation to each child's teacher in the fall to set up the daily home-school note and other programs to maintain treatment gains.

Fourth, the STP provides excellent motivation for children to change. Throughout the STP, children's behavior is carefully and systematically measured and recorded. This allows counselors the opportunity to give the children specific and immediate feedback and reinforcement. For example, children have the opportunity to earn playtime, which most children enjoy, twice per day if they achieve specific, individualized treatment goals. Similarly, children have the opportunity to earn a fun activity on Friday afternoons if they achieve their weekly treatment goals. Alternatively, children who have an exceptionally poor week, showing a decrease in adaptive behavior, receive minor negative consequences, such as having to do light chores or serve "detention" for a short period of time instead of going on a field trip. These procedures are in place to provide the children maximal motivation to change their behavior in an adaptive fashion, as well as to teach them the important lesson that what they do influences what happens to them. It is also likely that children are motivated to do well in the STP because they find the STP enjoyable and like spending time with the counselors.

EMPIRICAL SUPPORT

As noted above, the STP includes many different types of treatments that are interwoven in the context of summer camp activities. Hundreds of studies have evaluated these individual components and have found them to be effective. One review of treatments for ADHD found more than 100 studies supporting the efficacy of behavior modification (including 48 examining classroom situations and 80 examining parenting programs), hundreds supporting the efficacy of psychostimulant medication, and 10 supporting a combined (i.e., both behavior modification and stimulant medication) treatment approach. These same treatments are provided in the STP, providing some support for the STP.

At the same time, it cannot be assumed that combined interventions have the same effects as their component parts (17). Indeed, there are multiple ways that treatments may combine, some of which result in more positive treatment effects and some of which result in a reduction of treatment effects (18). Therefore, it is important to empirically examine combined treatment approaches such as the STP, and recent research has begun to do so.

One review of nearly 500 families that attended an STP (19) found that nearly 100% of them anonymously rated the STP as at least somewhat beneficial to themselves and their child, with the vast majority (80%) rating the STP as very beneficial. Moreover, 95% of parents indicated that their child enjoyed the STP. Ratings from the STP staff followed the same pattern, with 95% of children rated as at least somewhat improved by the STP. Finally, the authors found that less than 5% of families who started treatment failed to finish treatment. This is remarkable when one considers that the failure rate for typical treatments of ADHD are estimated closer to 50% (20,21).

The authors also examined whether ratings of children's behavior and impairment improve as a result of participating in the STP. Parent ratings of ADHD, oppositional defiant disorder (ODD), and conduct disorder (CD) symptoms showed a 24% improvement after the STP as compared to before the STP, and an 18% improvement in parent ratings of overall problems (19). In another study (22), teacher ratings of hyperactive-impulsive and ODD symptoms, conflict with the teacher, and dependency on the teacher all improved significantly after the STP as compared to before the STP. The change in ODD symptoms and conflict with the teacher are especially noteworthy because children were rated as significantly different from normal controls prior to the STP but were not significantly different after the STP, suggesting that they were "normalized" after participating in the STP.

An add-on to the Multimodal Treatment Study of Children with ADHD examined the effects of the STP by comparing children who received only the STP to those who received both the STP and medication (23). Results showed that children who received both the STP and medication were superior to children who received only the STP on five measures, whereas groups did not differ on the remaining 30 measures, with both groups showing a similarly positive response to the STP. This study also replicated the high satisfaction ratings and improvement ratings reported by Pelham and Hoza (19).

A recent series of investigations is providing a wealth of evidence for the efficacy of the STP treatment package as a whole, compared with a no-treatment condition (24–27). In a study of a 2-day withdrawal of the STP procedures (26), the withdrawal produced immediate and significant deterioration in behavior with very large effect sizes—regardless of whether or not children were receiving a medication regimen. A subsequent investigation removed the behavioral treatment for 2 weeks in a BABAB design (24,27) and again showed large and significant effects of the STP treatment.

These results have recently been replicated and extended in a program of research that examined the unimodal and interactive effects of behavior modification and stimulant medication by manipulating the intensity of the two treatments as administered in an STP setting The first published study in this program of research examined the classroom behavior of 44 boys and 4 girls (5–12 years old) who participated in a 9-week STP (28). Throughout the STP, children were administered different doses of treatment. Each child received a placebo, low dose (0.15 mg/kg), medium dose (0.30 mg/kg), or high dose (0.60 mg/kg) of immediate release methylphenidate in the morning, at noon, and in the midafternoon each day. These doses were randomly assigned across days in the program. At the same time, each group participated in a 3-week block of no behavior modification (NBM) treatment, low behavior modification treatment (LBM), and high behavior modification treatment (HBM). In the NBM treatment, classes were structured like a general education class—children received adult feedback in response to rule violations, and were asked to leave the classroom for severely disruptive behavior. In LBM treatment, children had a DRC that targeted academic and classroom behaviors, could earn weekly home and camp rewards for meeting DRC goals throughout the week, and staff were trained to provide high rates of praise and social reinforcement for meeting classroom goals. The HBM condition included a DRC that was backed by daily home and camp rewards for meeting DRC goals, a token economy point system linked to camp rewards and privileges, high rates of praise and social reinforcement delivered by staff, and individualized behavior modification programs as needed.

Results of the study supported the effectiveness of behavior modification, stimulant medication, and their combination in the classroom setting. LBM and HBM procedures were generally effective for classroom behavior and seatwork completion. For medication, a low dose resulted in a substantial increase in work completed, with modest increases obtained with increasing doses. Specifically, results showed that half (i.e., 0.15 mg/kg) of the standard dose used in most studies (i.e., 0.3 mg/kg) was effective. When behavior modification and medication were compared, LBM and HBM conditions alone were as good as or better than low, medium, and high doses of medication alone on measures of classroom rule violations. When medication and behavior modification were combined, many interactive effects were observed. For example, LBM combined with a low dose of medication was equivalent to a high dose of medication or high behavior modification alone. Similar results were found for recreational (29) and home (30) settings.

In summary, there is now clear evidence that the STP intervention is effective compared to an attention-control condition consisting of a summer camp where minimal or no treatment is provided. Further, there is now clear evidence that the blended treatment components offered in the STP result in significant improvement across domains, raters, and measures.

FUTURE DIRECTIONS

Although we have shown that the STP produces significant improvements in the behavior of children with ADHD, additional research will help to answer specific questions regarding the STP. One question concerns the mechanism(s) of action through which the STP has its effects. It has long been known that peer relationships are impaired in children with ADHD, and it has been speculated that peer problems may be a mediator of long-term functioning. It would be interesting to evaluate how the STP impacts peer relationships in children with ADHD and whether this influences the long-term outcome of children with ADHD. Similarly, recent theories of ADHD argue that cognitive impairments play a central role in ADHD (31,32). It would be useful to evaluate whether the STP impacts these purported deficits. It is likely that there are complementary effects of the different types of interventions offered in the STP. For example, the social interventions may help children get along better with peers and adults, whereas time-out procedures may improve children's levels of aggression, and the classroom intervention may improve children's ability to stay on task. In fact, a recent investigation (33) found that the time-out component of the STP produced significant improvement in noncompliant and aggressive behavior beyond the improvement induced by the point system and other treatment components of the STP, lending credence to the hypothesis that it is the combination of the component treatments that provide maximal benefit.

Second, just as with most other treatments, there is a need for more research on how to generalize treatment effects beyond the treatment setting. Many aspects of the STP are implemented to help ensure that the STP is the first step of a long-term intervention to help the child. Parents are included in the child's treatment as much as possible through daily meetings with the child's counselors and weekly parenting meetings that they are required to attend. Similarly, a DRC is developed for each child that can be easily adapted to the child's natural classroom after that STP. Further, we offer children's teachers considerable information about the STP (including a free tour of the STP) to increase the chance that the children's teachers implement effective behavioral treatments routinely in their classroom. In addition, many of the treatments provided in the STP (e.g., social reinforcement, time-out, point systems, etc.) are widely employed in home and school settings and therefore immediately generalize to these settings. The STP provides parents and teachers an excellent opportunity to refine the procedures they use when implementing these treatments. Further evaluation of these efforts in helping children maintain treatment gains that result from the STP would be both interesting and useful.

Finally, evaluation of the cost-effectiveness of the STP would be useful. A key consideration in implementing any intensive treatment such as the STP is whether it offers sufficient supplemental effectiveness (beyond more traditional interventions) to justify its use. The costs of conducting the STP, including comprehensive follow up for 1 year, ranges from US $ 3000 to US $ 5000 (in U.S. dollars) per child (19). This is roughly the same cost as 1 year of weekly individual outpatient therapy sessions. For the same cost, we believe that available evidence strongly supports the effectiveness of the STP over traditional outpatient therapy. Further, if the STP is effective in partially or wholly ameliorating the long-term negative outcomes associated with ADHD, the cost of the STP will be more than justified. Indeed, the incremental costs associated with ADHD have been conservatively estimated at US $ 14,576 per year (34). If participation in the STP leads to less use of special education services, less contact with the juvenile justice system, less use of medication, or less use of residential treatment services, then these costs would be considerably reduced. In light of these arguments, further examination of the cost-effectiveness of the STP seems warranted.

SUMMARY

Intensive summer day treatment is an effective approach for treating children with ADHD. Children are treated in their natural environments using a variety of interventions that have been demonstrated to be effective for children with ADHD and other disruptive behavior problems. Data from the STP suggests that children and families are likely to stay in treatment, are satisfied at the end of treatment, and show significant improvement on symptoms of ADHD and related impairments. Such effects are unique among treatments for child psychopathology and indicate that the STP approach to treating ADHD is one of the most effective available.

REFERENCES

1. MTA Cooperative Group. A 14-month randomized clinical trial of treatment strategies for attention-deficit/hyperactivity disorder. Arch Gen Psychiatry 1999; 56:1073–86.

2. Pelham WE, Gnagy EM, Greiner AR. Children's Summer Day Treatment Program Manual. Buffalo, NY: CTADD, 1998.
3. Pelham WE, Bender ME. Peer relationships in hyperactive children: description and treatment. In: Gadow K, Bailer I, eds. Advances in Learning and Behavioral Disabilities. Greenwich, CT: JAI, 1982:365–436.
4. Hoza B, Gerdes AC, Mrug S, et al. Peer-assessed outcomes in the Multimodal Treatment Study of Children with Attention Deficit Hyperactivity Disorder. J Clin Child Adolesc 2005; 34:74–86.
5. Bierman KL, Wargo JB. Predicting the longitudinal course associated with aggressive-rejected, aggressive (nonrejected), and rejected (nonaggressive) status. Dev Psychopathol 1995; 7:669–82.
6. Lahey BB, Green KD, Forehand R. On the independence of ratings of hyperactivity, conduct problems, and attention deficits in children: a multiple regression analysis. J Consult Clin Psychol 1980; 48:566–74.
7. Pope AW, Bierman KL. Predicting adolescent peer problems and antisocial activities: the relative roles of aggression and dysregulation. Dev Psychol 1999; 35:335–46.
8. Waschbusch DA, Willoughby MT, Pelham WE. Criterion validity and the utility of reactive and proactive aggression: Comparisons to Attention deficit hyperactivity disorder, oppositional defiant disorder, conduct disorder, and other measures of functioning. Journal of Clinical Child Psychology 1998; 27 (4):396–405.
9. Atkins MS, Pelham WE, Licht MH. The differential validity of teacher ratings of inattention/overactivity and aggression. J Abnorm Child Psychol 1989; 17: 423–35.
10. Hartup WW, Stevens N. Friendships and adaptation across the life course. Psychol Bull 1997; 121:355–70.
11. Parker JG, Asher SR. Peer relations and later personal adjustment: are low-accepted children at risk? Psychol Bull 1987; 102:357–89.
12. Pelham WE, Milich R. Peer relations in children with hyperactivity/attentions deficit disorder. J Learn Disabil 1984; 17:560–7.
13. Pelham WE, Schnedler RW, Bender ME, et al. The combination of behavior therapy and methylphenidate in the treatment of attention deficit disorders: a therapy outcome study. In: Bloomingdale L, ed. Attention Deficit Disorders III: New Research in Attention, Treatment, and Psychopharmacology. London: Pergamon, 1988:29–48.
14. Whalen CK, Henker B, Swanson JM, Granger D, Kliewer W, Spencer J. Natural social behavior in hyperactive children: dose effects of methylphenidate. J Consult Clin Psychol 1987; 55:187–93.
15. Whalen CK, Henker B. Social impact of stimulant treatment for hyperactive children. J Learn Disabil 1991; 24:231–41.
16. Martin G, Pear J. Behavior Modification: What It Is and How to Do It. 5th ed. Upper Saddle River, NJ: Prentice-Hall, 1996.
17. Kazdin AE. Combined and multimodal treatment in child and adolescent psychotherapy: issues, challenges, and research directions. Clin Psychol: Sci Pract 1996; 3:69–100.

18. Pelham WE, Murphy A. Attention deficit and conduct disorders. In: Hersen M, ed. Pharmacological and Behavioral Treatment: An Integrative Approach. New York: Wiley, 1986:108–48.
19. Pelham WE, Hoza B. Intensive treatment: a summer treatment program for children with ADHD. In: Hibbs E, Jensen PS, eds. Psychosocial Treatments for Child and Adolescent Disorders: Empirically Based Strategies for Clinical Practice. New York: APA Press, 1996:311–40.
20. Kazdin AE, Marciano PL. Childhood and adolescent depression. In: Mash EJ, Barkley RA, eds. Treatment of Childhood Disorders. 2nd ed. New York: Guilford Press, 1998:211–48.
21. Kazdin A. Current treatments. In: Conduct Disorders in Childhood and Adolescence. New York: Sage, 1995:75–98.
22. Waschbusch DA. How do children with ADHD think in social situations and what does it tell us about treatment? In: Center for Children and Families, Buffalo, NY: University at Buffalo, 2004.
23. Pelham WE, Gnagy EM, Greiner AR, et al. Behavioral vs. behavioral and pharmacological treatment in ADHD children attending a summer treatment program. J Abnorm Child Psychol 2000; 28:507–25.
24. Pelham WE, Burrows-Maclean L, Gnagy EM, et al. Behavioral, pharmacological, and combined treatment for children with ADHD. In: Annual Meeting of the American Psychological Association, Chicago, IL, 2002.
25. Pelham WE, Hoza B, Pillow DR, et al. Effects of methylphenidate and expectancy on children with ADHD: behavior, academic performance, and attributions in a Summer Treatment Program and regular classroom setting. J Consult Clin Psychol 2002; 70:320–35.
26. Chronis AM, Fabiano GA, Gnagy EM, et al. An evaluation of the summer treatment program for children with ADHD using a treatment withdrawal design. Behav Ther 2004; 35:561–85.
27. Coles EK, Pelham WE, Gnagy EM, et al. A controlled evaluation of behavioral treatment with children with ADHD attending a summer treatment program. J Emot Behav Disord 2005; 13:99–112.
28. Fabiano GA, Pelham WE, Gnagy EM, Burrows-MacLean L, Coles EK, Chacko A, Wymbs BT, Walker KS, Arnold F, Garefino A, et al. The single and combined effects of multiple intensities of behavior modification and multiple intensities of methylphenidate in a classroom setting. School Psychology Review, 36:195–26.
29. Pelham WE, Burrows-MacLean L, Coles EK, Wymbs BT, Chacko A, Walker KS, et al. A dose ranging study of behavioral and pharmacological treatment for children with ADHD. In: Paper presented at the Association for Advancement of Behavior Therapy. Boston, MA, November 2003.
30. Burrows-MacLean L, Pelham WE, Coles EK, Wymbs BT, Chacko A, Walker KS, et al. Behavioral and pharmacological treatment for children with ADHD in the home setting. In: Paper presented at the Association for Advancement of Behavior Therapy. Boston, MA, November 2003.
31. Barkley RA. Behavioral inhibition, sustained attention, and executive functions: constructing a unified theory of ADHD. Psychol Bull 1997; 121:65–94.

32. Schachar RJ, Mota V, Logan G, Tannock R, Klim P. Confirmation of an inhibitory control deficit in Attention-Deficit/Hyperactivity Disorder. J Abnorm Child Psychol 2000; 28:227–35.
33. Fabiano GA, Pelham WE, Manos M, et al. An evaluation of three time out procedures for children with attention-deficit/hyperactivity disorder. Behav Ther 2004; 35:449–69.
34. Pelham WE, Foster EM, Robb JA. The economic impact of Attention-Deficit/Hyperactivity Disorder in children and adolescents. Ambul Pediatr 2007; 7:121–31.

20

ADHD: Organizing and Financing Services

Abram Rosenblatt and Lisa Hilley
Department of Psychiatry, University of California San Francisco, San Francisco, California, U.S.A.

Mental disorders among children and adolescents constitute a serious public health and public policy problem in the United States. One in five children and adolescents has some level of impairment associated with a specific diagnosis, and the majority of these young people receive no mental health care (1). The delivery of mental health services to children and adolescents is complicated by the range of settings, including schools, juvenile justice, social welfare, and primary care, in which these youth may access and receive care. The most commonly diagnosed childhood psychiatric disorder is attention deficit hyperactivity disorder (ADHD), which is estimated to affect 3–5% of school age children (1–3). ADHD receives relatively more public attention than other mental disorders among children in part because it is more prevalent, in part because of well-publicized treatment controversies regarding the use of stimulants, and in part because of the impact of ADHD on the broader education and primary healthcare systems. This chapter examines the financing and organization of services to children and adolescents with ADHD from the perspective of current trends in children's mental health services research.

SYSTEMIC REFORMS AND EMPIRICALLY SUPPORTED TREATMENTS

Research on the organization, financing, and delivery of children's mental health services is currently dominated by two movements (4): (*i*) The systems of care philosophy and approach to service delivery (5) and (*ii*) The implementation and development of evidence-based or evidence-supported practices (6,7). Although these two sets of approaches developed independently out of different traditions, methods, and philosophies, they are increasingly becoming interrelated for scientific, pragmatic, and political purposes. The systems of care approach focuses largely on how to more effectively organize and finance services for youth who have severe emotional disturbance often involving multiple diagnosis (5), including ADHD as one of the more prevalent primary or secondary diagnoses (8). The system of care approach is, at its core, a systemic, policy-oriented change in the structure and delivery of services. Systems of care place a special emphasis on linkages between child-serving agencies such as mental health, juvenile justice, social welfare, and education, on community-based care in lieu of restrictive placements, on developing a continuum of services, and, in some cases, on measuring the costs and outcomes of care.

The term "systems of care" is part of the child, and often now adult, mental health lexicon, used both with and without any particular meanings or definitions in many states and localities to describe service systems and sometimes even programs or practice approaches. The growth in systems of care is remarkable and can only be considered a tremendous success in terms of its popularity across the United States. This growth occurred even in the context of equivocal findings regarding the effectiveness of these reforms (1,9,10).

Unlike systems of care, empirically based and supported treatments grew out of academic research centers and professional organizations. Empirically supported treatments (ESTs) exist predominantly at the practice level of service delivery. The American Academy of Pediatrics (11) and the American Academy of Child and Adolescent Psychiatry (12) followed the medical pharmaceutical (MP) model (13) utilizing efficacy treatment outcome findings and the consensus conference model (researchers and practitioners meetings to deliberate best practices) to reach agreement on practice guidelines and parameters.

Treatments are first developed in a university laboratory to assess the efficacy of the intervention and later implemented in the field to assess the effectiveness or public health impact. Using randomized controlled trials (RCTs), researchers work to isolate the utility of a treatment in direct comparison to an alternative treatment approach. RCTs can afford a unique opportunity to determine the efficacy of a treatment, the probability that the intervention will generate positive change under ideal circumstances (14). Treatments evaluated as efficacious within the context of an RCT earn the labels, "evidence-based practice" or EST. Pharmacological, psychosocial, and multimodal (15) treatments, which combine pharmacological and psychosocial interventions, have been studied using the MP model with regard to ADHD. Evidence-based or supported treatments constitute the backbone of academic research in mental health service delivery, though they traditionally have not been particularly popular methods of service delivery in community settings. This situation is rapidly changing, however, as NIH and other funding sources began to lay out roadmaps for bridging science, practice, and translational research (16).

Research on children with ADHD tends to focus largely in the arena of empirically based and supported treatments and their efficacy and effectiveness, with less attention to the questions of access or equity and efficiency or cost that constitute a primary focus of the systems of care approach. Although there is a growing body of research evidence for diagnosis based and increasingly sophisticated treatment approaches for ADHD, significant barriers to service delivery clearly exist. There is only the most limited information pertaining to how services can best be financed and organized to provide efficient and equitable services to youth with ADHD.

FINANCING SERVICES FOR ADHD

The U.S. Surgeon General (1) placed the overall cost of mental illness at $ 69 billion in 1996. Costs of childhood-specific disorders are not well documented; however Hinshaw et al. (17) place the estimated costs for ADHD treatment for children diagnosed with ADHD to be about 3.5 to 4.0 billion dollars. The researchers note that this figure is likely a low estimate as it only accounts for children eligible for special education services. Based on Medicaid data, the average reimbursement for total treatment costs of a child with ADHD in 1999 was estimated at $ 1795 and this disorder was the most common diagnosis for privately insured children. To date, the direct and indirect cost to society for ADHD has not been calculated. There is only limited research regarding the cost of ADHD to individuals, systems (e.g., education, foster care, health care, juvenile justice), or society (e.g., employment loss, disruption to families).

Estimating the treatment costs for ADHD is made more difficult due to the complexity of public and private mental health coverage and ongoing changes in how services are financed. Private health insurance remains problematic with regard to funding children's mental health services. Private health insurance is usually limited and will not cover long-term or more intensive treatment needs and typically limits access to mental health services. An increasing emphasis on managed care has resulted in attempts at "cost-effective" services by reducing inpatient hospitalizations and increased use of short-term therapies.

Within the public sector, access to and availability of services varies by location and type of payer. The federal Medicaid program is the primary mechanism for funding public mental health services to children and adolescents. In 1989 opportunities for accessing the federal Medicaid program increased significantly through the expansion of the Early Periodic

Screening, Diagnosis and Treatment (EPSDT) program (Omnibus Budget Reconciliation Act of 1989 [PL 101-239]). Most states have expanded their Medicaid Services through EPSDT; however, rules and regulations regarding EPSDT and Medicaid remain complicated and also are subject to change. In addition, states must provide matching funds to Medicaid, effectively limiting the degree to which states choose to participate in the program.

Accessing other public funds outside of Medicaid to provide mental health services is often possible; though doing so requires joint planning and may require federal waivers. Child welfare entitlement funds, for example, including Title IV-A, IV-B, and IV-E can be utilized to provide mental health services, particularly those who are at risk for separation from their families through out-of-home placement. Many states have become creative in utilizing a range of public funding sources to provide mental health services because of limitations to Medicaid funding and the joint public responsibility across public agencies of many youth with behavioral disorders. Nonetheless, funding restrictions in the public sector along with limited mental health coverage in the private sector lead to large numbers of youth not receiving mental health services as well as considerable variability across states with regard to access.

Historically, the schools have been considered a primary potential arena for providing mental health services, particularly for youth with ADHD which has a direct negative impact on educational attainment. Many children do receive services as a result of the Individuals with Disability Education Act (IDEA) passed in 1975, which mandates schools to provide services to children whose disability interferes with their education. Schools are legally obligated to evaluate all children suspected of having a disability. Under this federal law, services are also mandated for preschool age children. For those determined to be eligible for services, schools must provide appropriate and free special education and related services to meet each child's unique needs. Changes to the IDEA in 1991 broadened eligibility criteria to include children diagnosed with ADHD. The majority of eligible children diagnosed with ADHD are classified as "other health impaired," (18). Some children with ADHD who have coexisting problems may meet eligibility criteria under "learning disability, developmental delay," or "emotional disturbance" categories. Very recently in 2005, the most recent reauthorization of IDEA changed the name to the Individuals with Disabilities Education Improvement Act (IDEIA) that continued to alter criteria for eligibility. Finally, other federal legislation such as No Child Left Behind potentially intersects with IDEIA in how local districts and schools make decisions regarding authorizing and providing services (19).

Under the IDEAs requirements, states must ensure that schools identify and evaluate children suspected of having ADHD in public and private schools. States are obligated to provide "free appropriate public education" to eligible children with ADHD. Additionally, states must develop and implement an Individualized Education Plan (IEP), which includes educational goals and recommended behavioral interventions. Under this federal law, states are mandated to include parents in the process and to make every effort to keep children in a regular classroom environment.

States and school districts have a great deal of discrepancy in how they provide "free appropriate education" services to eligible children. All children who need services do not receive them. The U.S. Department of Education reported in 2004 that approximately 11.5% of school-aged children receive special education services. This is below the 20% estimates of the number of youth who receive psychiatric diagnoses and have sufficient impairment to require services. Many school systems are not prepared to provide direct services, some states have contracted services to county agencies. Several potential problems arise in the context of multiple agency involvement and current federal and state budget crises (19). As a result of contractual services, there often is a lack of clarity regarding who should provide the services and how these services should be monitored and evaluated.

The state of California is one example of increasing tensions between community agencies required to provide services and a decreasing state budget for mental health and special education services, often leaving mental health agencies with budgetary deficits. A recent superior court (July 2004) decision ruled in favor of several counties so they would not be mandated to provide services without adequate state funding. The public policy debate in California, as in many states, is ongoing regarding whether services mandated under IDEA should be funded and delivered by mental health, education, state, federal, or local sources.

In theory, the addition of ADHD services under the IDEA, would have the potential to: (1) address this prevalent disorder within a system that is convenient for children and families, (2) increase the number of qualified and trained educators to address the needs of children diagnosed with ADHD, and (3) provide integrated services, which would allow for attention to academic, behavioral, and emotional functioning. In practice, local communities often do not have adequately trained staff, or enough monetary or physical resources to address mental health needs for students. Thus, services available within one school district or state may be difficult to obtain in another.

The Youth and Education Law Clinic at Stanford Law School conducted an evaluation of California's mental health delivery system to special education students (Challenge and Opportunity, May, 2004). In California, these services are provided through government code, Chapter 26.5, which created an interagency system to address the needs of special education students throughout the state. The report concluded that "Although parents and teachers are looked to as the primary stakeholders responsible for identification and referral for Chapter 26.5 services, they may be ill-equipped to do so" (p. 39). The authors indicated several potential barriers to accessing services including shortage of appropriate school-based locations, lack of transportation to off-site services, and inconvenient appointment scheduling. Problems with accountability and responsibility for following special education plans (IEP plans) for students were also highlighted. There appears to be an inconsistent monitoring of actual service delivery for students, even those who may have outlined educational plans for ADHD services and no formal structured evaluation of the quality or effectiveness of the services.

The Stanford report highlights the detrimental impacts of federal, state, and county budget crises on the delivery of services to those most in need: "In the face of inadequate funding, eligibility criteria for Chapter 26.5 services are "narrowed" and the number of open slots and the types of services available are reduced. As a result, those students with less serious and/or less obvious mental health problems may go without any services at all, while others may receive services that are not appropriately tailored to individual needs" (p. 40).

Many of the potential barriers identified for mental health services in general also apply to children and adolescents in need of services for ADHD referred through the schools. For example, problems accessing appropriate and effective treatment, lack of transportation, limited clinic hours and no school-based services, differences between community mental health and educators regarding the importance of or approach to mental health problems, and difficulties with insurance coverage all impact delivering services to youth with ADHD.

Budget cuts have been a significant problem in providing the full range of services to special education students. In the context of extreme budget crises, parents may have even more difficulty navigating the system and obtaining the best services available. The authors conclude that "the system bears the full cost of providing the services, but students often do not receive or benefit from the services being provided" (p. 61, Challenge and Opportunity).

Children with disabilities who are determined not to be eligible for special education services under IDEA may still be protected and served under two other federal laws: Section 504 of the Rehabilitation Act of 1973 (Section 504) and the Americans with Disabilities Act of 1990 (ADA). The Office for Civil Rights in the U.S. Department of Education enforces the provisions of Section 504 and Title II of the ADA with respect to school districts, while the Department of Education administers IDEA.

Section 504 of the Rehabilitation Act of 1973 is a civil rights law designed to eliminate discrimination on the basis of disability in any program or activity receiving federal financial assistance (REFS). Eligibility for Section 504 is based on the existence of an identified physical or mental impairment that substantially limits a major life activity. Thus, ADHD symptoms must significantly impact a child's learning or behavior (National Resource Center on ADHD) appropriate accommodation for a student with a disability under Section 504 could entail education in regular classrooms, education in regular classrooms with supplementary services, modifications and/or accommodations, special education, and related services or any combination. Local school districts typically implement the provisions of Section 504; however, ultimate responsibility for enforcing these provisions resides with the Office of Civil Rights (OCR) of the U.S. Department of Education.

ORGANIZATION: STRUCTURING THE DELIVERY OF SERVICES FOR ADHD

ADHD services are delivered within broader systems that are structured and organized based in part, though not entirely, on how they are financed. There are many examples of systemic reform in health services. For example, managed care is predominantly a reform that occurs at the system level, where fiscal changes (such as capitation) and structural changes (such as utilization review) are put in place to provide more efficient service delivery. Over the past decade, systemic reform in the delivery of children's mental health services has been promulgated largely through the system of care approach (5). The system of care model emphasizes many systems-level alterations including: developing linkages between child-serving agencies (e.g., mental health, juvenile justice, child welfare, and education), using community-based care in lieu of restrictive placements, developing a continuum of services, restructuring service financing (i.e., blended funding pools), and creating interagency policy and treatment teams for coordinated care.

Two primary realities drive the need for considering systems factors in providing services to youth with ADHD: (1) As already described, services for ADHD are currently funded through multiple public agencies, especially the schools, primary health care, and specialty mental health services, requiring creative interagency strategies for assembling viable funding strategies; and (2) ADHD is often comorbid with other psychiatric disorders and results in a diverse range of problems in daily functioning, requiring collaborative approaches across agencies.

Comorbidity and the negative consequences of ADHD lead these youth to interact with other service sectors outside of mental health. Children with ADHD may have difficulty with working memory, organization, planning, problem-solving, motivation, social skills, emotion regulation, insight, rule-governed behavior, volition, will power, self-discipline, and even sense of time (2, 20–22). ADHD, therefore, puts children at risk for a variety of problems, including school failure, social rejection, antisocial behavior, substance abuse, psychiatric disorders including anxiety and depression, and involvement with the juvenile justice system (21). Approximately 50% of children diagnosed with ADHD also meet diagnostic criteria for conduct disorder or oppositional-defiant disorder (ODD) (2,23).

Clearly, youth with ADHD typically have problems in school, may be involved in the juvenile justice system, and may also be subject to abuse and neglect and consequently be involved with the social welfare system. ADHD does pose particular challenges for service delivery systems. Outside the school system, the majority of children diagnosed with ADHD are being treated by primary care physicians (3,24). Understanding service system delivery issues for youth with ADHD requires an understanding of how medications are delivered.

Stein and Orlando (3) report that increasingly a psychiatrist is responsible for medication management and other mental health professionals provide behavioral treatment. The researchers suggest that this change is a direct result of managed care policies to reduce the higher costs of psychiatrists by limiting their role. Recently researchers examined data from two national surveys to compare trends in the use of psychotropic medication for children over a 10-year period (1987 to 1996) (25). Olfson and colleagues (25) reported that stimulant medication use was four times higher in 1996 compared to 1987, with the exception that children without insurance were much less likely to use stimulant medication. Also, children from higher income families were more than twice as likely to receive ADHD services compared to children from low-income families in 1987, but no differences were found in 1997, suggesting an increase in public insurance expenditures for treatment of ADHD (25). The data from this study suggests that uninsured children may not have the same access to psychotropic treatments for ADHD.

Olfson et al. (18) reported a significant increase in outpatient treatment for ADHD between 1987 and 1997. The increased rate in treatment over the specified decade was greater for boys than girls and for older children (12 to 18 years) compared to younger children (3 to 11 years) (18). Also, Caucasian children were twice as likely to receive treatment as Hispanic or African-American children. Despite research findings suggesting positive treatment effects for behavioral approaches for ADHD, Olfson and colleagues (18) report a significant decrease in the number of treatment visits, with only a minority of children receiving psychotherapy as a treatment for ADHD. The researchers estimate that children who received psychotherapy received three fewer visits in 1997 than in 1987, which is likely a result of restrictions from managed care organizations.

Overall, physicians, rather than psychologists or other health care professionals, served as the provider for the majority of children treated for

ADHD. For the 1997 survey data, roughly one-third of children diagnosed with ADHD received special education services (18). The authors outlined several factors that may have influenced the increased use of ADHD services from 1987 to 1997. The inclusion of ADHD (as other health impaired) under the IDEA increased the number of students eligible for special education services and likely increased attention on ADHD in schools and school-based mental health programs. The public awareness of ADHD has led to the development of parent groups, community resources, and advocacy organizations (18).

BUILDING AND BLENDING SYSTEMS AND CLINICAL INTERVENTIONS: SPECIAL CONSIDERATIONS FOR ADHD

From the perspective of financing and organizing service systems, ADHD is similar to other disorders found in childhood such as conduct and ODD, depression, and anxiety. Because children live in complex social systems that include schools, parents, and potentially other service agencies, the coordination of varying service sectors remains both complex and essential to providing access to services and to providing mechanisms for treatment. ADHD is, however, unique in two primary ways that pose challenges for the financing and organization of services.

First, ADHD has more direct and immediate consequences on school performance that are often evident earlier in life when compared to other childhood psychiatric disorders. Consequently, many youth with ADHD receive special education services (18). Second, youth with ADHD also receive medication and though there remains considerable controversy regarding whether medication is appropriately prescribed, there is clear evidence that medication can provide reductions in symptoms and improvements in functioning, especially when combined with psychosocial interventions (15). Youth may receive medication at relatively young ages, including elementary school. Though medication may be helpful for other psychiatric disorders (especially depression and anxiety), they are relatively less frequently used, particularly for younger children and the evidence for effectiveness is not as strong (25).

The direct impacts of ADHD on school performance have lead states to experiment with innovative strategies to provide effective ADHD services to children under the IDEA. For example, the Kentucky Department of Education has included instructional strategies, accommodations, and modifications in their training programs and publications, implemented a behavior Web site with detailed information on ADHD, and developed an annual conference on ADHD. This information is designed to ensure that students with disabilities are able to participate in the general curriculum. The state of Tennessee sponsored an expert-led workshop for teachers to address ADHD topics including identification, evaluation, medication, parent training, social skills, classroom strategies, assessment, and intervention. Similarly, the West Virginia Department of Education has sponsored teacher trainings on the specifics of the IDEA and on state regulations for special education. These are just a few examples of state-based programs to inform educators and families on the laws and regulations, individual rights, and resources available to students with ADHD.

The use of stimulants for youth with ADHD raises numerous concerns regarding access to appropriate health care and particularly psychiatric care. In 2006, over 8 million children (about 11% of the total number of children in the United States) did not have any form of health insurance. Access to specialty mental health care is limited, with over three quarters of those youth with mental disorders not receiving any services from specialty providers (26). The shortage of child psychiatrist, particularly in rural areas, is well-documented. Family practitioners are less likely to provide adequate quality of care. Consequently, providing access to high-quality medical care and medication management for youth with ADHD is a major challenge.

EMPIRICALLY SUPPORTED TREATMENTS?

This chapter began by noting that ESTs are one of the two dominant trends in mental health services research for children and adolescents. Since that point, the majority of the chapter focused on organizational and financing concerns. Optimally, ESTs and innovations in the organization and financing of services are both essential components to providing equitable, efficient, and effective services (4). Historically, many ESTs were not tested in the community, and many reforms in systems structure did not consider clinical innovations developed in academic centers. This situation is rapidly changing as service reform efforts based in the community are embracing ESTs and these treatments are, in turn, being tested in the community. The relationships between community-based services, systems reform, and empirically based treatments are complex and the understanding of their interrelationships is undergoing considerable analysis (27).

The full scope of such discussions is beyond this chapter. However, many psychosocial interventions for youth with ADHD are community based in that they exist in part or in whole within schools. Schools are the primary system impacting on youth with ADHD, however these youth are also potentially subject to how services are financed and organized within the primary health care, juvenile probation, and even social welfare sectors. Ultimately, the delivery of effective services to youth with ADHD will rest on how services are organized and financed. Conversely, in an optimal system the organization and financing of services can be driven by those treatments that have empirical support. To this point, there is no evidence that the organization and financing of services to youth with ADHD promotes effective services. There is, however, discouraging evidence that access, equity, and efficiency are also not promoted by current organizational and systemic factors. The considerable progress in understanding how to provide more effective services to youth with ADHD has not been mirrored by similar progress in the financing and organization of services, and that ultimately will significantly hamper how many youth receive any services, let alone high quality or empirically supported care.

REFERENCES

1. U.S. Department of Health and Human Services. Children and Mental Health, in Mental Health: A Report of the Surgeon General, chap. 3. Rockville: MD: US Public Health Service, 1999.
2. Kutcher S, Aman M, Brooks SJ, et al. International consensus statement on attention-deficit/hyperactivity disorder (ADHD) and disruptive behavioral disorders (DBDs): clinical implications and treatment practice suggestions. Eur Neuropsychopharmacol 2004; 14:11–28.
3. Stein B, Orlando M. ADHD treatment in a behavioral health care carve-out: medications, providers, and service utilization. J Behav Health Ser Res 2001; 28:30–41.
4. Rosenblatt A, Compian L. Exchanging glances? Systems, practice and evidence in children's mental health services. In: Fisher WH, ed. Research in Community and Mental Health, Vol. 14—Research on Community Based Mental Health Services for Children and Adolescents: Oxford, UK. Elsevier, 2007.
5. Stroul BA, Friedman RM. The system of care concept and philosophy. In: Stroul BA, ed. Children's Mental Health: Creating Systems of Care in a Changing Society. Baltimore, MD: Paul H. Brookes Publishing, 1996.
6. Chambless DL, Ollendick TH. Empirically supported psychological interventions: controversies and evidence. Annu Rev Psychol 2001; 52:685–716.
7. Kazdin AE. Evidence-based treatments: challenges and priorities for practice and research. Child Adoles Psychiatr Clin N Am 2004; 13:923–40 [special issue].
8. Rosenblatt A, Rosenblatt J. Demographic, clinical and functional characteristics of youth enrolled in six California systems of care. J Child Fam Studies 2000; 9:51–66.
9. Rosenblatt A. Assessing the child and family outcomes of systems of care for youth with severe emotional disturbance. In: Epstein MH, Kutash K, Duchnowski A, eds. Outcomes for Children and Youth with Emotional and Behavioral Disorders and their Families: Programs and Evaluation Best Practices. Austin, TX: PRO-ED, 1998:329–62.
10. Farmer EMZ. Issues confronting effective services in systems of care. Child Youth Ser Rev 2000; 22:627–50.
11. American Academy of Pediatrics. Pediatric Clinical Practice Guidelines and Policies. 5th ed. Washington, DC: American Academy of Pediatrics. 2005.
12. American Academy of Child and Adolescent Psychiatry (n.d.). Practice parameters. Retrieved October 11, 2005 from American Academy of Child and Adolescent Psychiatry web site http://www.aacap.org/clinical/parameters/index.htm.

13. Greewald P, Cullen JW. The scientific approach to cancer control. CA Cancer J Clin 1984; 34:328–32.
14. Weisz JR, Jensen AL. Child and adolescent psychotherapy in research and practice contexts: review of the evidence and suggestions for improving the field. Eur Child Adolesc Psychiatry 2001; 10:12–8.
15. MTA Collaborative Group. A 14 Month Randomized Clinical Trial of Treatment Strategies for Attention Deficit Hyperactivity Disorder. Anaheim, CA: American Academy of Child and Adolescent Psychiatry, 1998.
16. National Advisory Mental Health Council. Bridging Science and Service: A Report By the National Advisory Mental Health Council's Clinical Treatment and Services Research Workgroup. Bethesda, MD: National Institute of Mental Health, 1999.
17. Hinshaw S, Peele P, Danielson L. Public Health Issues in ADHD: Individual, System, and Cost Burden of the Disorder. Workshop. Atlanta: National Center on Birth Defects and Developmental Disabilities, 1999.
18. Olfson M, Gameroff MJ, Marcus SC, Jensen PS. National trends in the treatment of attention deficit hyperactivity disorder. Am J Psychiatry 2003; 160: 1071–7.
19. Pearrow M, Whelley P. School based mental health services for children and adolescents. In: Fisher WH, ed. Research in Community and Mental Health, Vol. 14—Research on Community Based Mental Health Services for Children and Adolescents: Oxford, UK. Elsevier, 2007.
20. Castellanos X. Toward a pathophysiology of attention-deficit/hyperactivity disorder. Clin Pediatr 1997; 36:381–93.
21. Goldman L, Genel M, Bezman R, Slanetz P, for the Council on Scientific Affairs of the American Medical Association. Council report: diagnosis and treatment of attention-deficit/hyperactivity disorder in children and adolescents. J Am Med Assoc 1998; 279:1100–7.
22. Pennington B. Diagnosing Learning Disorders: A Neuropsychological Framework. New York: The Guilford Press, 1991.
23. Angold A, Costelo EJ, Erkanli A. Comorbidity. J Child Psychol Psychiatry 1999; 40:57–87.
24. Zarin DA, Tanielian TL, Suarez AP, et al. Treatment of attention-deficit hyperactivity disorder by different physician specialties. Psychiatr Serv 1998; 49:171.
25. Olfson M, Marcus SC, Weissman MM, Jensen PS. National trends in the use of psychotropic medications by children. J Am Acad Child Adolesc Psychiatry 2002; 41:514–21.
26. Bruns EJ, Burchard JD, Yoe JT. Evaluating the Vermont system of care: outcomes associated with community-based wraparound services. J Child Fam Studies 1995; 4:321–39.
27. Weisz JR, Jensen-Doss A, Hawley KM. Evidence-based youth psychotherapies versus usual care: a meta-analysis of direct comparisons. Am Psychol 2006; 61: 671–89.

21

Principles of Medication Titration

Steven R. Pliszka

Division of Child and Adolescent Psychiatry, University of Texas Health Science Center at San Antonio, San Antonio, Texas, U.S.A.

INTRODUCTION

The previous chapter outlined the wide variety of medications used in the treatment of attention deficit hyperactivity disorder (ADHD) and discussed their classification as first or second line agents. This chapter will focus on the clinical use of these medications, particularly the titration of each agent to its optimal dosage for the patient. Here the science of medication treatment, as established by clinical trials of these agents, interacts with the art of clinical care where conclusions from averaged data in studies do not always apply to the individual patient. The physician must be flexible in the dosing strategy used, carefully balancing control of the symptoms of ADHD with minimization of side effects.

STIMULANTS

Stimulants are by far the most commonly used medications in the treatment of ADHD. The American Academy of Child and Adolescent Psychiatry has recently published guidelines for their clinical use (1). The National Institutes of Mental Health Multimodality Study of ADHD (MTA) study also provides valuable guidance for the titration of stimulant medication (2,3). In this study, children were randomized to one of four long-term treatment groups: community controls, medication management, psychosocial intervention or combined treatment (medication management + psychosocial intervention). Those children in the two medication management groups received a double-blind placebo-controlled crossover trial of methylphenidate using the full range of methylphenidate doses (generally 0.3–1.0 mg/kg/dose). Teacher and parent ratings were obtained each week and blinded evaluators determined which dose of methylphenidate yielded the optimal response compared to the placebo week. This dose was selected for the child's long-term medication management. That dose was then adjusted at monthly medication visits. In contrast, those community controls treated with medication had more variable follow-up and no set titration of stimulant. At follow-up one year later, those in the medication management group had a significantly better outcome than those in the community control group (4). Children in the medication management group who received a significantly higher mean daily dose of methylphenidate, were more likely to receive a third, afternoon dose of methylphenidate, and received higher individual doses than those in the community control group (4,5).

These data suggest that doses commonly used in clinical practice (generally about 0.3 mg/kg/dose) may be too low to achieve full remission of ADHD symptoms. Typically, physicians will place a patient on a low-starting dose and schedule a follow-up within the first month of treatment. At this visit, the parent is usually queried about the child's progress. If the parent and physician are satisfied with the response, no further dose adjustment is made. The possibility that a higher dose of stimulant might lead to even greater improvement is not explored. The MTA study suggests that higher doses of stimulant should be administered if there is not near-complete remission of ADHD symptoms with the starting dose. Table 1 adopts this philosophy. The child's weight establishes the starting dose; the response of the child to each dose is assessed over a 1–2 week period. This need not necessarily be at an office visit. The parent and teacher can be provided with standardized rating scales (6) to fill out assessing the child's behavior, and these can be faxed to the office along with a scale rating side effects (Table 2). The physician can review these scales and order a dose increase for the next week if the child's symptom ratings do not fall within the normative range (7). This process continues for each week until the maximum dose is reached. If resolution of ADHD symptoms is not satisfactory or side effects are prohibitive, the given stimulant is discontinued and an alternative stimulant is tried. In general at least two different classes of stimulants should be tried before moving to any of the non-stimulant alternatives.

The advent of long-acting stimulants has made the titration of stimulant medication much easier (Table 2). Studies show that the long-acting stimulants are equally efficacious as their immediate release forms (8–11) thus there is no need to titrate the patient to a full dose of immediate release before moving the patient to a long-acting form. Side effects must be monitored closely when higher doses are used for younger children, as shown by the italicized cells in Table 1. Note that Focalin, the pure dextro

Table 1 Titration of Immediate Release Stimulant Medications

d, l-Methylphenidate (Ritalin®)

	35–50 lbs	51–70 lbs	70–90 lbs	>90 lbs
Week 1–2	2.5 am/noon	5 mg am/noon	10 mg am/noon	10 mg am/noon
Week 2–4	5 mg am/noon	10 mg am/noon	15 mg am/noon	20 mg am/12 noon
Week 3–6	10 mg am/noon	15 mg am/noon	20 mg am/noon	20 mg am/12 noon
Week 7	*15 mg bid*	*20 mg bid*		

Add third dose after school if necessary up to a maximum of 60–80 mg day.
For d-methylphenidate (Focalin®), doses are 1/2 those of the above.

Dextro (75%)/Levo (25%) Amphetamine (Adderall®)
Dextro (100%) Amphetamine (Dexedrine®, Dextrostat®)

	35–50 lbs	51–70 lbs	70–90 lbs	>90 lbs
Week 1–2	2.5 am & noon	2.5 mg am & noon	5 mg q am & noon	7.5 q am & noon
Week 2–4	5 mg am & noon	5 mg q am & noon	7.5 mg q am & noon	10 mg q am & noon
Week 3–6	7.5 mg q am & noon	7.5 mg q am & noon	10 mg q am & noon	15 mg q am & noon
Week 7	*10 mg q am & noon*	*7.5 mg q am & noon*	*20 mg q am/ 10 mg q noon*	20 mg q am & noon to 30 mg bid

form of methylphenidate, is given in doses one-half that of mixed racemic methylphenidate. The dosing of mixed salts amphetamine (Adderall, Adderall-XR) is the same as the pure dextroamphetamine (Dexedrine, Dextrostat, and Dexedrine Spansule). Most recently, a methylphenidate transdermal patch (Daytrana) and an amphetamine pro-drug (lisdexamfetamine dimesylate, Vyvanse) (12) have been approved by the Food and Drug Administration for use in children aged 6–12 years. These agents also show an average duration of action of 10–12 hr; their dosing is shown in Table 2. Weight-based dosing is not known for these agents, thus a standard titration is used for all children. Caution is warranted when using these agents in preschoolers as no study data has been gathered in that age group.

As the dose is titrated, the physician should assess the side effects (adverse events) listed in Table 3. A direct inquiry about the most common side effects is better than an open-ended question as it is likely to jog the parents' memory. It is, however, important to assess the frequency of these "side effect" symptoms at baseline, since many ADHD children evidence

(Text continues on page 215.)

Table 2 Titration of Long Acting Stimulant Medications

Adderall® XR, Dexedrene Spansules

	35–50 lbs	51–70 lbs	70–90 lbs	>90 lbs
Week 1–2	5 mg q am	5 mg q am	10 mg q am	10 q am
Week 2–4	10 mg q am	10 mg q am	15 mg q am	15 mg q am
Week 3–6	15 mg q am	15 mg q am	20 mg q am/10 mg q noon	20 mg to 30 mg q am
Week 7	15 mg q am	20 mg qm	20–40 mg q am	30–60 mg q am

Vyvanse (lisdexafetamine dimesylate)

	35–50 lbs	>51 lbs
Week 1–2	Unknown	30 mg q am
Week 2–4	Unknown	50 mg q am
Week 3–6	Unknown	70 mg q noon

Vyvanse (lisdexafetamine dimesylate)

	35–50 lbs	>51–70 lbs
Week 1–2	Unknown	30 mg q am
Week 2–4	Unknown	50 mg q am
Week 3–6	Unknown	70 mg q am

Concerta (Give as am dose only, average 12 hr duration)

	35–50 lbs	51–70 lbs	70–90 lbs	>90 lbs
Week 1–2	18 mg	18 mg	36 mg	36 mg
Week 2–4	27–36 mg	27–36 mg	54 mg	54 mg
Week 3–6	54 mg	54–72 mg	72 mg	72–108 mg

Daytrana (methylphenidate transdermal system)

	>51 lbs
Week 1–2	10 mg q am
Week 2–4	20 mg q am
Week 3–6	30 mg q am

Metadate-CD/Ritalin LA (Give as am dose only, average 8 hr) duration

	35–50 lbs	51–70 lbs	70–90 lbs	>90 lbs
Week 1–2	Use IR first	20 mg	20 mg	20 mg
Week 2–4	20 mg	40 mg	40 mg	40 mg
Week 3–6				60 mg

Supplement with pm immediate release methylphenidate if after school dose needed.
Focalin XR use am doses appropimately 1/2 of the above

Table 3 Side Effect Questionnaire

Is your child having any of the problems listed below?	How bad is problem?			How has medication affected the problem?		
	None	Some	Very much	Made it worse	No change	Made it better
Poor appetite						
Trouble sleeping						
Sleepiness in day						
Stomach aches						
Constipation						
Diarrhea/loose bowels						
Headaches						
Rash						
Muscle twitches						
Nervousness						
Grouchy, more angry						
Withdrawn, stares, "zombie"						
OTHER:						

poor appetite and sleeping difficulties at baseline. It also important to ask if the parent feels the symptoms has been affected by the medication. Older children, adolescents, and adults can report on side effects themselves. Height (for children and adolescents), weight, blood pressure, and pulse should be monitored at each visit. Blood pressure and pulse are particularly important to monitor in adult patients who may have asymptomatic hypertension. No laboratory monitoring of hematological measures, serum chemistry or electrocardiogram is required during stimulant treatment.

Once the most optimal dose has been established during the initial trial, the dose should remain fairly stable over the long term, except when the child grows substantially. There is little evidence of tolerance to stimulant treatment within the dose ranges described in Table 1, several studies show continued effectiveness of medication after one year of continuous treatment (13,14). The maximum dose of stimulant to be given to a patient is much debated. Initial research with long-acting stimulants was carried out in school aged children, but recent controlled trials of stimulants have focused on adolescents (15,16) and adults (17,18). These studies in older individuals show response rates to stimulants similar to that of children. Adults have been successfully managed on up to 60 mg a day of amphetamine (19) and 70–100 mg a day of methylphenidate (20,21). Thus it is permissible to exceed the maximum dose limits prescribed by the *Physician's Desk Reference*. Indeed, if amphetamine is twice as potent as methylphenidate, a dose of

120 mg a day would need to be given to achieve equivalence of methylphenidate with 60 mg of amphetamine (22). Doses in this range should be used only with extreme caution; the physician should be particularly suspicious of the adult patient who claims to need higher and higher doses of stimulant at each visit, or who insists on needing 60–100 mg doses several times a day. Such a patient may be involved in diversion, or may be developing tolerance to the stimulant.

How frequently do patients on stimulant medication require follow-up? MTA patients were seen monthly, but it is not clear that face-to-face physician contact was a key variable in improving outcome. Rather, physicians had access to detailed rating scale data that allowed them to fine-tune the child's dosages. The number of follow-ups per year may range from 2 to 12 depending on a variety of factors: robustness of stimulant response, existence of other comorbid psychiatric or medical conditions, chronic treatment with other medications or presence of psychosocial stressors. The more complicating factors are present, follow-up should occur more frequently. Height (for children and adolescents) weight, blood pressure and pulse should be monitored at each visit. Blood pressure monitoring is important in adults who may have asymptomatic hypertension. There is no need to monitor serum chemistries, hematological indices or electrocardiogram unless a medical condition other than ADHD is present (23).

Atomoxetine

Atomoxetine (Strattera®) is a non-tricyclic norepinephrine re-uptake inhibitor which has been approved for the treatment of ADHD. It shows clear superiority over placebo in several double-blind parallel group studies (24–27). In the latter study, atomoxetine dosed once-a-day was superior to placebo in reducing both parent and teacher ratings of ADHD symptoms in children and adolescents aged 6–16 years. The effect size of atomoxetine was calculated to be 0.71 (27), compared to an effect size of 1.0 that is commonly seen in stimulant studies (28). Atomoxetine was comparable to methylphenidate in a open-label trial (29), but no teacher ratings were obtained in that study and the mean mg/kg/dose of methylphenidate was not specified. Thus it is not clear that atomoxetine is equally efficacious as stimulant medications. Nonetheless, the availability of a new non-stimulant for the treatment of ADHD is important, as it will be a valuable option for those who do not tolerate stimulant medications or who have comorbid substance abuse problems.

The starting dose of atomoxetine is 0.5 mg/kg/day given as a single AM dose for 3 days, and then increased over a 1-week period to a maximum of 1.2 mg/kg/day. Side effects are generally mild and most commonly consist of gastrointestinal complaints, decreased appetite and sedation. The dose can be divided twice a day (12 hr apart) for those who cannot tolerate a single daily dose or experience wearing off of the medication in the evening. For older adolescents and adults, the starting dose is 40 mg a day, increasing to 60 or 80 mg a day after the first week of treatment. Atomoxetine (Strattera®) comes in 10, 18, 25, and 40 mg capsules. It should be used with caution in persons taking medications which are metabolized by the 2D6 CYP 450 system. Since atomoxetine is an inhibitor of this system, the action of the other medications could be potentiated. Due to the emergence of suicidal ideation (but no completed suicides) in a small number of patients taking atomoxetine in the clinical trials, a boxed warning regarding suicidal thoughts as an adverse event is included in the package label (30).

Bupropion

Bupropion is agent which blocks the reuptake of dopamine; its metabolite blocks the reuptake of norepinephrine; it may also enhance the function of the noradrenergic system though mechanisms other than re-uptake blockade (31). Conners and colleagues (32) showed bupropion to be superior to placebo in the treatment of ADHD in children, though the effect size was lower than that seen in stimulant studies. Wilens et al. (33,34) showed bupropion to be efficacious in adults with ADHD. It is an effective second line agent for the treatment of ADHD. In children, its starting dose is 3 mg/kg/day in divided doses. After 2 weeks, its dose can be increased to 6 mg/kg/day or 300 mg/day, whichever is smaller. In adults or older adolescents the slow release or extended release form of bupropion is more convenient. The slow release form of 150 mg is given in the morning only for 3–5 days, after that it is given twice a day. The XL form is given once a day, and is available in 150 and 300 mg capsules.

Tricyclic Antidepressants

Tricyclic antidepressants (TCAs) were once the principle second–line agent after methylphenidate in the treatment of ADHD. With the advent of multiple stimulants, bupropion and atomoxetine, their use for the treatment of ADHD has declined considerably over the last decade. The TCA desipramine was associated with several cases of sudden death in children in the late 1980s (35,36), and while a causative relationship was never established, the use of desipramine for treating ADHD was effectively ended. Furthermore, the experience with desipramine lead to standards regarding electrocardiogram monitoring in any children treated with any other of the tricyclics (imipramine, nortriptyline). This had made their use cumbersome, but TCAs may still have uses in children who have not responded to stimulants and patients with comorbid tic disorders. In such patients, tricyclics will reduce tics as well as ADHD symptoms (37).

Imipramine is typically started at doses of 1 mg/kg/day in divided doses, with titration to doses of 2.0–2.5 mg/kg/day over a 1–2 week period. If the ADHD symptoms respond to this dose, no further titration is required. If there is non-response or an inadequate response, then the imipramine dose should be increased at a rate 1 mg/kg/day per week up to a maximum of 5.0 mg/kg/day. At doses above 2.0 mg/kg/day, serum levels should be obtained to document that the level has not exceeded 200 ng/mL. If the level is below the therapeutic level for depression treatment, but the ADHD symptoms have adequately responded, there is no need to raise the dose further. Once stable, blood levels and EKG should be repeated annually or whenever a dose adjustment is made. Nortriptyline is used in doses one-half that of imipramine.

During treatment with a TCA, resting heart rate should be less than 130 bpm, the PR interval less than 200 msec, the QRS interval should not be widened over 30% of the baseline value, and the QTc interval should be less than 460 msec (37). Most TCAs are metabolized by cytochrome P450 2D system. Thus medications which inhibit this system such as cimetidine, many SSRIs, phenothiazines, aspirin, oral contraceptives, and phenytoin may raise TCA levels and EKG abnormalities that correlate with higher TCA levels.

Alpha-Agonists

The alpha-agonists clonidine and guanfacine were widely used despite relatively little published data on their efficacy and safety. There has been an ongoing debate as to their safety with regard to cardiovascular side effects (38,39). Alpha agonists have also been used for a variety of indications apart from the treatment of ADHD per se. Clonidine, the more sedative of the two alpha agonists, has often been given a single dose at bedtime to treat stimulant-induced insomnia or evening rebound when the last stimulant dose of the day has worn off (40). There are no controlled trials of this practice. Clonidine has also been combined with stimulant to treat comorbid aggression, although the first small controlled trial of this practice was negative (41). A subsequent, larger study did show clonidine was superior to placebo when added to methylphenidate for the treatment of aggression (42). While studies of the efficacy of clonidine in ADHD are limited in number and have numerous methodological problems, a metaanalysis of these studies did show a significant effect size relative to placebo (43). Guanfacine has been shown to be efficacious in the treatment of ADHD in children with comorbid tics, though with an effect size for reducing ADHD symptoms less than that of stimulants (44).

The dose titration of both clonidine and guanfacine is shown in Table 4. Guanfacine is only one-tenth as potent as clonidine. Blood pressure and pulse must be monitored carefully. Alpha-agonists should not be terminated abruptly, as rebound hypertension may occur (31). This raises

Table 4 Titration of Alpha-Agonists

Preadolescent doses	Clonidine	Guanfacine
Day 1–4	0.05 q hs	0.5 q hs
Day 5–9	0.05 q am & hs	0.5 q am and q hs
Day 10–14	0.05 tid	0.5 mg tid
Day 14 and up	0.05 qid	1 mg bid
Adolescent (> 100 lbs)		
Day 1–4	0.05 q hs	0.5 q hs
Day 5–9	0.1 q hs	1 mg hs
Day 10–14	0.1 bid	1 mg bid
Day 14 and up	0.1 tid/qid	1 mg tid

Note: Need baseline BP and pulse (standing, lying), repeat when dose stable or cardiovascular symptoms presence. Reduce dose if patient complains of dizziness, cheat pain, palpitations, sedation.

questions about the safety of such medications used as one time dose in the evening for sleep, as they are wearing off in every morning as the child awakes. Nonetheless, nearly all adverse events with clonidine were reported in children taking multiple doses per day (38).

CONCLUSION

A wide variety of psychopharmacological agents are available for the treatment of ADHD. The physician should be guided by a number of key principles: (1) Quantify the ADHD symptoms at baseline, (2) use the appropriate starting dose of the agent and follow-up with parent and teacher ratings to document response, (3) continue to titrate the agent upward until full remission of ADHD symptoms occurs (unless discomforting side effects prevent this), (4) switch to alternative agent if a given medication does not achieve remission, and (5) monitor long progress once the acute symptoms are in remission. By careful use of the many therapeutic agents discussed here, the physician will be able to substantially improve the quality of life for patients with ADHD.

REFERENCES

1. Greenhill LL, Pliszka S, Dulcan MK et al. Practice parameter for the use of stimulant medications in the treatment of children, adolescents, and adults. J Am Acad Child Adolesc Psychiatry 2002; 41(2 suppl.):26S–49S.
2. Greenhill LL, Swanson JM, Vitiello B et al. Impairment and deportment responses to different methylphenidate doses in children with ADHD: the MTA titration trial. J Am Acad Child Adolesc Psychiatry 2001; 40(2):180–7.

3. Greenhill LL, Abikoff HB, Arnold LE et al. Medication treatment strategies in the MTA study: relevance to clinicians and researchers. J Am Acad Child Adolesc Psychiatry 1996; 35:1304–13.
4. MTA Cooperative Group. Moderators and mediators of treatment response for children with attention deficit hyperactivity disorder: The MTA study. Arch Gen Psychiatry 1999; 56:1088–96.
5. Jensen PS, Hinshaw SP, Swanson JM et al. Findings from the NIMH Multimodal Treatment Study of ADHD (MTA): implications and applications for primary care providers. J Dev Behav Pediat 2001; 22(1):60–73.
6. Conners CK. Conners' Rating Scales-Revised. Toronto: Multi-Health Systems, Inc., 1997.
7. Pliszka SR, Greenhill LL, Crismon ML et al. The Texas children's medication algorithm project: report of the Texas consensus conference panel on medication treatment of childhood attention deficit/hyperactivity disorder. Part II: Tactics. J Am Acad Child Adolesc Psychiatry 2000; 39:920–7.
8. Wolraich ML, Greenhill LL, Pelham W et al. Randomized, controlled trial of oros methylphenidate once a day in children with attention-deficit/hyperactivity disorder. Pediatrics 2001; 108(4):883–92.
9. Swanson J, Greenhill L, Pelham W et al. Initiating Concerta (OROS methylphenidate HCI) qd in children with attention-deficit hyperactivity disorder. J Clin Res 2000; 3:59–76.
10. Pelham WE, Gnagy E, Burrows-MacLean L et al. Once-a-day Concerta methylphenidate vs three-times-daily methylphenidate in laboratory and natural settings. Pediatrics 2001; 107:e105.
11. Biederman J, Lopez FA, Boellner SW, Chandler MC. A randomized, double-blind, placebo-controlled, parallel-group study of SLI381 (Adderall XR) in children with attention-deficit/hyperactivity disorder. Pediatrics 2002; 110(2 pt 1):258–66.
12. Childress AC, Krishman S, McGough JJ, Findling RL. Interim analysis of a long-term, open-label, single-arm study of lisdexamfetamine (LDX), an amphetamine prodrug, in children with ADHD. Presented at the 53rd Annual Meeting of the American Academy of Child and Adolescent Psychiatry (Oct 27), San Diego, CA. 2006.
13. Gillberg C, Melander H, von Knorring AL et al. Long-term stimulant treatment of children with attention-deficit hyperactivity disorder symptoms. A randomized, double-blind, placebo-controlled trial. Arch Gen Psychiatry 1997; 54(9):857–64.
14. MTA Cooperative Group. 14 month randomized clinical trial of treatment strategies for children with attention deficit hyperactivity disorder. Arch Gen Psychiatry 1999; 56:1073–86.
15. Spencer TJ, Wilens TE, Biederman J, Weisler RH, Read SC, Pratt R. Efficacy and safety of mixed amphetamine salts extended release (Adderall XR) in the management of attention-deficit/hyperactivity disorder in adolescent patients: a 4-week, randomized, double-blind, placebo-controlled, parallel-group study. Clin Ther 2006; 28(2):266–79.
16. Wilens TE, McBurnett K, Bukstein O et al. Multisite controlled study of OROS methylphenidate in the treatment of adolescents with attention-deficit/hyperactivity disorder. Arch Pediatr Adolesc Med 2006; 160(1):82–90.

17. Biederman J, Mick E, Surman C et al. A randomized, placebo-controlled trial of OROS methylphenidate in adults with attention-deficit/hyperactivity disorder. Biol Psychiatry 2006; 59(9):829–35.
18. Weisler RH, Biederman J, Spencer TJ et al. Mixed Amphetamine salts extended-release in the treatment of adult ADHD: A randomized, controlled trial. CNS Spectr 2006; 11(8):625–39.
19. Spencer T, Biederman J, Wilens T et al. Efficacy of a mixed amphetamine in adults with attention deficit/hyperactivity disorder. Arch Gen Psychiatry 2001; 58:775–82.
20. Spencer T, Wilens T, Biederman J, Faraone SV, Ablon JS, Lapey K. A double-blind, crossover comparison of methylphenidate and placebo in adults with childhood-onset attention-deficit hyperactivity disorder. Arch Gen Psychiatry 1995; 52(6):434–43.
21. Spencer T, Biederman J, Wilens T et al. A large, double-blind, randomized clinical trial of methylphenidate in the treatment of adults with attention-deficit/hyperactivity disorder. Biol Psychiatry 2005; 57(5):456–63.
22. Biederman J. Practical considerations in stimulant drug selection for the attention-deficit/hyperactivity disorder patient- efficacy, potency and titration. Today's Therapeutic Trends 2002; 20:311–28.
23. American Academy of Child and Adolescent Psychiatry. Practice parameter for the assessment and treatment of children and adolescents with attention-deficit/hyperactivity disorder. J Am Acad Child Adolesc Psychiatry. In press.
24. Heiligenstein J, Biederman J, Faries D et al. Atomoxetine efficacy versus placebo in school-age girls with ADHD. Presented at the 48th Annual Meeting of the American Academy of Child and Adolescent Psychiatry, Honolulu, HI (Oct 23–28), 2001.
25. Kratochvil C, Heiligenstein JH, Dittmann R et al. Atomoxetine and methylphenidate treatment in ADHD children: a randomized, open-label trial. Presented at the 48th Annual Meeting of the American Academy of Child and Adolescent Psychiatry, Honolulu, HI (Oct 23–28), 2001.
26. Michelson D, Faries D, Wernicke J et al. Atomoxetine in the treatment of children and adolescents with attention-deficit/hyperactivity disorder: a randomized, placebo-controlled, dose-response study. Pediatrics 2001; 108(5):1–9.
27. Michelson D, Allen AJ, Busner J et al. Once-daily atomoxetine treatment for children and adolescents with attention deficit hyperactivity disorder: a randomized, placebo-controlled study. Am J Psychiatry 2002; 159(11): 1896–901.
28. Pliszka SR, Browne R, Olvera RL, Wynne SK. A double-blind placebo controlled trial of Adderall and methylphenidate in the treatment of Attention deficit hyperactivity disorder. J Am Acad Child Adolesc Psychiatry 2000; 39: 619–26.
29. Kratochvil CJ, Heiligenstein JH, Dittmann R et al. Atomoxetine and methylphenidate treatment in children with ADHD: a prospective, randomized, open-label trial. J Am Acad Child Adolesc Psychiatry 2002; 41(7):776–84.
30. Food and Drug Administration. FDA Alert [09/05]: Suicidal thinking in children and adolescents. Available at Food and Drug Administration Website. 2005. 12-29–2005.

31. Pliszka SR. Comparing the effects of stimulant and non-stimulant agents on catecholamine function: implications for theories of ADHD. In: Solanto MV, Arnsten AFT, Castellanos FX, eds. Stimulant Drugs and ADHD Basic and Clinical Neuroscicncc. New York: Oxford University Press, 2001:332–52.
32. Conners CK, Casat CD, Gualtieri CT et al. Bupropion hydrochloride in attention deficit disorder with hyperactivity. J Am Acad Child Adolesc Psychiatry 1996; 35(10):1314–21.
33. Wilens TE, Spencer TJ, Biederman J et al. A controlled trial of bupropion for attention deficit hyperactivity disorder in adults. Am J Psychiatry 2001; 158: 282–9.
34. Wilens TE, Prince J, Spencer TJ et al. Bupropion SR for attention deficit hyperactivity disorder (ADHD) in adults with bipolar disorder (BPD) and ADHD. Presented at the 47th Annual Meeting of the American Academy of Child and Adolescent Psychiatry, New York, October 24–29, 2000.
35. Riddle MA, Geller B, Ryan N. Another sudden death in a child treated with desipramine. J Am Acad Child Adolesc Psychiatry 1993; 32:792–7.
36. Riddle MA, Nelson JC, Kleinman CS et al. Sudden death in children receiving Norpramin: a review of three reported cases and commentary. J Am Acad Child Adolesc Psychiatry 1991; 30:104–8.
37. Daly JM, Wilens T. The use of tricyclics antidepressants in children and adolescents. Pediatr Clin North Am 1998; 45:1123–35.
38. Swanson JM, Flockhart D, Udrea D, Cantwell D, Connor D, Williams L. Clonidine in the treatment of ADHD: questions about safety and efficacy. J Child Adolesc Psychopharmacol 1995; 5(4):301–4.
39. Wilens TE, Spencer TJ. Combining methylphenidate and clonidine: a clinically sound medication option. J Am Acad Child Adolesc Psychiatry 1999; 38(5): 614–22.
40. Wilens TE, Biederman J, Spencer T. Clonidine for sleep disturbances associated with attention-deficit hyperactivity disorder. J Am Acad Child Adolesc Psychiatry 1994; 33:424–6.
41. Connor DF, Barkley RA, Davis HT. A pilot study of methylphenidate, clonidine, or the combination in ADHD comorbid with aggressive oppositional defiant disorder or conduct disorder. Clin Pediatrics 2000; 39:15–25.
42. Hazell PL, Stuart JE. A randomized controlled trial of clonidine added to psychostimulant medication for hyperactive and aggressive children. J Am Acad Child Adolesc Psychiatry 2003; 42(8):886–94.
43. Connor DF, Fletcher KE, Swanson JM. A meta-analysis of clonidine for symptoms of attention-deficit hyperactivity disorder. J Am Acad Child Adolesc Psychiatry 1999; 38(12):1551–9.
44. Scahill L, Chappell PB, Kim YS et al. A placebo-controlled study of guanfacine in the treatment of children with tic disorders and attention deficit hyperactivity disorder. Am J Psychiatry 2001; 158(7):1067–74.

Section V: Special Populations

22

Clinical Assessment of Preschoolers: Special Precautions

Laurie Miller Brotman and Kathleen Kiely Gouley

NYU Child Study Center, New York University School of Medicine, New York, New York, U.S.A.

INTRODUCTION

The clinical assessment of preschoolers poses several challenges. These challenges relate primarily to the evaluation of symptoms relative to behavior considered to be within the normal range, understanding symptoms relative to the child's developmental status, and the assessment of functional impairment for children who are not in school and have limited social encounters outside of the family. These issues are exacerbated by the limited developmentally informed clinical research in preschoolers with attention deficit hyperactivity disorder (ADHD). Additionally, clinicians must consider differential diagnosis with other disorders of early childhood, including oppositional defiant disorder (ODD), speech and language disorders, and developmental disorders.

ADHD IN PRESCHOOLERS

Although the diagnostic criteria for ADHD require that the symptoms onset prior to 7 years of age (20), and community-based studies report rates of ADHD in preschoolers ranging from 2% to 6% (1,2), the overwhelming majority of research in ADHD has been conducted with school-aged children. The few systematic studies of clinically-referred preschool children suggest that ADHD preschoolers, relative to non-ADHD preschoolers, have difficulties with peer and family interactions, language impairments, and academic difficulties (3–6). Preschoolers with ADHD, like older children with ADHD, have also been shown to have problems in working memory (7), and high rates of comorbid disorders (8). Existing data suggest that ADHD in preschoolers parallels ADHD in school-aged children in terms of symptom expression, functional correlates, and comorbid disorders. However, there are important differences in cognitive, behavioral, motor, and social development in preschoolers relative to older children that need to be considered in the evaluation process (22,23).

Developmentally Informed Assessments

A comprehensive and developmentally sensitive evaluation of ADHD in preschoolers is critical so that children with levels of inattention, impulsivity and activity that are within the normal range for the preschool period are not inaccurately diagnosed with ADHD. A proper evaluation can also ensure that an appropriate diagnosis is made in cases where behavioral symptoms significantly interfere with development and social functioning. The delay in diagnosis and treatment of preschoolers with ADHD that is functionally impairing might result in additional developmental problems, the onset of comorbid disorders, and other consequences of untreated mental health problems. This is of particular concern because ADHD that onsets in the preschool period may, in fact, represent a potent version of the disorder (5,9).

Although there have been only a limited number of clinical studies with preschoolers with ADHD, studies of developmental psychopathology and normal development during the preschool period provide a basis for consideration of special issues related to assessing preschoolers. Developmental studies suggest that relative to older children, the behavior of preschoolers is highly sensitive to context, and the normal variation for attention, activity level and impulsivity is wide. Furthermore, symptoms must be considered in relation to the child's cognitive developmental status, speech and language development, and motor development. Preschoolers have rapidly emerging skills in these three areas; each area of development is also highly variable within the preschool period. Functional impairment must also be considered in light of the child's developmental status as well as in the context of important relationships and demands of the preschool period. During the preschool period, there are growing expectations regarding compliance and independence. Additionally, early educational settings add demands for attention, impulse control, and regulation of behavior (6). Thus, clinicians must be aware of developmentally appropriate expectations for a preschooler. Finally, due in part to the convergence of certain aspects of development in the preschool period, certain comorbid disorders, (e.g., ODD, speech and language disorders, and pervasive developmental disorders) are more likely to onset in the preschool period.

Therefore, special consideration should be given to comorbid disorders in the evaluation of a preschooler with ADHD.

Context Matters

Preschooler's behavior, as well as neurobiological functioning, has been shown to vary according to context (10). Accordingly, the clinical assessment of preschoolers requires consideration of behavior across contexts, taking into account factors such as time of day, peer composition (same or mixed sex peer group), relationship factors (preschoolers tend to behave differently with mothers vs. fathers), and social, cognitive, and behavioral demands of the setting. For example, child behavior is likely to vary significantly between relatively structured settings with high demands for attention and impulse control (e.g., preschool circle time, church services) and those that are unstructured yet socially challenging (e.g., neighborhood playground).

Gathering information from multiple informants (such as mother, father, teacher, daycare provider, and older sibling) who observe and relate to the child in different contexts is important for achieving a comprehensive picture of the child's behavior. Each informant is likely to observe the child in different settings and under different environmental conditions. Context-sensitive information from multiple informants can then be integrated to inform diagnostic conclusions and tailor treatment planning (24). For example, different treatment plans would be developed for an ADHD preschooler whose symptoms are exacerbated at daycare when he is tired or hungry versus a preschooler who is able to follow verbal directions at school when provided in a low stimulation environment but has trouble when there are too many visual or auditory distractions. Evaluations that provide this level of detail about symptom expression related to contextual variables are likely to be highly useful for treatment planning.

Observations in Naturalistic Settings

In addition to obtaining information from multiple informants, clinicians should consider observing the child in a naturalistic setting. This is especially important if discrepant information is provided by different informants, or if questions about functional impairment exist. A range of core ADHD behaviors can be observed in naturalistic settings such as the home or school environment, including spontaneous verbalizations, fidgeting, excessive motor behavior, and off-task behaviors. School observation measures of ADHD symptoms originally designed for school-aged children have been used successfully with preschoolers (11). The clinician should select the setting for observation that is most likely to allow for observation of the specific presenting problem behavior(s) of interest. Observations in familiar settings not only permit clinicians to evaluate core symptoms, but they also can inform treatment planning by helping the clinician to understand how core behaviors impair academic or social functioning, and whether there are features of the environmental context that elicit, maintain, or exacerbate symptoms.

Distinguishing Symptoms from Normal Variation

Another challenge in assessing preschoolers concerns differentiating ADHD symptoms from behaviors that may be considered developmentally appropriate. Developmental variability is one of the hallmarks of the preschool period. To determine whether a specific child behavior (e.g., inattention, distractibility, or hyperactivity), meets criteria as a symptom of ADHD, the clinician must compare the behavior to developmental expectations or normative behavior for the preschooler. This is complicated by the fact that there is a wide range of "normal" or "acceptable" levels of inattention, activity, and impulsivity during the preschool period (12,13).

There are a few parent and teacher DSM-IV (20) referenced ratings scales of ADHD symptoms, such as the Conners Rating Scales (14) and the Early Childhood Inventory-4 (ECI-4; 15) with norms specific to the preschool period that can be helpful in this aspect of evaluation (16,17). However, the options are much more limited for evaluating preschoolers with ADHD relative to older children. This is unfortunate, and may result in the underdiagnosis of preschoolers by clinicians who are reluctant to view the behavior of preschoolers as atypical without a solid empirical basis for making this conclusion. The assessment of inattention in preschoolers can be particularly difficult and even fewer psychometrically sound rating scales capture this core feature of ADHD in preschoolers (18).

Developmental Status

An understanding of the child's cognitive developmental level, language skills and social and motor development are necessary for evaluating individual symptoms of ADHD as well as functional impairment. For example, consideration of the child's level of receptive language skills is important for establishing whether a child is "not listening" or "not following directions." Similarly, consideration of the child's play skills is critical for evaluating whether the child is "having difficulty playing quietly," and understanding of the child's level of social awareness is necessary for determining if the child is "having difficulty waiting his or her turn."

There are several cognitive tests currently available for preschoolers, some of which can be completed in fewer than 60 min, which can provide a basis for evaluating cognitive developmental status [e.g., Differential Abilities Scale; Ref. (19)]. Many cognitive tests are accompanied by observational ratings to be completed by a psychometrician during testing. These observations of behavior during structured cognitive testing (e.g., out-of-seat, requiring multiple directives, difficulty following directions) can also be informative as part of the comprehensive assessment of preschoolers.

Evaluating Functional Impairment

A diagnosis should only be made if the ADHD behaviors are causing "clinically significant distress or impairment in social, occupational or other important areas of functioning" (20). The evaluation of clinical impairment in preschoolers can be particularly challenging. The impact on academic or school functioning is difficult to evaluate in children who have not yet entered school; similarly the impact on peer relations and social functioning can be hard to assess in children who have not had opportunities to engage with same-age peers on a regular basis (25). In cases where children are not yet in school or have not had much peer exposure, clinicians should consider distress or impairment as related to parent–child relationships, sibling relationships, developing sense of self and self-esteem. When possible, functional impairment should be assessed in whatever social environments are relevant (e.g., play with same age peers, playdates, informal peer group play).

Differential Diagnosis

Finally, the clinical assessment of preschoolers requires consideration of issues of differential diagnosis with disorders of the early childhood period. Disorders of early childhood to be considered in the evaluation of ADHD include ODD, autism-spectrum disorders, and speech and language disorders. The differentiation of ODD and ADHD symptoms in the preschool period can be particularly challenging, especially for children who are not in school-like settings. Sole reliance on parent report to make such distinctions can be highly problematic (21). Observations of the child in multiple contexts may be essential for making this distinction. Differential diagnoses involving speech and language problems or autism-spectrum disorders may require a multidisciplinary team approach. If a team approach is not feasible, consultation with a speech-language therapist or a developmental specialist in disorders of early childhood may be helpful.

CONCLUSION

The assessment of preschoolers requires attention to developmental issues that influence all aspects of behavior and functioning during the preschool period. Given the considerable variability and degree of contextual influence on behavior during the preschool period, a multimethod, multiinformant approach to evaluation is required. This involves collecting data from parents, teachers, and other caregivers who observe the child in multiple naturalistic settings. Furthermore, the assessment of ADHD during the preschool period raises particular challenges, not unique to the disorder, regarding how behavior is evaluated in light of developmental status and normal individual variation. Differential diagnoses of ODD, speech and language problems, and autism-spectrum disorders are of particular relevance to the evaluation of ADHD during the preschool period. Clinicians must consider these issues as part of an informative and comprehensive clinical assessment of ADHD in preschoolers.

REFERENCES

1. Keenan K, Shaw DS, Walsh B, et al. DSM-III-R disorders in preschool children from low-income families. J Am Acad Child Adolesc Psychiatry 1997; 36:620–7.
2. Lavigne JV, Gibbons RD, Christoffel KK, et al. Prevalence rates and correlates of psychiatric disorders among preschool children. J Am Acad Child Adol Psychiatm 1996; 35:204–14.
3. Byrne JM, DeWolfe NA, Bawden HN. Assessment of attention-deficit hyperactivity disorder in preschoolers. Child Neuropsychol 1998; 4:49–66.
4. DuPaul GJ, McGoey KE, Eckert TL, VanBrakle J. Preschool children with attention-deficit/hyperactivity disorder: impairments in behavioral, social, and school functioning. J Am Acad Child Adolesc Psychiatry 2001; 40:508–15.
5. Wilens TE, Biederman J, Brown S, et al. Psychiatric comorbidity and functioning in clinically referred preschool children and school-age youths with ADHD. J Am Acad Child Adolesc Psychiatry 2002; 41:262–8.
6. Cunningham CE, Boyle MH. Preschoolers at risk for attention-deficit hyperactivity disorder and oppositional defiant disorder: family, parenting, and behavioral correlates. J Abnorm Child Psychol 2002; 30:555–69.
7. Mariani MA, Barkley RA. Neuropsychological and academic functioning in preschool boys with attention deficit hyperactivity disorder. Dev Neuropsychol 1997; 13:111–29.
8. Keenan K, Wakschlag LS. More than the terrible twos: the nature and severity of behavior problems in clinic-referred preschool children. J Abnorm Child Psychol 2000; 28:33–46.
9. Wilens TE, Biederman J, Brown S, Monuteaux M, Prince J, Spencer TJ. Patterns of psychopathology and dysfunction in clinically referred preschoolers. J Dev Behav Pediatr 2002; 23:S31–6.
10. Brotman LM, Gouley KK, Klein RG, Castellanos F, Pine DS. Children, stress, and context: integrating basic, clinical, and experimental prevention research. Child Dev 2003; 74:1053–7.
11. Abikoff H, Martin D. School Observations: Procedure Manual for Preschool Attention-Deficit Hyperactivity Disorder Treatment Study (PATS). 2001. Unpublished manuscript; New York University School of Medicine, New York. NY
12. Campbell SB. Behavior problems in preschool children: a review of recent research. J Child Psychol Psychiatry 1995; 36:113–49.

13. Barkley RA. Attention-deficit/hyperactivity disorder, self-regulation, and time: toward a more comprehensive theory. J Dev Behav Pediatr 1997; 18:271–9.
14. Conners CK. Conners Rating Scales–Revised. In: Maruish ME, ed. The Use of Psychological Testing for Treatment Planning and Outcomes Assessment. 2nd ed. Mahwah, NJ: Lawrence Erlbaum Associates, 1999:467–95.
15. Sprafkin J, Volpe RJ, Gadow KD, Nolan EE, Kelly K. A DSM-IV-referenced screening instrument for preschool children: The Early Childhood Inventory-4. J Am Acad Child Adolesc Psychiatry 2002; 41:604–12.
16. Miller LS, Koplewicz HS, Klein RG. Teacher ratings of hyperactivity, inattention, and conduct problems in preschoolers. J Abnorm Child Psychol 1997; 25:113–9.
17. Fantuzzo J, Grim S, Mordell M, McDermott P, Miller L, Coolahan K. A multivariate analysis of the revised Conners' Teacher Rating Scale with low-income, urban preschool children. J Abnorm Child Psychol 2001; 29:141–52.
18. DeWolfe NA, Byrne JM, Bawden HN. Early clinical assessment of attention. Clin Neuropsychol 1999; 13:458–73.
19. Elliott CD. Differential Abilities Scale. San Antonio, TX: The Psychological Corporation, 1990.
20. American Psychiatric Association. Diagnostic and Statistical Manual of Mental Disorders. 4th ed. Washington, D.C.: American Psychiatric Publishing, 1994.
21. Gadow KD, Nolan EE. Differences between preschool children with ODD, ADHD and ODD+ADHD symptoms. J Child Psychol Psychiatry 2002; 43: 191–201.
22. Dennis T, Brotman LM, Huang KY, Gouley KK. Effortful control, social competence, and adjustment problems in children at risk for psychopathology. J Clin Ch Adol Psy 2007; 36:442–54.
23. Gouley KK, Brotman LM, Huang KY, Shrout P. Construct validation of the Social Competence Scale in preschool-age children. Social Development, in press.
24. Sonuga-Barke EJS, Thompson M, Abikoff H, Klein R, Brotman LM. Nonpharmacological interventions for preschoolers with ADHD. The case for specialized parent training. Inf & Young Child 2006; 2:142–53.
25. Brotman LM, Gouley KK, Chesir-Teran D. Assessing peer entry and play in preschoolers at risk for maladjustment. J Clin Ch Adol Psy 2005; 34:671–80.

23

Psychosocial Treatment for Adolescents with ADHD

Steven W. Evans, Carey B. Dowling, and Ruth C. Brown
Alvin V. Baird Attention and Learning Disabilities Center, James Madison University, Harrisonburg, Virginia, U.S.A.

OVERVIEW

Epidemiological data suggest that attention deficit hyperactivity disorder (ADHD) affects between 2% and 4% of adolescents in the general population. Similar to children with ADHD, problems for adolescents with the disorder typically include academic difficulties, discipline problems at school and at home, and conflict with peers; however, adolescents tend to experience more serious consequences than children. For example, problems such as school dropout, substance abuse, and legal problems become more common among youth with ADHD as they mature. In addition, between 25% and 75% of adolescents with ADHD meet diagnostic criteria for other disruptive behavior disorders (1), resulting in significant additional impairments. Treatment for these youth therefore requires a comprehensive, multimodal approach that addresses impairment across multiple domains and contexts (2).

The most widely used treatment for adolescents with ADHD is stimulant medication, but many questions and concerns still surround the use of stimulants among adolescents. Professional literature is replete with studies of stimulant treatment for children with ADHD (3); however, as of 2000 we found only 20 controlled studies of the use of stimulants with adolescents (4–6). Overall, the research on stimulant treatment with children suggests that stimulants are efficacious, but result in improvement rather than a normalization of functioning. The current literature on adolescents suggests a similar conclusion, with one study reporting that between 9% and 29% of the adolescent participants demonstrated no benefit from taking small, medium, or large dosages of methylphenidate on measures of academic performance and classroom behavior (4). In addition, stimulant medication appears insufficient for treating the common problems of parent-teen conflict (7) and social functioning (8). Other limitations of medication treatment include the lack of sustained adherence to medication regimens and resistance by some families and youth to taking medication. Medication is an effective treatment option for many adolescents with ADHD; however, it has limitations and additional treatments are needed in order to address the problems frequently associated with adolescents with ADHD.

Although some studies suggest that benefits due to medication treatment may indeed generalize from childhood to adolescence (9), the continuity of efficacy for psychosocial treatment from childhood to adolescence is largely untested. Since the vast majority of literature on the treatment of ADHD has focused on elementary school-aged children, the temptation exists to simply extrapolate psychosocial treatments from studies of children with ADHD and apply them to the treatment of adolescents. However, the independence, differing social influences, greater ability to defy adult directives, and dramatically different school environment associated with adolescence influence the feasibility and effectiveness of treatments that may have proved effective with children. As a result, investigations into psychosocial treatments specifically designed for the adolescent population are important and some studies have begun to address this deficiency in the literature. The following review describes psychosocial interventions for adolescents with ADHD and is organized in terms of domains and providers. Since physicians are frequently the initial and primary caregiver for adolescents with ADHD and their role in psychosocial treatment is increasing, interventions physicians can implement are described first. Most other psychosocial treatments developed for adolescents have included school interventions and/or family treatment and the literature pertaining to each is reviewed in subsequent sections.

PHYSICIANS

Physicians are increasingly called to play important roles in the delivery of universal and selective psychosocial mental health services (1), and represent a primary source of contact with the health care system for most adolescents and their families. Diagnostic evaluations and medication treatment are typically provided by physicians, as well as psychoeducation regarding other mental health treatment options (1). Basic psychoeducational interventions are well suited to a physician's office where families can learn about the disorder and the available treatments. Given the wide range of impairments associated with adolescents with ADHD, many treatments may be appropriate and necessary, so physicians are often the primary source of referrals to other mental health professionals. Collaborating with a qualified psychologist or mental health counselor with the expertise of working with adolescents and using behavioral techniques can enhance care by making available coordinated multimodal treatment; however, there are a large number of communities that do not have providers with behavioral health expertise. As an alternative, school counselors and teachers at secondary schools may provide many of these services in active collaboration with the primary physician.

As other providers become involved, the coordination of care is a central issue and can be facilitated by the sharing of information about the services and measures of progress. Although collaborative treatment planning between physicians, mental health counselors, parents, and educators is recommended, it is difficult to achieve due to the demands placed on each of these individuals. Web-based systems that allow for efficient information sharing between parents, schools, physicians, and others have been developed and are currently being field tested (10) although early attempts have proven problematic (11). Clearly, much more work is needed to improve collaboration to achieve truly interprofessional mental health care coordination.

An area that has received little attention in the psychosocial literature is the potential supporting role that psychosocial interventions may play in increasing adherence to medication regimens. While this is a common approach with other chronic disorders, such as asthma and diabetes as well as bipolar disorder and schizophrenia, it has not been studied for adolescents with ADHD. Such interventions appear warranted since children with ADHD frequently discontinue their use of stimulant medication when they reach adolescence (12,13). The lack of medication compliance is not always obvious to the prescribing physician since it is usually manifested as the absence of visits. Unless the physician is monitoring in such a manner as to note omissions and actively follow up when they occur, the discontinuation of medications may go unnoticed. In our experience, we have found that when children with ADHD reach adolescence they often believe that they do not have a problem and therefore do not need medication. Unlike young children, adolescents are often effective at actively defying their parents' requests, so struggles around medication can develop within families. Physicians, nurses, or other staff may provide appropriate education and counseling to adolescents and their parents that can help increase adherence to medication regimens. In order for this to be successful, the omission of a follow-up visit would have to be noticed and prompt additional interventions have to be made.

FAMILY

Family-based interventions are frequently recommended for adolescents with ADHD (14) and Barkley and colleagues have conducted two studies that have examined their efficacy (15,16). In the first, three types of family-based treatments were compared: (1) parent training in behavior management skills, (2) structural family therapy, and (3) problem-solving and communication training. The three treatments performed about equally well and produced statistically significant improvements in parent-child communication, school adjustment, and child and mother symptoms as assessed by a variety of rating scales completed by parents and adolescents. However, few subjects exhibited clinically significant improvement and the authors concluded that long-term, multimodal treatments were needed. Subsequently, Barkley and colleagues (16) reported that increasing the dosage (doubling the number of sessions), and combining behavioral management training with problem-solving communication therapy led to lower rates of dropout from family therapy than problem-solving communication therapy alone; however, combination treatment did not improve outcomes above that of problem-solving communication therapy alone. Overall, neither treatment produced reliable change in the majority of families who received therapy leading the authors to conclude that the family may not be the preferred target in interventions for adolescents with ADHD.

Although Barkley and colleagues (15,16) concluded that family therapy provides little benefit to families of adolescents with ADHD, others have reported benefits from family treatment. For example family therapy (FFT) is effective for many of the problems experienced by adolescents with ADHD, including substance abuse, poor peer relations, and strained family relationships (17). FFT is a family systems oriented, behaviorally based prevention and intervention program that requires anywhere from 8 to 30 sessions depending on the severity of the problems, and consists of two to five phases. A common description of this treatment indicates that there are three phases: (1) engagement and motivation, (2) behavior change, and (3) generalization. Early sessions focus on engaging the family and maximizing their motivation to change. Assessment procedures targeting interactional and functional aspects of behavior are completed in order to gain an understanding of the family system and the individual relationships. Later sessions focus on changing behaviors and generalizing these changes. Waldron and colleagues (18) found that participants who received 12-hr of FFT, either alone or combined with individual Cognitive-Behavioral Therapy (CBT), showed significant decreases in marijuana use. Bolstering these findings are numerous studies that demonstrate that FFT significantly reduces recidivism and the cost of treatment (19). As such, FFT has been deemed by many to be an effective treatment and prevention model, but it has yet to be studied with a sample of families with an adolescent with

ADHD. Since many of the areas of impairment successfully treated through FFT frequently occur among adolescents with ADHD, FFT may be a viable treatment modality for adolescents with ADHD.

Another example of a comprehensive prevention and treatment program that targets problems similar to those experienced by adolescents with ADHD is the Adolescent Transitions Program (ATP). The ATP is a multilevel ecological intervention and prevention program that includes direct interaction with youth, consultation and training, and the media (20). There are three levels of the ATP strategy: (1) universal, (2) selected, and (3) indicated family interventions. The first level reaches the most people, involves the least amount of professional support, and typically takes the form of a family resource center (FRC) in a school system. The FRC staff typically involved in multiple activities which include implementing curriculum in classrooms, conducting parent nights, presenting an introduction of the FRC at parent orientation, utilizing public access television and newsletters to teach family management techniques, conducting summer check-ins with families to plan for the next academic year, and conducting workshops for school staff. The second level, the family check-up broadly targets at-risk families and is designed to build motivation for change. The family check-up consists of an initial interview, an assessment, and a feedback session, each based on motivational interviewing techniques. The assessment involves gathering many types of data from the adolescent, parents, and teachers that indicate how the adolescent is performing in multiple domains and some versions of the family check-up include structured observations of family interactions. The feedback session utilizes the stages-of-change model and motivational interviewing and typically ends with the therapist and parent(s) collaborating to develop a menu of change options.

The third level of the ATP reaches the least amount of families and requires the highest level of professional support as it involves providing direct treatment and intervention services to at-risk families. At this level, practitioners specifically address three broad parent skill areas: (1) using incentives to encourage behavioral change, (2) setting limits for and monitoring adolescents, and (3) improving relationship skills such as listening, problem solving, and negotiation. Intervention options include parent training, establishing a school/home communication and monitoring system, periodic telephone calls from the therapist, family management therapy, and parent networking (e.g., parents meet with their adolescent's friends' parents and the group problem-solves how to keep their adolescents safe and out of trouble).

To our knowledge, there are currently no published studies evaluating the FFT or ATP with a sample of adolescents with ADHD; however, both treatments target youth with problems similar to many of those experienced by teens with ADHD and have yielded beneficial results. It is very likely that youth with ADHD have comprised some portion of the samples in studies given the inclusion criteria that have been used; however, research on families of adolescents with ADHD using these family therapy techniques is needed. Given the lack of positive findings reported by Barkley and colleagues with respect to family therapy (15,16), along with the positive findings reported for FFT and ATP (18–20), these family interventions merit some attention as potential components of an effective psychosocial treatment approach.

SCHOOL

Adolescents with ADHD continue to have serious problems at school and the consequences of these problems frequently lead to dropouts, long-term suspensions, and academic failure (21). While medication can be effective in improving academic performance and social functioning at school (4,22), school problems are still very common among adolescents taking stimulant medication (23) and they do not appear to have a long-term beneficial effect on academic functioning (24). Furthermore, since 1991 schools have been required to provide psychosocial and educational interventions for adolescents with ADHD who meet eligibility criteria for special education services (25), but there has been very little empirical literature to guide the implementation of these interventions. As a result, there continues to be a need to develop and evaluate psychosocial and educational interventions for problems at school for these youth.

Fortunately, treatment development work in this area is advancing and there is a set of psychosocial treatment studies with small sample sizes that have reported encouraging findings. One promising intervention for adolescents with ADHD was demonstrated in a case study that evaluated the effects of self-monitoring for a student who received social and tangible reinforcement for on-task behavior (26). The result of this treatment was a large improvement in on-task behavior. In another study, self-management procedures were found to improve the classroom preparation skills of three middle school-aged youth with ADHD (27). Students were taught to be on time for class, have all of their materials, complete work, and self-monitor their proficiency achieving these goals on a daily basis. Outcome data suggested that this intervention maintained behavior gains over time and was acceptable to teachers and students. Thus, self-monitoring training for adolescents with ADHD may bolster the effects of classroom-based behavioral interventions, especially in the context of heightened structure imposed by contingencies for accurate monitoring and appropriate behavior.

Another promising intervention involves the use of a functional assessment followed by classroom-based interventions. In a case study that utilized this approach in a middle school setting (28), functional hypotheses were developed for chronic off-task behavior observed for two boys. Based on the results of the functional assessment, recommendations were offered to classroom teachers who selected intervention strategies based on practicality and perceived effectiveness. Following implementation, the investigators found large improvements in the on-task behavior of both boys in the targeted classrooms. Thus, teacher consultation for behavioral interventions delivered in the classroom may be an effective component in a multimodal program.

Many interventions for adolescents with ADHD have targeted education outcomes. In their comprehensive review of the relevant literature, Raggi and Chronis (29) described a series of academic interventions that have targeted impairment frequently associated with youth with ADHD. For example, in one study adolescents were taught to take structured notes while they listened to a lecture-format American history class (30). Following this note-taking training, adolescents with ADHD showed improvement on measures of comprehension and increased levels of on-task behavior compared to when they simply listened to the lectures. The effect size for the note-taking intervention was in the moderate range. Other interventions have been developed and assessed only on adolescents with related disorders (e.g., learning disabilities) and, as a result, may need modifications to effectively address the needs of adolescents with ADHD. Although these interventions alone may not deal with the full range of problems exhibited by adolescents with ADHD, they each may be a useful component in a multimodal treatment.

Some research has examined the possibility of combining intervention strategies in a comprehensive fashion to address multiple areas of home and school impairments associated with ADHD. For example, the Challenging Horizons Program (CHP) was designed to be a comprehensive school-based treatment program for middle school students with ADHD targeting behavioral, academic, and social functioning. Initially developed and piloted in 1999 (31), there has been continuous treatment development and evaluation work completed across three sites and two distinct models of the CHP have emerged.

The first model of the CHP is as an after-school program that operates two to four times per week for just over 2 hr/day. The second model that was developed was a consulting model that involved classroom teachers providing CHP interventions during the school day. Both models of CHP included interventions targeting academic problems. Organization and task completion are two of the most problematic areas of impairment at school. To target these problems, program staff help students set up a system to organize and maintain their binders, bookbags, and lockers. The system included frequent monitoring, supervised adherence, and behavioral contingencies to help students advance toward independence. All students in the CHP are required to use an assignment notebook provided by the school. Students are required to record homework assignments for each class, or write "none" if homework is not assigned. Teacher signatures are usually required in the early phases of this intervention to ensure accurate recording. The requirement for signatures may be tapered as students progress toward independent mastery of this skill. The CHP counselors or mentors check the assignment notebook frequently and school and home contingencies are used to improve performance. These organization interventions are provided to all participants in both models of the CHP.

Many other interventions are provided to middle school-aged youth who participate in the after-school model of the CHP. Some of these interventions target academic problems and are provided during education group and include note taking and study skills. During education group students are taught how to make and use flash cards, acronyms, and other tools for preparing for tests. Students learn methods of note taking from lecture and text (30), how to prepare written summaries of text, and how to create and use outlines to help them write coherent papers. After demonstrating mastery within the CHP, students are required to bring examples of having used the study skills and notes at home and in their classes. Complete mastery of a skill is not achieved until competency was demonstrated both within the CHP and in their regular classrooms.

To address difficulties with homework, three individual sessions are offered to help parents develop and implement an individualized Homework Management Plan (HMP). The HMP manual includes procedures for teaching parents how to use behavior management techniques to create a homework routine for their adolescent. Parents set a mandatory homework time, typically 30 min to 1 hr, that the student must complete 5 days/week. The student is required to to work the entire time regardless of the amount of homework assigned. If the student does not have homework or does not bring home the necessary materials to complete homework, he/she is required to use the time to study for upcoming tests, read, prepare written summaries of reading material, or parents assign the student work such as writing summaries of newspaper articles. The most common rewards are access to privileges, such as phone, television, and video games. This system removes parents from battles over things they cannot control such as the child knowing what is assigned, when it is due, and bringing materials home. It allows parents to focus their effort on things that they can control such as time spent studying at home.

The after-school model of the CHP also includes interventions to target disruptive, defiant, and annoying behaviors frequently exhibited by adolescents with ADHD. When a student exhibits a targeted behavior in the after-school program, a counselor announces (calls) the behavior aloud to the child and records it on a behavior-tracking card. These behaviors include both positive behaviors, such as contributing and complimenting, and negative behaviors such as teasing, complaining, blurting, and repeated noncompliance. The calls draw students' attention to these behaviors, raises their awareness of problematic behaviors, and serves as praise or reprimand. Many behaviors are successfully modified without explicit contingencies beyond the consistent behavior calls. When the rate or intensity of a behavior needs to be modified and it is not sufficiently responding to the behavior calls, individualized contingencies are applied. Following successful behavior change at the CHP, interventions shift focus to modifying these behaviors in other settings. One frequently used technique to achieve this generalization involves the use of a daily or weekly report card (32). Report cards are lists of two to four operationally defined behaviors that briefly describe a problem the adolescent is experiencing in a school setting. These descriptions are defined in positive terms and space is provided next to each item for an adult to rate the behavior as achieved/not achieved or on an incremental scale (e.g., not at all, just a little, pretty much, and very much). Report cards for classroom teachers are completed at the end of class or the end of the week to reflect behavior exhibited over the defined time interval, and parents or CHP counselors provide contingencies based on these ratings. Point systems are used to reinforce appropriate behavior. These report cards are also used at home so parents may complete the ratings and students receive contingencies within the CHP. In addition to providing a mechanism to reliably provide rewards and consequences, the data produced by these cards may be used to measure progress.

Because the social problems of children and adolescents with ADHD are so pervasive, persistent, and detrimental for long-term prognosis, investigators include interventions to improve the social functioning of middle school-aged children as part of the treatment provided in the after-school CHP. The majority of the programs that are currently available utilize a Social Skills Training (SST) approach that teaches participants new social behaviors. Unfortunately, most SST programs have failed to demonstrate efficacy in improving the social problems of children with ADHD (33–35). There is little reason to believe that they would be beneficial to a slightly older sample of children (ages 11–14) who are the focus of the CHP. As a result, the interventions targeting social impairment in the CHP have been developed and piloted over the last 8 years.

One component of the social interventions that remains consistent throughout this treatment development process is the instruction and practice with social problem solving. Previous studies have reported consistent benefits to these procedures over time with samples that were likely to include many participants with ADHD (36,37). Although potentially helpful, these procedures are unlikely to be adequate for most children with ADHD. Considering the findings from the social cognition literature and recommendations regarding generalization of treatment gains (38) the investigators incorporated children reviewing videos of themselves in social situations, live coaching during social activities, and instruction and practice on reading social cues into their treatment development work. Outcome data on the various iterations of this development process are not yet available. Given the debilitating effects of social impairment (39), treatment development and research on causes of social deficits in youth with ADHD is an area requiring extensive resources and effort.

Whatever is learned through this research and treatment development, it seems that coaching generalization will likely be an activity that persists in successful interventions targeting social impairment. Counselors working in the CHP are trained to use subtle and direct prompts to facilitate appropriate social behaviors in as many settings as possible. One activity during the CHP that specifically targets this is a 30-min recreation period. Adolescents spend time playing sports such as soccer, basketball, and American football and counselors modeled, prompted, and promoted appropriate social interactions. These activities challenged the adolescents' social skills because it is difficult to implement appropriate social behavior in the "heat of a game" when one may perceive that a child has fouled him/her and no one is making a corrective call. It also provides a context to practice positive skills such as complimenting. In addition, students are provided instruction and practice in how to play these popular sports. The goal is to help them gain sufficient knowledge, confidence, and skill mastery so they are able to participate in neighborhood pick-up games or recreation league activities. It has been our experience that these adolescents' history of social impairment and difficulty with organized group activities contributed to a lack of sufficient skill to engage in sports activities, thereby reducing the number of available social opportunities.

A series of pilot studies were conducted to investigate the feasibility and outcomes of the after-school model of the CHP (23,31,40–42). These studies were conducted in a variety of middle schools across three different cities. When the CHP was provided for at least one semester, the outcome data were in the moderate to large effect size range. In one pilot study where implementation was less than one semester (10 weeks) the outcomes were less favorable, although parent satisfaction was still high (42). Operating the CHP in these settings was feasible assuming that there was university-school collaboration. This collaboration has been necessary due to the expense of operating a fairly labor intensive after-school program between 2 and 4 days/week.

In an attempt to develop a less expensive model of the CHP, the developers modified many of the treatment procedures so they could be provided by educators and other school staff during the school day (43). Not all of the CHP interventions were able to be provided in this manner. In a study of the school consultation model of the CHP, teachers, administrators, and school counselors implemented interventions similar to those used in the after-school model; however, school staff provided the interventions during the school day in collaboration with a CHP consultant. Similar to the role of the counselor in the after-school model, a school staff member functioned as a mentor for a child with ADHD. Students met regularly with their mentors to implement and evaluate the educational and behavioral interventions. The consulting model was designed to provide services similar to the after-school model without the need for as many staff. In the initial study, the interventions were provided over a 3-year period and small but meaningful gains across the 3 years were reported. In addition, grades improved by approximately one letter grade for the treatment group during the second semester and grades for students in the control group remained the same or declined (44). Treatment fidelity by the educators was variable as some provided the interventions with great integrity and consistency, others ignored their agreement to provide the services to the targeted child, and some claimed that ADHD did not really exist and attempting to help these children was a waste of time. Although costing much less to provide than the after-school model of the CHP, there are implementation costs involved in the consultation model related to quality that may compromise outcomes.

Preliminary results of a randomized trial of the after-school version of the program indicate that effect sizes for symptoms and impairment are notably larger for this version of the CHP than the consultation model. Nevertheless, there may be children with ADHD for whom the consultation model is adequate. Future research on the CHP should focus on moderators of treatment response and relative benefits of differences in costs and treatment intensity of the two models.

SUMMARY AND CONCLUSIONS

Continued research and development is needed for the CHP as well as for other psychosocial interventions for this population. The current lack of empirically supported psychosocial treatment leads to many problems in the health care and education system. For example, for many providers it is easier to get payment from most health insurance companies to provide play therapy to treat the impulsivity of a child or adolescent with ADHD than it is to get payment for a school-based behavioral intervention. Unfortunately, this creates incentives for providing treatment that is unlikely to work while discouraging the use of practices with an increasing amount of empirical support. The absence of empirically supported psychosocial treatments also negatively impacts the public education system. Since 1991 schools have been obligated to provide accommodations for students with ADHD who meet criteria for special education (25). Given the lack of effective techniques, many educators have adopted techniques that actually have the effect of reducing expectations instead of helping students achieve increased independence and improved functioning. Temporary relief of expectations may be necessary while providing instruction, training, or some other form of intervention prior to reestablishing the normal expectation once the individual has progressed; however, many times these accommodations take the form of permanent reductions in expectations or a "lowering of the bar."

This approach is rewarded because it reduces problems and may improve grades without a need to do the work to produce a commensurate improvement in functioning. For example, one common practice by those trying to help adolescents with ADHD in school is to relieve them of the responsibility for keeping track of classroom assignments. The well-intentioned teachers gather the assignment information for the students and keep track of assignment completion by communicating directly with the students' teachers. This can help a student keep track of assignments because someone does it for him or her, but this strategy alone does nothing to improve the functioning of the student. When there are not empirically supported psychosocial and educational interventions available and the schools are required to make accommodations for these youth, the temptation to placate situations by lowering expectations has appeal.

Policies and procedures related to the provision of psychosocial interventions for adolescents with ADHD are vague and inefficient in our current health care and education systems resulting in compromised care and few alternatives for families. Further evidence of these problems can be gleaned from state education records on due process hearings. Due process hearings are grievance procedures related to special education that are managed by a state's department of education. A review of recent records in Virginia revealed that almost half of all due process hearings in a recent year were related to children with behavioral and emotional problems (including ADHD) when these youth (emotionally disturbed and other health impaired) represent approximately 13% (45) of the special education population. This overrepresentation of cases with behavioral and emotional problems is another sign that our system of caring for these children is not working.

Finally, almost all of the studies reviewed in this chapter were conducted with young adolescents (i.e., middle school ages). There is a real need for treatment development and evaluation of older adolescents (ages 14–18) with ADHD as the impairment continues and these youth encounter even greater potential problems as they begin to drive, become sexually active (46), and experience a greater exposure to drugs and alcohol. Schools and the health care system are the sources of care for most adolescents with ADHD (47) and the systems in place are fraught with problems. Continuing to develop and evaluate effective psychosocial interventions for these youth is an important part of remediating these systems and providing treatment that can make a positive difference.

REFERENCES

1. Wolraich M, Wibbelsman CJ, Brown TE, et al. Attention-deficit hyperactivity disorder among adolescents: a review of the diagnosis, treatment, and clinical implications. Pediatrics 2005; 115:1734–46.

2. Faraone S, Biederman J, Monuteaux MC. Further evidence for the diagnostic continuity between child and adolescent ADHD. J Attent Disord 2002; 6: 5–13.
3. Swanson JM, McBurnett K, Christian DL, Wigal T. Stimulant medication and treatment of children with ADHD. In: Ollendick TH, Prinz RJ, eds. Advances in Clinical Child Psychology, Vol 17. New York: Plenum Press, 1995:265–322.
4. Evans SW, Pelham WE, Smith BH, et al. Dose-response effects of methylphenidate on ecologically valid measures of academic performance and classroom behavior in adolescents with ADHD. Exp Clin Psychopharmacol 2001; 9:163–75.
5. Findling RL, Short EJ, Manos MJ. Developmental aspects of psychostimulant treatment in children and adolescents with attention-deficit/hyperactivity disorder. J Am Acad Child Adolesc Psychiatry 2001; 40:1441–7.
6. Smith BH, Waschbusch DA, Willoughby M, Evans SW. The efficacy, safety, and practicality of treatments for adolescents with attention-deficit/hyperactivity disorder (ADHD). Clin Child Fam Psychol Rev 2000; 3: 243–67.
7. Meichenbaum DL, Pelham WE, Gnagy E, Smith BH, Bukstein OG. Effects of methylphenidate on parent-adolescent interactions in families with an ADHD teenager. In: 33rd Association for the Advancement of Behavior Therapy Annual Convention, Ontario, Canada, November 1999.
8. Bagwell CL, Molina BSG, Pelham WE, Hoza, B. Attention-deficit hyperactivity disorder and problems in peer relations: predictions from childhood to adolescence. J Am Acad Child Adolesc Psychiatry 2001; 40:1285–92.
9. Smith BH, Pelham WE, Gnagy E, Yudell RS. Equivalent effects of stimulant treatment for Attention-Deficit Hyperactivity Disorder during childhood and adolescence. J Am Acad Child Adolesc Psychiatry 1998; 37: 314–21.
10. Evans SW, Timmins B, Sibley M, White LC, Serpell ZN, Schultz B. Developing coordinated, multimodal, school-based treatment for young adolescents with ADHD. Educ Treat Child 2006; 29:195–214.
11. Wolraich ML, Bickman L, Lambert EW, Simmons T, Doffing MA. Intervening to improve communication between parents, teachers, and primary care providers of children with ADHD or at high risk for ADHD. J Attent Disord 2005; 9:354–68.
12. Pelham WE, Molina BSG, Meichenbaum DL, Gnagy EM, Greenhouse J. Stimulant effects on long term outcomes in ADHD individuals. Invited address at the 43rd Annual Meeting of New Clinical Drug Evaluation Unit Program (NCDEU), Boca Raton, FL, 2003.
13. Barkley RA, Fischer M, Smallish L, Fletcher JM. Does the treatment of attention-deficit/hyperactivity disorder with stimulants contribute to drug use/abuse? A 13-year prospective study. Pediatrics 2003; 111:97–109.
14. Robin AL. ADHD in Adolescents. New York: The Guilford Press, 1998.
15. Barkley RA, Guevremont DC, Anastopoulos AD, Fletcher KE. A comparison of three family therapy programs for treating family conflicts in adolescents with Attention-Deficit Hyperactivity Disorder. J Consult Clin Psychol 1992; 60: 450–62.

16. Barkley RA, Edwards G, Laneri M, Fletcher K, Metevia L. The efficacy of problem-solving communication training alone, behavior management training alone, and their combination for parent-adolescent conflict in teenagers with ADHD and ODD. J Consult Clin Psychol 2001; 69:926–41.
17. Alexander JF, Pugh C, Parsons BV. Functional family therapy. In: Elliott D, Series ed. Blueprints for Violence Prevention, Golden, CO: Venture, 2000.
18. Waldron HB, Slesnick N, Brody JL, Turner CW, Peterson TR. Treatment outcomes for adolescent substance abuse at 4- and 7-month assessments. J Consult Clin Psychol 2001; 69:802–13.
19. Sexton TL, Alexander JF. Family-based empirically supported interventions. Couns Psychol 2002; 30:238–61.
20. Dishion TJ, Kavanagh K. Intervening in Adolescent Problem Behavior: A Family Centered Approach. New York: The Guilford Press, 2003.
21. Klein RG, Mannuzza S. Long-term outcome of hyperactive children: a review. J Am Acad Child Adolesc Psychiatry 1991; 30:383–7.
22. Smith BH, Pelham WE, Evans SW, et al. Dosage effects of methylphenidate on the social behavior of adolescents diagnosed with attention-deficit hyperactivity disorder. Exp Clin Psychopharmacol 1998; 6:187–204.
23. Evans SW, Langberg J, Raggi V, Allen J, Buvinger E. Evaluation of a school-based treatment program for middle school youth with ADHD. J Attent Disord 2005; 9:343–53.
24. MTA Cooperative Group. National Institute of Mental Health multimodal treatment study of ADHD follow-up: changes in effectiveness and growth after the end of treatment. Pediatrics 2004; 113:762–9.
25. Davila R, Williams M, MacDonald J. Clarification of Policy to Address the Needs of Children with Attention Deficit Disorders Within General and/or Special Education. Washington, D.C.: Department of Education, 1991.
26. Stewart KG, McLaughlin TF. Self-recording: effects on reducing off-task behavior with a high school student with an attention deficit hyperactivity disorder. Child Fam Behav Ther 1992; 14:53–9.
27. Gureasko-Moore S, DuPaul GJ, White GP. The effects of self-management in general education classrooms on the organizational skills of adolescents. Behav Modif 2006; 30:159–83.
28. Ervin RA, DuPaul GJ, Kern L, Friman PC. Classroom-based functional and adjunctive assessments: proactive approaches to intervention selection for adolescents with Attention Deficit Hyperactivity Disorder. J Appl Behav Anal 1998; 31:65–78.
29. Raggi V, Chronis AM. Interventions to address the academic impairment of children and adolescents with ADHD. Clin Child Fam Psychol Rev 1006; 9: 85–111.
30. Evans SW, Pelham WE, Grudberg MV. The efficacy of notetaking to improve behavior and comprehension of adolescents with Attention Deficit Hyperactivity Disorder. Exceptionality 1995; 5:1–17.
31. Evans SW, Axelrod J, Langberg J. Efficacy of a school-based treatment program for middle school youth with ADHD: pilot data. Behav Modif 2004; 28:528–47.

32. Evans SW, Youngstrom E. Evidence based assessment of attention-deficit hyperactivity disorder: measuring outcomes. J Am Acad Child Adolesc Psychiatry 2006; 45:1132–7.
33. Hoza B, Gerdes AC, Mrug S, et al. Peer-assessed outcomes in the multimodal treatment study of children with attention deficit hyperactivity disorder. J Clin Child Adolesc Psychol 2005; 34:74–86.
34. Hoza B. Peer functioning in children with ADHD. Suppl Ambul Pediatr 2007; 7:101–6.
35. Kavale KA, Mathur SR, Forness SR, Rutherford RB, Quinn MM. Effectiveness of social skills training for students with behavioral disorders: a meta-analysis. In: Scruggs T, Mastropieri M, eds. Advances in Learning and Behavioral Disabilities, Vol 11. Greenwich, CT: JAI Press, 1996.
36. Lochman JE, Wells KC. Effectiveness of the Coping Power Program and of classroom intervention with aggressive children: outcomes at a 1-year follow-up. Behav Ther 2003; 34:493–515.
37. Pfiffner LJ, McBurnett K. Social skills training with parent generalization: treatment effects for children with attention deficit disorder. J Consult Clin Psychology 1997; 65:749–57.
38. Evans SW, Langberg J, Williams J. Treatment generalization in school based mental health. In: Weist M, Evans S, Lever N, eds. Handbook of School Mental Health: Advancing Practice and Research. New York: Kluwer/Plenum, 2003:335–48.
39. Greene RW, Biederman J, Faraone SV, Wilens TE, Mick E, Blier HK. Further validation of social impairment as a predictor of substance use disorders: findings from a sample of siblings of boys with and without ADHD. J Clin Child Psychol 1999; 28:349–54.
40. Langberg J, Smith BH. Developing evidence-based interventions for deployment into school settings: a case example highlighting key issues of efficacy and effectiveness. Eval Program Plan 2006; 29:323–34.
41. Langberg J, Smith BH, Bogle KE, Schmidt JD, Cole WR, Pender CAS. A pilot evaluation of small group Challenging Horizons Program (CHP): a randomized trial. J Appl Sch Psychol 2006; 23:31–58.
42. Molina BSG, Flory K, Bukstein O, Greiner A, Baker J, Evans SW. Feasibility of a randomized study of the CHP model of treatment for ADHD in a large Pittsburgh middle school. In: Evans SW, Chair. School Based Treatment of Middle School Aged Children With ADHD. Symposium Presented at the Annual Meeting of the Association for Behavioral and Cognitive Therapies, Chicago, IL, 2006.
43. Evans SW, Green A, Serpell ZN. Community participation in the treatment development process using assessment and Community Development Teams. J Clin Child Adolesc Psychol 2005; 34:765–71.
44. Evans SW, Serpell ZN, Schultz B, Pastor D. Cumulative benefits of secondary school-based treatment of students with ADHD. Sch Psychol Rev 2007; 36: 256–73.
45. Special Education Programs. To Assure the Free Appropriate Public Education of All Children with Disabilities: Annual Report to Congress on the Implementation of the Individuals with Disabilities Education Act. Washington, D.C.: U.S. Department of Education, 2002.

46. Flory K, Molina BSG, Pelham WE, Gnagy EM, Smith B. Childhood ADHD predicts risky sexual behavior in young adulthood. J Clin Child Adolesc Psychol 2006; 35:571–7.
47. Jensen PS, Kettle L, Roper MT, et al. Are stimulants overprescribed? Treatment of ADHD in four U.S. communities. J Am Acad Child Adolesc Psychiatry 1999; 38:797–804.

24

ADHD in Girls

Amori Yee Mikami
Department of Psychology, University of Virginia, Charlottesville, Virginia, U.S.A.

Stephen P. Hinshaw
Department of Psychology, University of California Berkeley, Berkeley, California, U.S.A.

Although attention deficit hyperactivity disorder (ADHD) has garnered considerable research, controversy, and even notoriety among researchers as well as the popular media in recent years, only a small amount of our knowledge is based on studies of girls. Boys with ADHD outnumber girls with ADHD at a ratio of approximately 3:1 in community samples, and often at a far higher ratio in clinical samples (1,2). Nonetheless, the vast predominance of male-dominated samples in the ADHD literature extends beyond these ratios. Several key samples comprising a large percentage of the literature on ADHD are, in fact, exclusively male, and most mixed-sex samples have too few girls for separate analysis of female manifestations and mechanisms. There has been a surge of research on girls with ADHD in the past decade (3–7), but the field's predominant models still reflect what is known largely about males. Because ADHD is potentially underrecognized in girls and clearly underinvestigated in female populations, despite its significant impairments and influences on key life domains, investigation of ADHD in girls and women is a priority.

In this chapter, we first provide some historical perspective on the roots of this male-dominated literature in the field. We then summarize what we know about both the prevalence rates and manifestations of ADHD among girls versus boys and the processes and mechanisms through which

ADHD affects girls. Finally, we address the clinical relevance of these points, concluding with some theoretical implications and future directions for research.

HISTORICAL PERSPECTIVE

Girls with ADHD have been neglected both scientifically and clinically for several reasons. First, like most other developmental disorders that become salient prior to adolescence, ADHD more often appears in boys than in girls, making males with ADHD simply more visible (8). Second, boys with ADHD tend to have more concurrent aggression, oppositional behavior, and conduct problems than do girls with ADHD (3,5,9). Such externalizing symptoms were previously seen as part of the ADHD spectrum, so boys were more often selected for research investigations. Additionally, these externalizing symptoms are likely to attract the attention of parents and teachers, making boys prone to be referred for treatment, and then to become study participants in clinic-referred samples. However, recent assessment instruments that disentangle ADHD from externalizing behaviors (10), as well as formal recognition of the Inattentive type of ADHD (11), suggest that the field is beginning to recognize forms of the disorder that are more salient for females. Finally, we note that that there has been a general historical tendency for all biomedical sciences to prioritize research with males. However, this too has changed recently. Since the early 1990s the National Institutes of Health have explicitly required that grant applicants address adequate representation of females and ethnic minorities (and now children) in all proposals. Because of these changes, the door seems to be open for increasing recognition of ADHD in girls and women.

EPIDEMIOLOGY

Although definitive data on the prevalence of ADHD are limited, the best available evidence suggests that preadolescent boys outnumber girls by a ratio of approximately 3:1 in community samples but by 9:1 in clinic-referred samples (2), again because boys with ADHD are more likely to display concurrent aggressive behavior that elicits concern from parents and teachers. By adolescence, however, sex ratios in community samples may lower somewhat, with boys outnumbering girls 2:1. Furthermore, there is some suggestion that sex ratios may become equal by adulthood (12,13). However, because these latter data are cross-sectional, we cannot draw valid conclusions about developmental progressions. For example, females with ADHD could be more likely to persist in their symptoms; they could simply be more veridical in terms of self-report; or females with ADHD could be more likely to develop their symptoms later than do males. The field needs a larger number of prospective longitudinal studies to answer these sorts of process-oriented questions.

Regarding subtypes of ADHD, girls appear relatively more likely to display the inattentive type of ADHD than do boys, in both clinical as well as community samples (14,15). Indeed, the Inattentive type of ADHD may be particularly salient for girls, and so long as parents, teachers, and clinicians focus on the more noticeable and disruptive hyperactive/impulsive symptom cluster (11), girls will continue to be overlooked.

COMORBIDITY AND IMPAIRMENT

Results from meta-analytic reviews on the topic of sex differences and ADHD suggest several trends regarding comorbidity and impairment. Referral source appears to moderate a number of key findings. Among clinic-referred samples, boys and girls with ADHD are largely indistinguishable on most measures of comorbidity and impairment, with some suggestion that clinical samples of girls have lower IQ scores (5) and greater amounts of inattention (9) than clinic-referred boys. By contrast, in community (nonclinic referred) samples, girls with ADHD often seem less impaired than their male counterparts, although most sex differences are small in effect (5).

Most notably, girls with ADHD appear to have lower rates of comorbid disruptive behavior disorders (e.g., ODD, CD), than do boys with ADHD (5,9,14), but still demonstrate higher rates of disruptive comorbidity than do girls without ADHD (3,6). Additionally, girls may be more likely to display relational aggression as opposed to overt forms of aggression more typical of boys (Crick and Grotpeter, 1995); this form of aggression has been found to be more prevalent among girls with ADHD relative to girls without ADHD as assessed by adult-informant rating scales, peer nominations, and observation in a computerized game (16,17).

Findings are mixed regarding comorbidities with internalizing disorders (e.g., depression, anxiety). Whereas some studies suggest girls with ADHD have higher rates of internalizing comorbidities than do boys with ADHD (9), others in fact suggest the opposite (5), especially for community-based samples. Girls with ADHD, however, do appear to demonstrate higher rates of internalizing disorders than do girls without ADHD (6). Of note, few studies have examined sex differences in comorbidities past childhood. Rucklidge and Tannock (18) found that, particularly for internalizing symptomatology, adolescent girls with ADHD were more impaired than males with ADHD. Relatedly, other all-female samples have found girls with ADHD to have more internalizing comorbidities in adolescence than do girls without ADHD (4,7). An implication is that, by adolescence, ADHD may become an increasing burden for girls compared to boys, although prospective longitudinal studies comparing both sexes are needed to test this hypothesis.

Despite suggestive evidence that girls with ADHD have lower IQ scores than boys with ADHD (5), it may be the case that girls with ADHD have fewer diagnosable learning disabilities, as defined by discrepancy-based reading or math disabilities (14). Still, it is clear that girls with ADHD, relative to girls without ADHD, have significantly more school-related problems (e.g., special education placement, grade retention, speech/language difficulties) as well as lower academic and cognitive performance, including IQ and achievement test scores (3,6,7,19).

Some preliminary evidence also suggests that girls with ADHD are at risk for developing several problems specifically relevant to adolescence. First, girls with ADHD may be at higher risk for comorbid substance use disorders than are boys with ADHD (14,20), and girls without ADHD (4,7). Preliminary evidence also suggests adolescent girls with ADHD may display more bulimia nervosa symptoms and diagnoses than boys with ADHD (21) or than girls without ADHD (53).

Regarding neuropsychological functioning, girls with ADHD appear to demonstrate relatively comparable deficits to boys with ADHD in a wide variety of domains. First, when tested without medication, girls with ADHD show significant executive function deficits (e.g., response organization, planning, and set shifting), in contrast to girls without ADHD, and such deficits are similar in magnitude to those found in boys with ADHD (22–25). Executive function deficits (as well as other neuropsychological problems) have been found to persist in girls with ADHD as evidenced via longitudinal studies; such problems are particularly strong in girls who continue to meet criteria for ADHD from childhood to adolescence (4,26). On the continuous performance test, however, an objective measure of inattention and impulsivity, another study found that girls with ADHD were in fact less impulsive than were boys (27).

Regarding actual neural deficits, a magnetic resonance imaging study showed that, similar to boys with ADHD in relation to male controls, girls with ADHD had significantly smaller total cerebral volumes than did comparison girls. However, most other brain regions that had differed between boys with and without ADHD did not differ for girls. Exceptions to this trend were noted for the caudate and posterior-inferior cerebellar vermis, which were reduced in volume for girls with ADHD relative to the control group. Finally, adolescent girls with ADHD appear to have less efficient prefrontal processing on working memory tasks than do girls without ADHD, as indicated through functional MRI (29).

Next, girls with ADHD show clear impairment in their social relationships with peers, family members, and nonparental adults such as teachers and camp counselors. Although not part of the diagnostic criteria for ADHD, impairments in the social domain have been consistently demonstrated for children with ADHD (30). Girls with ADHD are highly peer rejected relative to girls without ADHD both in childhood (6) and adolescence (7). Some scant existing evidence suggests that girls with ADHD may in fact be more likely to be peer rejected than boys with ADHD (31), although other studies have found no sex differences in the high level of rejection associated with ADHD (30). Yet the symptoms of ADHD (e.g., intruding into a conversation, having trouble waiting one's turn in line, being inattentive to social cues) are perhaps more unusual in a normative sense when displayed by girls, and more disruptive within female peer groups than in male peer groups. Additionally, children with ADHD tend to have cognitive and language deficits, which may put girls at a particular disadvantage given the strong focus on verbal interchange in female peer groups (32). We also note that a critical distinction exists between children's general status in the peer group (i.e., acceptance or rejection) and their participation in dyadic friendships. Girls with ADHD also have trouble making and keeping stable friendships, and their friendships tend to be marked by high conflict (33).

In addition to their troubles with peers, girls with ADHD suffer impairment in their relationships with adults. First, girls with ADHD were found to be less popular with nonparental adults such as camp teachers and camp counselors than were comparison girls (34). This population also reports more contentious relationships with classroom teachers (18). Second, like their male counterparts (35), girls with ADHD have substantially impaired relationships with parents. Relative to those of comparison girls, the parent–child relationships of girls with ADHD appear to be marked by high levels of authoritarian parenting, verbal conflict during laboratory tasks, as well as high levels of "expressed emotion"—i.e., hostility/criticism and overinvolvement (6,36). Additionally, girls with ADHD (particularly the combined type) have been found to exhibit higher rates of abuse histories than do comparison girls, with such histories associated with externalizing behavior and peer rejection (37).

In sum, although there is a dearth of research about girls with ADHD, a body of emerging literature suggests that girls with ADHD suffer clinically significant impairments in functioning in a wide variety of domains. Indeed, the findings from Biederman et al. (3, p. 966) "...stress the severity of the disorder in females." The limited amount of prospective longitudinal data currently available strongly suggests that such impairments persist at least though adolescence in girls with this condition (7).

DEVELOPMENTAL PROCESSES

Realizing, however, that girls with ADHD are symptomatic and impaired in multiple domains does not inform us of the processes by which such problems emerge or by which some girls may show resilience. A developmental psychopathology perspective can address these questions, often via prospective longitudinal studies through which relevant mechanisms can be evaluated (38,39). As just noted, the field is only beginning to collect evidence about the longitudinal course of symptoms, comorbidity, and impairment of girls with ADHD, as well as process-oriented studies to examine the mediators and moderators of these effects. In this section, we attempt to address what we know about sex differences in the developmental process.

First, it appears that family and genetic loading exerts relatively similar influences on ADHD in girls as in boys. In both sexes, ADHD is moderately to strongly heritable (40). Whereas girls with ADHD are substantially more likely than non-ADHD girls to have relatives with ADHD, the rates of familial disorder seem comparable to those of boys with ADHD (41,42).

Additionally, it appears that whereas nongenetic risk factors such as low birth weight and maternal use of tobacco and other drugs during pregnancy are risk factors for ADHD, the effect of such factors does not seem to differ based on child sex. In other words, these risk factors seem equally likely to predispose girls as well as boys to ADHD (43,44).

What is the developmental course of ADHD? Again, our knowledge about this in girls is restricted by the few prospective follow-up studies of this topic. Studies of boys suggest a gradual reduction, over time, of the core symptoms of hyperactivity and impulsivity; however, inattentive symptoms seem more likely to persist (45). This pattern appears to be similar in girls with ADHD followed into adolescence (7). Nonetheless, up to 80% of children with ADHD still suffer from impairing symptoms of ADHD in adolescence. Rates of persistence into adulthood are more controversial, with several methodological factors (e.g., unsuitability of extant criteria for adults; need for multi-informant adult evaluations) highly influential in determination of exact rates of diagnostic persistence (46,47). Because girls with ADHD tend to display more inattentive symptoms than do boys with ADHD, it may be that ADHD is particularly likely to persist in girls as they reach adolescence and adulthood. Indeed, this fact could explain why the male: female sex ratio tends to become more equal in adolescent and adult samples.

Additionally, adult males with childhood histories of ADHD are at high risk for externalizing disorders (including antisocial personality disorder), academic failure, and employment problems (48). Even though girls with ADHD are somewhat less likely than their male ADHD counterparts to display these aggressive comorbidities in childhood, preliminary evidence suggests that girls do remain at high risk for both externalizing as well as internalizing problems in adolescence (4,7). This finding suggests that girls with ADHD may display multifinality with regards to adolescent and young adult outcomes, similar to what is found in follow-up studies of girls with aggression. That is, aggressive behavior in boys is more stable across time than aggressive behavior in girls, but girls with conduct problems are likely to develop disparate negative adult outcomes, including serious relationship problems and a propensity for internalizing symptomatology (49–51). The same pattern could hold for girls with ADHD, who may show higher risk than boys with ADHD for depression, anxiety, eating pathology, substance abuse, and serious relationship problems later in life. This provocative hypothesis awaits clearer tests via long-term prospective research.

Longitudinal work on mechanisms predicting competence and impairment among girls with ADHD has been conducted in our laboratories. First, we have found that both childhood ADHD and peer rejection independently (and additively) predict (1) girls' lower adolescent academic achievement, after controlling for childhood achievement, and (2) adolescent eating pathology symptoms (52,53). Similarly, ADHD status and peer rejection predict adolescent externalizing and internalizing behaviors (but not after controlling for baseline levels of those constructs). Importantly, childhood self-perceived scholastic competence (with control of actual academic achievement) is associated with resilient outcomes in several domains, for both girls with ADHD and without ADHD (52). Both ADHD and harsh/critical parenting practices in childhood independently predict girls' adolescent eating pathology, and the predictive relationship between parenting practices and eating pathology is stronger for girls with ADHD than for girls without ADHD (53), suggesting a mechanism that may operate differently for girls with ADHD.

Second, Lee and Hinshaw (53) found that girls' adolescent conduct problems, internalizing problems, and substance abuse were best predicted by childhood hyperactivity and noncompliance. A similar pattern had emerged for boys with ADHD, in that, childhood noncompliance and covert antisocial behavior outweighed early ADHD in predicting later delinquency (54). However, girls' adolescent academic achievement and school suspensions/expulsions were predicted only by childhood inattention problems. Overall, the field is just beginning to understand the predictors of, and mechanisms underlying, the longitudinal outcomes of girls with ADHD.

CLINICAL RELEVANCE

Investigations of girls with ADHD raise several crucial issues regarding assessment and intervention with this population. First, regarding assessment, we believe that clinicians, parents, and teachers need to increase their awareness that ADHD exists in girls and that, when it occurs, significant impairment is likely. Indeed, in one survey, 97% of people reported that they knew a male with ADHD, but 50% said they did not know ADHD even existed in women (P. Quinn, personal communication, February 11, 2003). Girls may be especially likely to escape detection if they have the Inattentive type of ADHD, which is marked less by disruptive behavior and more by disorganized, unfocused performance that may not come to professional attention (11). Standard parent and teacher reports of symptoms, which focus on observable behaviors that are externalizing in nature (including hyperactivity/impulsivity), may not be as sensitive for assessing girls who display inattentive and/or internalizing symptomatology. When girls with ADHD are referred, they are more likely to be older than boys, and the primary concern is more often a comorbid disorder rather than ADHD symptomatology per se. In addition, the diagnostic criteria for ADHD insist that symptoms must appear by the time the child is seven years of age; this particular criterion, however, may be overly restrictive for children with primarily inattentive symptomatology (55), a disproportionate number of whom are girls (14,15). Nonetheless, as indicated throughout this chapter, ADHD is substantially impairing in girls; underdiagnosis may well lead to a lack of appropriate services and interventions.

Related to the issue of assessment, debate exists about whether sex-specific clinical cutoffs should be used when diagnosing ADHD. Like many mental disorders, ADHD represents a cluster of behaviors (inattention, hyperactivity/impulsivity) that fall in a continuum across the population. With respect to genetic etiology, there is no single gene linked to the disorder, and the heritable contribution to ADHD appears across the entire continuum of relevant symptomatology (56). In short, there is no one gene, nor cutoff score, which clearly denotes ADHD versus its absence. As a result, one line of argument maintains that because girls in the population have lower rates of the core symptoms of ADHD, diagnostic thresholds should be sex specific (57). Having a lower threshold for girls would ensure that girls with high rates of sex-specific symptomatology would not be missed just because they happened to have less symptomatology than the most extreme boys. Counterarguments maintain that sex-specific cutoff scores may not yield truly impairing levels of symptomatology (58,59).

Clearly, this is an empirical question, and one that is a priority for future research. At present, we note that several large clinical investigations in the field have used a two-pronged screening strategy: (1) initial rating scales and checklists feature sex-specific norms (to ensure that potentially diagnosable girls are not missed as "false negatives" in the preliminary assessment phase), and (2) sex-neutral diagnostic interviews for the final phase of determining "caseness," to ensure that truly impaired participants are included (6,60).

With respect to treatment and intervention implications, the limited data in the field suggest that there are few, if any, differences in intervention response for boys versus girls. In three treatment studies, sex failed to moderate the effectiveness of medication as well as behavioral treatment, across a range of outcomes (61–63). However, these studies have primarily focused on prepubertal girls and girls with the Combined type of ADHD. First, if sex differences in medication effectiveness exist, they may be most likely to emerge during adolescence when differences in hormones and metabolism increase. Clinical anecdotes support this contention (64), although the limited existing data on medication effectiveness among postpubertal adolescents has not found sex differences (65). Second, it may be the case that different treatments are associated with maximum effectiveness for the Inattentive type of ADHD, a subtype that, once again, may be more salient for girls. Individuals with the inattentive type of ADHD may show a preferential response to relatively low doses of stimulant medication (66,67), suggesting that girls with ADHD may need lower doses of medication or more careful medication management to ensure that they are not overmedicated. Also, to the extent that girls with ADHD may be at least somewhat more likely to show associated internalizing symptomatology than their male counterparts, they may respond better to behavioral treatments. Indeed, children with ADHD who displayed comorbid anxiety disorders showed a relatively greater response to an intensive behavioral treatment program than did children without such comorbidity, in the Multimodal Treatment Study of Children with ADHD (62). However, we emphasize that systematic, empirically based investigations of the effectiveness of different treatments are needed before the field can draw any conclusions about sex differences in treatment response.

THEORETICAL IMPLICATIONS AND FUTURE DIRECTIONS

The study of girls with ADHD is a growing endeavor, but it is still relatively new. Overall, we can confidently assert that ADHD does exist as a real and substantially impairing condition in girls. However, we are in need of greater numbers of longitudinal, prospective studies that explore the course of ADHD throughout the life span, including adulthood. We note that ADHD seems to be particularly salient for adult women (at least according to self-report), so that the developmental precursors and concurrent manifestations of this phenomenon are an especially fruitful area for future study (68,69). Additionally, prospective longitudinal studies can elucidate mechanisms through which girls with ADHD develop impairment, as well as the mechanisms through which some girls with ADHD show resilience. Such knowledge has great potential to inform conceptual models of ADHD. For instance, if it continues to be confirmed that girls with ADHD are relatively more likely to display the inattentive type of the disorder than are boys, this finding would call into question the model of ADHD as a disorder characterized by faulty inhibitory processes that lead to predominantly impulsive behavior patterns (70,71). Additionally, the model of childhood ADHD as associated with early externalizing behavior patterns, inevitably leading to conduct disorder or serious aggressive problems in adulthood, may not apply for girls or at least may not apply as saliently as it does for boys. Finally, it is our hope that this deeper understanding of sex differences in ADHD will lead to both conceptual advances and more specific and fruitful assessment and treatment recommendations for boys and girls with this condition. The study of sex differences is essential for theoretical and practical reasons; relevant basic research and treatment research have the potential to improve both domains.

ACKNOWLEDGMENTS

Work on this chapter was supported by National Institute of Mental Health Grants R01 MH45064 and U01 MH50461. We gratefully acknowledge the many girls, and their families, who have participated in our research projects over the years.

REFERENCES

1. American Psychiatric Association. Diagnostic and Statistical Manual of Mental Disorders. 4th ed. text revision. Washington, D.C.: Author, 2000.
2. Lahey BB, Miller TL, Gordon RA, Riley AW. Developmental epidemiology of the disruptive behavior disorders. In: Quay HC, Hogan AE, eds. Handbook of Disruptive Behavior Disorders. New York: Kluwer Academic/Plenum, 1999: 23–48.
3. Biederman J, Faraone SV, Mick E, et al. Clinical correlates of ADHD in females: findings from a large group of girls ascertained from pediatric and psychiatric referral sources. J Am Acad Child Adolesc Psychiatry 1999; 38:966–75.
4. Biederman J, Monuteaux M, Mick E, et al. Psychopathology in females with Attention-Deficit/Hyperactivity Disorder: a controlled, five-year prospective study. Biol Psychiatry 2006; 60:1098–105.
5. Crick NR, Grotpeter JK. Relational aggression, gender, and social-psychological adjustment. Child Development 1995; 66:710–22.
6. Gaub M, Carlson CL. Gender differences in ADHD: a meta-analysis and critical review. J Am Acad Child Adolesc Psychiatry 1997; 36:1036–45.
7. Hinshaw SP. Preadolescent girls with attention-deficit/hyperactivity disorder. I. Background characteristics, comorbidity, cognitive and social functioning, and parenting practices. J Consult Clin Psychol 2002; 70:1086–98.
8. Hinshaw SP, Owens EB, Sami N, Fargeon S. Prospective follow-up of girls with Attention-Deficit/Hyperactivity Disorder into Adolescence: evidence for Continuing Cross-Domain Impairment. J Consult Clin Psychol 2006; 74: 489–99.
9. Eme RF. Selective female affliction in the developmental disorders of childhood: a review. J Child Clin Psychol 1992; 21:354–64.
10. Gershon J. A meta-analytic review of gender differences in ADHD. J Atten Disord 2002; 5:143–54.
11. Hinshaw SP, Nigg JT. Behavior rating scales in the assessment of disruptive behavior in childhood. In: Shaffer D, Lucas PT, eds. Diagnostic Assessment in Child and Adolescent Psychopathology. New York: Guilford Press, 1999: 91–126.
12. Milich R, Balentine A, Lynam D. ADHD combined type and ADHD predominantly inattentive type are distinct and unrelated disorders. Clin Psychol: Sci Pract 2001; 8:463–88.

13. Cohen P, Cohen J, Kasen S, et al. An epidemiological study of disorders in late childhood and adolescence. I. Age- and gender-specific prevalence. J Child Psychol Psychiatry 1993; 34:851–67.
14. DuPaul GJ, Schaughency EA, Weyandt LJ, et al. Self-report of ADHD symptoms in university students: cross-gender and cross-national prevalence. J Learn Disabil 2001; 34:370–9.
15. Biederman J, Mick E, Faraone SV, et al. Influence of gender on attention deficit hyperactivity disorder in children referred to a psychiatry clinic. Am J Psychiatry 2002; 159:36–42.
16. Lahey BB, Applegate B, McBurnett K, et al. DSM-IV field trials for attention deficit/hyperactivity disorder in children and adolescents. Am J Psychiatry 1994; 151:1673–85.
17. Ohan JL, Johnston C. What is the social impact of ADHD in girls? A multi-method assessment. J Abnorm Child Psychol 2007; 35:239–50.
18. Zalecki CA, Hinshaw SP. Overt and relational aggression in girls with Attention Deficit Hyperactivity Disorder. J Clin Child Adolesc Psychol 2004; 33:125–37.
19. Rucklidge JJ, Tannock R. Psychiatric, psychosocial, and cognitive functioning of female adolescents with ADHD. J Am Acad Child Adolesc Psychiatry 2001; 40:530–40.
20. Greene RW, Biederman J, Faraone SV, et al. Social impairment in girls with ADHD: patterns, gender comparisons, and correlates. J Am Acad Child Adolesc Psychiatry 2001; 40:704–10.
21. Disney ER, Elkin IJ, McGue M, Iacono WG. Effects of ADHD, conduct disorder, and gender on substance use and abuse in adolescence. Am J Psychiatry 1999; 156:1515–21.
22. Surman CBH, Randall ET, Biederman J. Association between attention-deficit/hyperactivity disorder and bulimia nervosa: analysis of 4 case-control studies. J Clin Psychiatry 2006; 67:351–4.
23. Hinshaw SP, Carte ET, Sami, N, Treuting JJ, Zupan BA. Preadolescent girls with attention-deficit/hyperactivity disorder. II. Neuropsychological performance in relation to subtypes and individual classification. J Consult Clin Psychol 2002; 70:1099–111.
24. Sami N, Carte ET, Hinshaw SP. Performance of girls with ADHD on the Rey-Osterrieth Complex Figure: evidence for executive processing deficits. Child Neuropsychol 2003; 9:237–54.
25. Seidman LJ, Biederman J, Monuteaux M, Valera E, Doyle A, Faraone SV. Impact of gender and age on executive functioning: do girls and boys with and without Attention Deficit Hyperactivity Disorder differ neuropsychologically in preteen and teenage years? Dev Neuropsychol 2005; 21:79–105.
26. Seidman LJ, Biederman J, Valera E. Neuropsychological functioning in girls with Attention-Deficit/Hyperactivity Disorder with and without learning disabilities. Neuropsychology 2005; 20:166–77.
27. Hinshaw SP, Carte ET, Fan C, Jassy JS, Owens EB. Neuropsychological functioning of girls with Attention-Deficit/Hyperactivity Disorder followed prospectively into adolescence: evidence for continuing deficits? Neuropsychology 2007; 21:263–73.

28. Newcorn JH, Halperin JM, Jensen PS, et al. Symptom profiles in children with ADHD: effects of comorbidity and gender. J Am Acad Child Adolesc Psychiatry 2001; 40:137–46.
29. Castellanos FX, Giedd JN, Berquin PC, et al. Quantitative brain magnetic resonance imaging in girls with attention-deficit/hyperactivity disorder. Arch Gen Psychiatry 2001; 58:289–95.
30. Sheridan M, Hinshaw SP, D'Esposito M. (in press). Efficiency of the prefrontal cortex during working memory in attention-deficit/hyperactivity disorder. J Am Acad Child Adolesc Psychiatry.
31. Hoza B, Mrug S, Gerdes AC, et al. What aspects of peer relationships are impaired in children with attention-deficit/hyperactivity disorder? J Consult Clin Psychol 2005; 73:411–23.
32. Carlson CL, Tamm L, Gaub M. Gender differences in children with ADHD, ODD, and co-occurring ADHD/ODD identified in a school population. J Am Acad Child Adolesc Psychiatry 1997; 36:1706–14.
33. Maccoby EE. The Two Sexes: Growing Up Apart, Coming Together. Cambridge, MA: Harvard University Press, 1998.
34. Blachman DR, Hinshaw SP. Patterns of friendship among girls with and without attention-deficit/hyperactivity disorder. J Abnorm Child Psychol 2002; 30:625–40.
35. Mikami AY, Hinshaw SP. Buffers of peer rejection among girls with and without ADHD: the role of popularity with adults and goal-directed solitary play. J Abnorm Child Psychol 2003; 31:381–97.
36. Johnston C, Mash EJ. Families of children with attention-deficit/hyperactivity disorder: review and recommendations for future research. Clin Child Fam Psychol Rev 2001; 4:183–207.
37. Peris TS, Hinshaw SP. Family dynamics and preadolescent girls with ADHD: the relationship between expressed emotion, ADHD symptomatology, and comorbid disruptive behavior. J Child Psychol Psychiatry 2003; 44:1177–90.
38. Briscoe-Smith A, Hinshaw SP. Linkages between child abuse and attention-deficit/hyperactivity disorder in girls: behavioral and social correlates. Child Abuse Neglect 2006; 30:1239–55.
39. Cicchetti D, Cohen DJ. Developmental Psychopathology, Vol 1: Theory and Method 2nd ed. Hoboken: John Wiley & Sons, 2006.
40. Hinshaw SP. (in press). Developmental psychopathology as a scientific discipline: relevance to behavioral and emotional disorders of childhood and adolescence. In: Beauchaine TP, Hinshaw SP, eds. Child and Adolescent Psychopathology: Developmental and Psychobiological Perspectives. New York: Wiley.
41. Rhee SH, Waldman I, Hay DA, Levy F. Aetiology of the sex difference in the prevalence of DSM-III-R ADHD: a comparison of two models. In: Levy F, Hay DA, eds. Attention, Genes, and ADHD. Philadelphia: Brunner-Routledge, 2001:139–56.
42. Doyle A, Faraone SV, DuPre EP, Biederman J. Separating attention deficit hyperactivity disorder and learning disabilities in girls: a familial risk analysis. Am J Psychiatry 2001; 158:1666–72.
43. Faraone SV, Biederman J, Mick E, et al. Family study of girls with attention deficit hyperactivity disorder. Am J Psychiatry 2000; 157:1077–83.

44. Mick E, Biederman J, Faraone SV, Sayer J, Kleinman S. Case-control study of attention-deficit hyperactivity disorder and maternal smoking, alcohol use, and drug use during pregnancy. J Am Acad Child Adolesc Psychiatry 2002; 41: 378–85.
45. Mick E, Biederman J, Prince J, Fischer MJ, Faraone SV. Impact of low birth weight on attention-deficit hyperactivity disorder. J Dev Behav Pediatr 2002; 23:16–22.
46. Hart EL, Lahey BB, Loeber R, Applegate B, Green SM, Frick PJ. Developmental change in attention-deficit hyperactivity disorder in boys: a four-year longitudinal study. J Abnorm Child Psychol 1995; 23:729–49.
47. Barkley RA, Fischer M, Smallish L, Fletcher K. The persistence of attention-deficit/hyperactivity disorder into young adulthood as a function of reporting source and definition of disorder. J Abnorm Psychol 2002; 111:279–89.
48. Mannuzza S, Klein RG. Adolescent and adult outcomes of attention-deficit/hyperactivity disorder. In: Quay HC, Hogan AE, eds. Handbook of Disruptive Behavior Disorders. New York: Kluwer Academic, 1999:279–94.
49. Barkley RA. Attention Deficit Hyperactivity Disorder: A Handbook for Diagnosis and Treatment 2nd ed. New York: Guilford Press, 1998.
50. Kratzer L, Hodgins S. Adult outcomes of child conduct problems: a cohort study. J Abnorm Child Psychol 1997; 25:65–81.
51. Pajer KA. What happens to "bad" girls? A review of the adult outcomes of antisocial adolescent girls. Am J Psychiatry 1998; 155:862–70.
52. Zoccolillo M, Pickles A, Quinton D, Rutter M. The outcome of childhood conduct disorder: implications for defining adult personality disorder and conduct disorder. Psychol Med 1992; 22:971–86.
53. Mikami AY, Hinshaw SP, Patterson KA, Lee JC. Resilient adolescent adjustment among girls: buffers of childhood peer rejection and Attention-Deficit/Hyperactivity Disorder. J Abnorm Child Psychol 2006; 26:823–37.
54. Lee SS, Hinshaw SP. Predictors of adolescent functioning in girls with attention deficit hyperactivity disorder (ADHD): the role of childhood ADHD, conduct problems, and peer status. J Clin Child Adolesc Psychol 2006; 35:356–68.
55. Lee SS, Hinshaw SP. Severity of adolescent delinquency among boys with and without Attention Deficit Hyperactivity Disorder: predictions from early antisocial behavior and peer status. J Clin Child Adolesc Psychol 2004; 33:705–16.
56. Barkley RA, Biederman J. Toward a broader definition of the age-of-onset criterion for attention-deficit-hyperactivity disorder. J Am Acad Child Adolesc Psychiatry 1997; 36:1204–10.
57. Levy F, Hay DA, McStephen M, Wood C, Waldman I. Attention-Deficit Hyperactivity Disorder: a category or a continuum? Genetic analysis of a large-scale twin study. J Am Acad Child Adolesc Psychiatry 1997; 36:737–44.
58. Barkley RA. Attention-deficit/hyperactivity disorder. In: Mash EJ, Barkley RA, eds. Child Psychopathology. 2nd ed. New York: Guilford Press, 2003:75–143.
59. Arnold LE. Sex differences in ADHD: conference summary. J Abnorm Child Psychol 1996; 24:555–69.
60. Zahn-Waxler C. Warriors and worriers: gender and psychopathology. Develop Psychopathol 1993; 5:79–89.

61. MTA Cooperative Group. Fourteen-month randomized clinical trial of treatment strategies for attention-deficit hyperactivity disorder. Arch Gen Psychiatry 1999; 56:1073–86.
62. Barkley RA. Hyperactive girls and boys: stimulant drug effects on mother–child interactions. J Child Psychol Psychiatry 1989; 30:379–90.
63. MTA Cooperative Group. Moderators and mediators of treatment response for children with ADHD: the MTA Study. Arch Gen Psychiatry 1999; 56: 1088–96.
64. Pelham WE, Walker JL, Sturges J, Hoza B. Comparative effects of methylphenidate on ADD girls and ADD boys. J Am Acad Child Adolesc Psychiatry 1989; 28:773–6.
65. Quinn PQ. Treating adolescent girls and women with ADHD: gender-specific issues. J Clin Psychol 2005; 61:579–87.
66. Wilens TE, McBurnett K, Bukstein O, et al. Multisite controlled study of OROS methylphenidate in the treatment of adolescents with attention-deficit/hyperactivity disorder. Arch Pediatric Adolesc Med 2006; 160:82–90.
67. Barkley RA, DuPaul GJ, McMurray MB. Attention deficit disorder with and without hyperactivity: clinical response to three dose levels of methylphenidate. Pediatrics 1991; 87:519–31.
68. McBurnett K. Ritalin treatment for DSM-IV Types of Attention-deficit Hyperactivity Disorder. In: Greenhill LL, Osman BB, eds. Ritalin: Theory and Patient Management. 2nd ed. New York: Mary Ann Liebert, 2000:253–63.
69. Arcia E, Conners CK. Gender differences in ADHD? J Dev Behav Pediatr 1998; 19:77–83.
70. Quinn PQ, Nadeau KG. Understanding Women with AD/HD. Silver Spring, MD: Advantage Books, 2002.
71. Barkley RA. ADHD and the Nature of Self-control. New York: Guilford, 1997.
72. Martinussen R, Tannock R. Working memory impairments in children with attention-deficit hyperactivity disorder with and without comorbid language learning disorders. J Clin Exp Neuropsychol 2006; 28:1073–94.

25

ADHD in Adults

Timothy E. Wilens, Jefferson Prince, and Joseph Biederman
Clinical Research Program in Pediatric Psychopharmacology, Massachusetts General Hospital, Harvard Medical School, Boston, Massachusetts, U.S.A.

INTRODUCTION

Adults with attention deficit hyperactivity disorder (ADHD) are increasingly presenting for diagnosis and treatment in psychiatric and primary settings. ADHD affects 4–5% of adults and is characterized by childhood-onset and persistent symptoms of inattention, hyperactivity, and impulsivity. Many adults with ADHD suffer from co-occurring depressive, anxiety, antisocial, and addictive disorders. Research has documented familial and genetic underpinnings, neuropsychological deficits, frontal-striatal, and catecholaminergic dysfunction. Treatment strategies include stimulant and non-stimulant medications as well as structured psychotherapies.

ADHD is a prevalent disorder worldwide estimated to affect 3–9% of school age children worldwide (1). Converging data on prevalence in adults suggests that 4–5% of college-aged students and adults have ADHD (2,3). Although historically ADHD was not thought to continue beyond adolescence, long-term controlled follow-up studies have shown the persistence of the disorder or prominent symptoms of the disorder plus impairment in approximately half of adults diagnosed as having ADHD in childhood (4). Although the diagnosis of adult ADHD has been questioned (5), evidence supports the syndromatic continuity of the disorder from childhood into adulthood as well as descriptive, face, predictive, and concurrent validity of diagnosing ADHD in adults (6,7).

Longitudinal studies in ADHD youth growing up show that, though the symptom clusters of hyperactivity and impulsivity decay over time, inattention tends to persist (8–10). Studies of clinically referred adults with

ADHD show that about half endorse clinically significant levels of hyperactivity/impulsivity and 90% endorse prominent attentional symptoms (11). Like some youth with ADHD, adults with ADHD tend to have additional cognitive deficits (known as executive function deficits) including problems in encoding and manipulating information; and difficulties with organization and time management (12).

Compared to adults without ADHD, adults with ADHD typically have childhood histories reflecting school dysfunction including deficits in educational performance, discipline problems, and higher rates of repeated grades, tutoring, placement in special classes, and reading disabilities (13,14). School problems faced by ADHD children often continue or worsen in college resulting in academic underachievement, low-grade point averages, lower completion rates, and more time to complete degrees (15). Adults with ADHD tend to have lower socioeconomic status, lower rates of professional employment, more frequent job changes, more work difficulties, and high rates of separation and divorce (16). Similarly, adults with ADHD have more speeding violations, drivers license suspensions, accidents, and poorer performance in driving simulators (3,17). Individuals with ADHD may have sleep disturbances both exacerbating ADHD symptoms (underarousal, poor attention) and being aggravated by the presence of ADHD (18). Adults with addictions (e.g., drugs or alcohol, smoking, gambling), repeated traffic violations (speeding, failure to renew license), and recurrent life failures (occupational, managing finances, academic)—especially in context to a family history of ADHD-should be screened for ADHD (see below).

DIAGNOSIS

ADHD can be diagnosed reliably in adults by carefully querying for developmentally appropriate symptoms from the DSM-IV attending to the childhood-onset, persistence, and current presence of these symptoms. Research shows that diagnosing ADHD based on the retrospective self-reports of adults is a valid method of diagnosing the disorder. For example, Murphy and Schachar reported high correlation (*R*'s>0.75) between childhood ADHD reports from adults with ADHD and their parents, and between current self- and partner-reported ADHD symptoms (19), however the use of rating scales alone may lead to underreporting in ADHD adults and overreporting in non-ADHD adults (20), necessitating a clinical interview for the diagnosis. Adult self-report scales such as the ADHD rating scale and the Conner's rating scales are valid and reliable instruments that have embedded the DSM criteria for ADHD; whereas the Brown-ADD and Wender-Reimherr scales are also used commonly to diagnose ADHD (and comorbidity) in adults (21). Clinical interview remains necessary in the final diagnosis of ADHD.

Common Histories of Adults with ADHD

- Difficulties in elementary and/or secondary school
  - Behavioral issues: Fidgety, hyperactive, disruptive, inability to stay seated
  - Reports of "Not living up to potential," spacey, forgetful, or overactive
  - Academics: Underperforming, discrepancy in abilities versus achievement
- College Performance
  - Poor study skills, procrastination on larger projects
  - Incomplete or longer duration to complete degree, difficulty engaging in further education
- Occupational Difficulties
  - Underachievement (mixed reviews), more absences, frequent job changes
  - Low efficiency: requiring more time to complete tasks than peers
- Home Problems
  - Disorganized, shifts activities prematurely, does not complete tasks
  - Procrastination
  - Poor time management
  - Strained relationships with spouse and children
  - General interpersonal disruption

Co-occurring psychiatric and learning problems exist in a majority of adults with ADHD. Adults with ADHD manifest higher rates of anxiety, depression, cigarette smoking, and substance use disorders than adults without ADHD (16). Conversely, approximately 15–20% of adults with substance abuse disorders, anxiety, depressive disorders, and bipolar disorders have ADHD (22–26). One comorbidity of great concern in adults with ADHD are the substance use disorders (27). Untreated adults with ADHD are at increased risk for an earlier onset, higher risk (50%), and longer duration of substance use disorders (28–30); conversely, substance abusers with ADHD have more severe substance problems and more difficulty going into remission (26,31,32). Since attentional dysfunction may be evident in a host of other disorders (e.g., depression, anxiety, dementias), careful attention to the existence of longitudinal symptoms and impairment of ADHD coupled with the possibility that the manifest cognitive deficits may be related to another co-occurring disorder are necessary for an accurate diagnosis. Adults presenting with diagnostic dilemmas or clinically significant co-occurring disorders such as depression, bipolar disorder, panic disorder, and substance abuse should be referred to a practitioner with experience in treating ADHD.

Assessment and Diagnosis

- DSM-IV is gold standard
- Several scales are available to aid assessment including the ADHD Rating Scale (RS), Brown Attention Deficit Disorder Scales, Conner's Adult Attention Deficit Scale, and the Wender Utah Rating Scale
- Reports validate reliability of data collected from adults with ADHD
- Neuropsychological testing to identify cognitive abilities, information processing, learning disabilities—not diagnostic of ADHD
- Potential use of neuroimaging and genetic testing to identify certain subtypes of ADHD—not diagnostic of ADHD
- Disentangling comorbidities and associated impairments are clinically derived

NEUROBIOLOGY OF ADHD IN ADULTS

Genes in ADHD in Adults

There is robust data suggesting biological underpinning of ADHD in adults (7,33,34). Family, twin, adoption, and molecular genetic studies show that genes influence the etiology of ADHD. The heritability of the disorder, about 70%, is among the highest within psychiatry (35). Family studies show that ADHD is more prevalent among the relatives of ADHD children, and the children of ADHD adults are at high risk for having ADHD themselves (36). For example, from 25% to 50% of children of parents with ADHD have ADHD (36,37). This high familial loading of adult ADHD led to the notion that biological factors may be stronger in adults than in pediatric ADHD (33).

Studies of children and adults have found evidence for the involvement of several genes in the etiology of ADHD: the D2 dopamine receptor gene, the dopamine-beta-hydroxylase gene, the dopamine transporter (DAT) gene, the SNAP 25, and the D4 dopamine receptor gene and others (38–40). The data for the D4 receptor are especially compelling because the gene variant associated with ADHD is known to mediate a blunted response to the neurotransmitters norepinephrine and dopamine (41), important neurotransmitters associated with the pathophysiology of ADHD.

Adults With ADHD Have Brain Anomalies

A substantial body of literature implicates abnormalities of brain structure and function in the pathophysiology of both childhood and adult ADHD (42–45). We have known for decades that ADHD youth show impaired performance on tasks assessing vigilance, motoric inhibition, organization, planning, complex problem solving, and verbal learning and memory. A recent meta-analysis has demonstrated that a smaller but substantial literature shows similar problems also impair adults with ADHD (43).

Consistently neuropsychological deficits have been documented in studies of adults with ADHD (44). These adults tend to have impaired performance on tasks assessing vigilance, motoric speed, response inhibition, verbal learning, and working memory (42,43). Age, learning disabilities, psychiatric comorbidity, and gender do not account for these impairments (43). While neuropsychological testing is not used clinically to diagnose ADHD in adults, such testing aids in identifying learning disabilities, subaverage intelligence, and specific information processing deficits.

As recently reviewed (34), current thinking suggests that a network of interrelated brain areas are involved in the attentional—executive impairments of ADHD children. The cingulate cortex plays a role in motivational aspects of attention and in response selection and inhibition. A system mainly involving the right prefrontal and parietal cortex is activated during sustained and directed attention across sensory modalities (34,46). The inferior parietal lobule and superior temporal sulcus are polymodal sensory convergence areas that provide a representation of extrapersonal space which plays an important role in focusing and selecting a target stimulus. The brain stem reticular activating system and reticular thalamic nuclei regulate attentional tone and filter interference, respectively. Working memory deficits implicate a distributed network including the anterior hippocampus, ventral anterior, and dorsolateral thalamus, anterior cingulate, parietal cortex, and dorsolateral prefrontal cortex (34,46).

Neuroimaging Studies of Adult ADHD

Reviews of the neuroimaging literature show that nearly all the structural imaging studies, using either computerized tomography or magnetic resonance imaging, found group evidence of structural brain abnormalities among ADHD individuals (46). The most common findings are smaller volumes in frontal cortex, cerebellum, and subcortical structures (45).

Functional imaging studies are consistent with the structural studies in implicating fronto-subcortical systems in the pathophysiology of ADHD (47). For example, in a positron emission tomography (PET) study of adult ADHD, Zametkin et al. (48) found reduced global and regional glucose metabolism in the premotor cortex and the superior prefrontal cortex. Three subcortical structures implicated by the imaging studies, caudate, putamen, and globus pallidus, are part of the neural circuitry underlying motor control, executive functions, inhibition of behavior, and the modulation of reward pathways. These frontal-striatal-pallidal-thalamic circuits provide feedback to the cortex for the regulation of behavior. Adults with ADHD also demonstrate less activation of the anterior cingulate than adults without ADHD (49). Of interest, functional imaging studies in children with ADHD show that stimulant medications do not affect brain growth adversely (50,51).

ADHD is thought to be mediated by catecholaminergic dysregulation- of dopamine and norepinephrine. While discrepancies remain, studies have shown increased DAT density in the striatum (52,53)—particularly important given that the DAT in the striatum is the site of action of stimulant medications used to treat ADHD (54).

Neurobiology and Genetics of ADHD

- ADHD is a highly familial disorder with heritability estimated to be 0.8
- Primary disturbance of catecholamine neurotransmission
- Anterior cingulate, frontal cortex, basal ganglia, corpus callosum, and cerebellum manifest decreased size in ADHD
- Variations in genes that code for DAT protein and dopamine D4 receptor (DRD4), SNAP 25, associated with distinct ADHD subtypes
- No current role for neuroimaging or genetic testing currently in diagnosis of ADHD

TREATMENT

Despite increased recognition that children with ADHD commonly grow up to be adults with the same disorder, the treatment of this disorder in adults remains under intense study. In addition, complicating the diagnostics and treatment strategy, many adults with ADHD have depressive and anxiety symptoms, as well as histories of drug and alcohol dependence or abuse. Thus, with the increasing recognition of the complex presentation of adults with ADHD, there is a need to develop effective therapeutic strategies. Formal guidelines on the treatment of adults with ADHD are lacking. Support groups (e.g., www.chadd.org) assist the newly diagnosed adult by providing ADHD education, available resources, and peer support. Coaching and organization training appear useful but remain unstudied (14). In general, it is important to set clear realistic treatment goals with the patient. Identify specific symptoms and problematic areas of functioning as targets of treatment. Response-based rating scales such as the Conner's and ADHD RS can be used to monitor outcome. Use additional therapies to support and compliment the effects of medication. As with children, college students, and adults returning to school may require additional educational services to succeed. Prioritize treatment if clinically significant psychiatric comorbidities are present with ADHD—typically sequencing treatment for the most severe disorder initially .

Although the efficacy of various psychotherapeutic interventions remains to be established, limited data suggests that standard interpersonal psychotherapies may not be particularly useful (55). In contrast, recent data suggests that specific cognitive-behavioral therapies adapted for medicated adults with ADHD may be useful (56). One open and one controlled trial have demonstrated efficacy of cognitive-behavioral therapies for medicated adults with ADHD showing improvement in not only ADHD but comorbidity and functioning outcomes (57,58).

Although medication therapy is well studied in treating ADHD in children, the use of pharmacotherapeutic agents for adults with ADHD remains less established. The medications used to treat ADHD largely affect catecholaminergic neurotransmission including dopamine and norepinephrine. A recent review of the literature (59) identified 15 studies ($N = 482$ subjects) of stimulants, and 28 studies of nonstimulant medications ($N = 1179$ subjects) including noradrenergic reuptake inhibitors, antidepressants, and cholinergic agents that may be useful for the treatment of ADHD in adults (Table 1).

Stimulants

The only FDA approved agents to date in adults with ADHD include the mixed amphetamine compounds, and the noradrenergic specific reuptake inhibitor, atomoxetine. Mechanistically, the stimulant medications—amphetamine, methylphenidate, and pemoline—block the presynaptic reuptake of dopamine (54) and norepinephrine while amphetamine additionally releases directly dopamine and norepinephrine (60); all resulting in accumulation of norepinephrine and dopamine in the synaptic cleft (61). Controlled clinical trials with stimulants (62–64), atomoxetine (65), and the catecholaminergic antidepressants (66,67) demonstrated significant short-term improvement in ADHD symptoms compared to placebo in adults (60). The stimulants methylphenidate and amphetamine are the most commonly used and highly effective in a dose-dependent manner for ADHD in adults (62–64,68). The stimulants have an immediate onset of action and may last from 4 to 12 hr based on the formulation of the agent (immediate, extended release). Longer term trials with methylphenidate in adults support the ongoing effectiveness and tolerability of stimulants (60,69). The most common side effects with stimulants include edginess, insomnia, headache, and mild increases in heart rate/blood pressure necessitating monitoring (62–64,70).

The side effects of the stimulants in ADHD adults have been reported to be mild with the following side effects most frequently reported: dry mouth, insomnia, edginess, diminished appetite, weight loss, dysphoria, and headaches (62–63,70). Mild increases in heart rate (+2–4 beats) and blood pressure (2–4 mmHg) occur necessitating monitoring blood pressure prior to and periodically with treatment (70). While the stimulants have an abuse liability (71); few reports of stimulant abuse in controlled or retrospective studies of adults with ADHD have emerged. Nevertheless, because of the potential for diversion (72) and misuse, careful monitoring and the use of extended release stimulants should be considered (73). For adults who manifest edginess or minor blood pressure problems with stimulants, the

Table 1 Medications Used in Adults With Attention Deficit Hyperactivity Disorder

Medication (generic)	Medication (brand)	Daily dose[a] (mg)	Daily dosage schedule	Common adverse effects
Stimulants				
Methylphenidate		20–100		Insomnia
	Ritalin		Twice to four times	Decreased appetite/weight loss
	Focalin			Headaches
	Metadate CD		Once	Edginess
	Concerta			Mild increases in pulse/blood pressure
	Ritalin LA			
Amphetamine		10–60		
Dextroamphetamine	Dexedrine		Twice or three times	
Mixed amphetamine salts	Adderall			
	Adderall XR[b]		Once	
Magnesium Pemoline	Cylert	75–150	Once or twice	Same as other stimulants Abnormal liver function tests
Noradrenergic Agent				
Atomoxetine	Strattera[b]	40–120	Once or twice	Sleep disturbance GI distress, nausea Headache Mild increase in pulse/blood pressure

Antidepressants				
Tricyclics (TCA) desipramine; imipramine	Norpramin, Tofranil,	100–300	Once or twice	Dry mouth, constipation
nortriptyline	Pamelor	50–200		Vital sign and ECG changes Insomania
Bupropion	Wellbutrin Wellbutrin SR/Xl	150–450	Three times once or twice	Risk of seizures (in doses >6 mg/kg) Contraindicated in bulimics
Venlafaxine	Effexor	75–225	Twice	Nausea Sedation GI distress

[a] Denotes typical daily doses.
[b] FDA approved for ADHD in adults.

addition of low-dose beta-blockers (i.e., propranolol at 10 mg up to three times daily) or busipirone (5–10 mg up to three times daily) may be helpful (74). The interactions of the stimulants with other prescription and non-prescription medications are generally mild and not a source of concern (75).

Stimulants

- First-line pharmacotherapy for ADHD in adults
- Two main types of stimulants, methylphenidate and amphetamine compounds have different effects and are metabolized differently
- Methylphenidate does not show up on urine drug screens
- Stimulants are not effective for comorbidities within ADHD
- Stimulants generally have few medication interactions (except with MAOIs)

Atomoxetine

Another FDA approved agent for ADHD in adults, atomoxetine, has been demonstrated in two large multisite trials to be effective in adults with ADHD (65). Atomoxetine specifically inhibits presynaptic norepinephrine reuptake resulting similarly in increased synaptic norepinephrine (65) with some increase in dopamine in the prefrontal cortex (76). In addition to the treatment of both inattention and hyperactivity/impulsivity in adults with ADHD, atomoxetine may be particularly useful when anxiety, mood, or tics co-occur with ADHD. Although untested, because of its lack of abuse liability (77), atomoxetine may be particularly of use in adults with current substance use issues. Atomoxetine should be initiated slowly (0.5 mg/kg/day for 2 weeks) and increased to therapeutic dosing over 1 month. Dosing of up to 100 mg/day is indicated, though increases up to 1.8 mg/kg/day may be necessary in refractory cases. Common side effects include dry mouth, gastrointestinal upset, sleep changes, and sexual dysfunction (males) (65). Additionally, because of mild increases in cardiac vital signs, adults should be checked prior to initiating treatment and periodically thereafter.

Antidepressants

Other available medications shown effective in adults with ADHD though not FDA approved for this indication include bupropion, desipramine, and pemoline—the latter two requiring serum level (desipramine) or frequent liver function test monitoring (pemoline) (60). Bupropion has been demonstrated in multiple open and controlled trials (78,79) to be useful for ADHD. Dosing of 400 to 450 mg (sustained release) appears optimal for best efficacy. Side effects include insomnia, edginess, and a theoretical risk for seizures with immediate release preparations. While a large literature suggests positive effects of tricyclic antidepressants in children and adolescents with ADHD (80), only one controlled trial exists in adults. Dosing of up to 200 mg daily of desipramine resulted in dry mouth, constipation, and sedation as the main side effects. Bupropion and desipramine may be particularly useful in adults with ADHD with comorbid anxiety, depression, tics, and substance use disorders (81).

Recent data suggest that procholinergic medications (e.g., nicotinic) may have a particular role in improving areas of inattention and executive functioning but data are limited. Modafinil, while shown useful in children with ADHD, has limited data suggesting efficacy in adults (82). Serotonergic antidepressants (e.g., fluoxetine) while useful for comorbid mood and anxiety, do not appear useful for ADHD in adults. A limited data suggest that pharmacotherapeutics of ADHD improve driving performance (83) and are associated with the prevention of substance abuse (84). Monitoring of treatment includes monthly visits initially until stable and then periodic reassessments subsequently (14). Although treatment is chronic, yearly reappraisals of the need to continue therapy are recommended.

Nonstimulants

- Atomoxetine is among first-line pharmacotherapy for ADHD in adults
- Atomoxetine may be particularly useful in treating comorbidity in ADHD
- Few drug interactions exist with atomoxetine; increasing use concomitantly with stimulants
- Tricyclic antidepressant and bupropion are second-line therapies
- Antidepressant dosing of the agents appears necessary for ADHD efficacy
- Empiric use of combinations may be appropriate in refractory and comorbid patients

Refractory Cases

Despite the availability of various agents for adults with ADHD, there appears to be a number of individuals who either do not respond, or are intolerant to adverse effects of medications used to treat their ADHD. In managing difficult cases, several therapeutic strategies are available. If psychiatric adverse effects develop concurrent with a poor medication response, alternate treatments should be pursued. Severe psychiatric symptoms that emerge during the acute phase can be problematic, irrespective of the efficacy of the medications for ADHD. These symptoms may require reconsideration of the diagnosis of ADHD and careful reassessment of the presence of comorbid disorders. For example, it is common to observe depressive symptoms in an ADHD adult which are independent of the ADHD or treatment. If reduction of dose or change in preparation (i.e., regular vs. slow-release stimulants) do not resolve the problem, consideration should be given to alternative treatments. Neuroleptic medications should be considered as part of the overall treatment plan in the face of comorbid bipolar disorder or extreme agitation. Concurrent nonpharmacologic interventions such as behavioral or cognitive therapy may assist with symptom reduction.

SUMMARY

ADHD in adults is a valid and reliably diagnosed disorder with clinical features highly reminiscent of the pediatric form of the disorder. Diagnosis is based on clinical assessment using the DSM-IV criteria with helpful ancillary information derived from diagnostic rating scales and neuropsychological testing. Many adults with ADHD suffer from co-occurring disorders and manifest academic, occupational, driving, and interpersonal impairments. Studies of biological features support a genetic etiology for the disorder, associated neuropsychological deficits, brain abnormalities, and catecholaminergic dysregulation. Treatment strategies are emerging that include structured psychotherapies, stimulant, and nonstimulant medications.

ACKNOWLEDGMENT

This work was supported by NIH grant R01 DA14419 (T. Wilens).

REFERENCES

1. Faraone SV, Sergeant J, Gillberg C, Biederman J. The worldwide prevalence of ADHD: is it an American condition? World Psychiatry 2003; 2:104–13.
2. Kessler R. The prevalence and correlates of adult ADHD in the United States: results from the National comorbidity Survey Replication. Am J Psychiatry 2006; 163:716–23.
3. Murphy K, Barkley RA. Prevalence of DSM-IV symptoms of ADHD in adult licensed drivers: implications for clinical diagnosis. J Atten Disord 1996; 1: 147–61.
4. Weiss G, Hechtman L, Milroy T, Perlman T. Psychiatric status of hyperactives as adults: a controlled prospective 15 year followup of 63 hyperactive children. J Am Acad Child Adolesc Psychiatry 1985; 24:211–20.
5. Hill JC, Schoener EP. Age-dependent decline of attention deficit hyperactivity disorder. Am J Psychiatry 1996; 153:1143–6.
6. Spencer T, Biederman J, Wilens T, Faraone S. Adults with attention-deficit/ hyperactivity disorder: a controversial diagnosis. J Clin Psychiatry 1998; 59 (Suppl. l):59–68.
7. Wilens T, Faraone SV, Biederman J. Attention-deficit/hyperactivity disorder in adults. J Am Med Assoc 2004; 292:619–23.

8. Achenbach TM, Howell C, McConaughy S, Stanger C. Six-year predictors of problems in a national sample: IV. Young adult signs of disturbance. J Am Acad Child Adolesc Psychiatry 1998; 37:718–27.
9. Biederman J, Faraone S, Mick E. Age dependent decline of ADHD symptoms revisited: impact of remission definition and symptom subtype. Am J Psychiatry 2000; 157:816–7.
10. Hart EL, Lahey BB, Loeber R, Applegate B, Frick PJ. Developmental change in attention-deficit hyperactivity disorder in boys: a four-year longitudinal study. J Abnorm Child Psychol 1995; 23:729–49.
11. Millstein RB, Wilens TE, Biederman J, Spencer TJ. Presenting ADHD symptoms and subtypes in clinically referred adults with ADHD. J Atten Disord 1997; 2:159–66.
12. Barkley RA. Behavioral inhibition, sustained attention, and executive functions: constructing a unifying theory of ADHD. Psychol Bull 1997; 121:65–94.
13. Wender P. The hyperactive Child, Adolescent, and Adult: Attention Deficit Disorder Through the Lifespan. New York: Oxford University Press, 1987.
14. Wilens T, Dodson W. A clinical perspective of ADHD into adulthood. J Clin Psychiatry, 2004; 65:1301–13.
15. Heiligenstein E, Conyers LM, Berns AR, Miller MA, Smith MA. Preliminary normative data on DSM-IV attention deficit hyperactivity disorder in college students [published erratum appears in J Am Coll Health 1998 Mar; 46:213]. J Am Coll Health 1998; 46:185–8.
16. Biederman J, Faraone SV, Spencer T, et al. Patterns of psychiatric comorbidity, cognition, and psychosocial functioning in adults with attention deficit hyperactivity disorder. Am J Psychiatry 1993; 150:1792–8.
17. Barkley RA, Murphy KR, Dupaul GI, Bush T. Driving in young adults with attention deficit hyperactivity disorder: knowledge, performance, adverse outcomes, and the role of executive functioning. J Int Neuropsychol Soc 2002; 8:655–72.
18. Stein MA. Unravelling sleep problems in treated and untreated children with ADHD. J Child Adolesc Psychopharmacol 1999; 9:157–68.
19. Murphy P, Schachar R. Use of self-ratings in the assessment of symptoms of attention deficit hyperactivity disorder in adults. Am J Psychiatry 2000; 157: 1156–9.
20. Mannuzza S, Klein RG, Klein DF, Bessler A, Shrout P. Accuracy of adult recall of childhood attention deficit hyperactivity disorder. Am J Psychiatry 2002; 159:1882–8.
21. Adler L, Cohen J. Diagnosis and evaluation of adults with ADHD. In Spencer T, ed. Psychiatric Clinics of North America, Vol. 27. Philadelphia, PA: Saunders Press, 2004:187–202.
22. Alpert J, Maddocks A, Nierenberg A, et al. Attention deficit hyperactivity disorder in childhood among adults with major depression. Psychiatry Res 1996; 62:213–9.
23. Fones CS, Pollack MH, Susswein L, Otto M. History of childhood attention deficit hyperactivity disorder (ADHD) features among adults with panic disorder. J Affect Disord 2000; 58:99–106.

24. Levin FR, Evans S, Kleber HD. Prevalence of adult attention-deficit/hyperactivity disorder among cocaine abusers seeking treatment. Drug Alcohol Depend 1998; 52:15–25.
25. Nierenberg A, Yan LJ, McMurrich SL, et al. ADHD in adults with bipolar disorder in the systematic treatment enhancement program for bipolar disorder. Paper Presented at the 156th Annual Meeting of the American Psychiatric Association, San Francisco, CA, 2002, May 17–22, 2003.
26. Schubiner H, Tzelepis A, Milberger S, et al. Prevalence of attention-deficit/hyperactivity disorder and conduct disorder among substance abusers. J Clin Psychiatry 2000; 61:244–51.
27. Wilens T. Attention-deficit/hyperactivity disorder and the substance use disorders: the nature of the relationship, subtypes at risk and treatment issues. In: Spencer T, ed. Psychiatric Clinics of North America, Vol. 27. Philadelphia, PA: Saunders Press, 2004:283–302.
28. Biederman J, Wilens TE, Mick E, Milberger S, Spencer TJ, Faraone SV. Psychoactive substance use disorders in adults with attention deficit hyperactivity disorder (ADHD): effects of ADHD and psychiatric comorbidity. Am J Psychiatry 1995; 152:1652–8.
29. Wilens T, Biederman J, Mick E. Does ADHD affect the course of substance abuse? Findings from a sample of adults with and without ADHD. Am J Addict 1998; 7:156–63.
30. Wilens TE, Biederman J, Mick E, Faraone SV, Spencer T. Attention deficit hyperactivity disorder (ADHD) is associated with early onset substance use disorders. J Nerv Ment Dis 1997; 185:475–82.
31. Carroll KM, Rounsaville BJ. History and significance of childhood attention deficit disorder in treatment-seeking cocaine abusers. Compr Psychiatry 1993; 34:75–82.
32. Levin FR, Evans SM. Diagnostic and treatment issues in comorbid substance abuse and adult attention-deficit hyperactivity disorder. Psychiatric Ann 2001; 31:303–12.
33. Faraone SV. Genetics of adult attention deficit hyperactivity disorder. In: Spencer T, ed. Psychiatric Clinics of North America, Vol. 27. Philadelphia, PA: Saunders Press, 2004:303–21.
34. Faraone SV, Biederman J. Pathophysiology of attention-deficit/hyperactivity disorder. In: Davis KL, Charney D, Coyle JT, Nemeroff C, eds. Neuropsychopharmacology: The Fifth Generation of Progress. Philadelphia, PA: Lippincott Williams & Wilkins, 2002:577–96.
35. Hudziak J, Heath A, Madden P, et al. Latent class and factor analysis of DMS-IV ADHD: a twin study of female adolescents. J Am Acad Child Adolesc Psychiatry 1998; 37:848–57.
36. Biederman J, Faraone SV, Mick E, et al. High risk for attention deficit hyperactivity disorder among children of parents with childhood onset of the disorder: a pilot study. Am J Psychiatry 1995; 152:431–5.
37. Wilens T, Hahesy A, Biederman J, et al. Influence of parental SUD and ADHD on ADHD in their offspring: preliminary Results from a Pilot Controlled Family Study. Am J Addict, 2005; 14:179–87.

38. Cook EH, Stein MA, Krasowski MD, et al. Association of attention deficit disorder and the dopamine transporter gene. Am J Hum Genet 1995; 56:993–8.
39. Faraone SV. Report from the third international meeting of the attention-deficit hyperactivity disorder molecular genetics network. Am J Med Genet 2002; 114:272–6.
40. LaHoste GJ, Swanson JM, Wigal SB, et al. Dopamine D4 receptor gene polymorphism is associated with attention deficit hyperactivity disorder. Mol Psychiatry 1996; 1:121–4.
41. Lanau F, Zenner M, Civelli O, Hartman D. Epinephrine and norepinephrine act as potent agonists at the recombinant human dopamine D4 receptor. J Neurochem 1997; 68:804–12.
42. Epstein JN, Conners CK, Erhardt D, March JS, Swanson JM. Asymmetrical hemispheric control of visual-spatial attention in adults with attention deficit hyperactivity disorder. Neuropsychology 1997; 11:467–73.
43. Hervey AS, Epstein J, Curry JF. The neuropsychology of adults with attention deficit hyperactivity disorder: a meta-analytic review. Neuropsychology, 2004; 18:485–503.
44. Johnson DE, Epstein JN, Waid LR, Latham PK, Voronin KE, Anton RF. Neuropsychological performance deficits in adults with attention deficit/hyperactivity disorder. Arch Clin Neuropsychol 2001; 16:587–604.
45. Seidman L, Doyle A, Fried R, Valera E, Crum K, Matthews L. Neuropsychological functioning in adults with attention-deficit/hyperactivity disorder. Psychiatric Clinics of North America, Vol 27. 2004:261–82.
46. Seidman LJ, Valera E, Bush G. Brain function and structure in adults with attention-deficit/hyperactivity disorder. In: Spencer T, ed. Psychiatric Clinics of North America, Vol 27. Philadelphia, PA: Saunders Press, 2004: 323–47.
47. Schweitzer JB, Faber TL, Grafton ST, Tune L, Hoffman JM, Kilts CD. Alterations in the functional anatomy of working memory in adult ADHD. Am J Psychiatry 2000; 157:278–80.
48. Zametkin AJ, Nordahl TE, Gross M, et al. Cerebral glucose metabolism in adults with hyperactivity of childhood onset. N Engl J Med 1990; 323: 1361–6.
49. Bush G, Frazier JA, Rauch SL, et al. Anterior cingulate cortex dysfunction in attention-deficit/hyperactivity disorder revealed by fMRI and the Counting Stroop. Biol Psychiatry 1999; 45:1542–52.
50. Castellanos FX, Giedd JN, Berquin PC, et al. Quantitative brain magnetic resonance imaging in girls with attention-deficit/hyperactivity disorder. Arch Gen Psychiatry 2001; 58:289–95.
51. Castellanos FX, Lee PP, Sharp W, et al. Developmental trajectories of brain volume abnormalities in children and adolescents with attention-deficit/hyperactivity disorder. JAMA 2002; 288:1740–48.
52. Dougherty D, Bonab A, Spencer T, Rauch S, Madras, B, Fischman A. Dopamine transporter density in patients with attention deficit hyperactivity disorder. Lancet 1999; 354:2132–3.
53. Krause K, Dresel SH, Krause J, Kung HF, Tatsch K. Increased striatal dopamine transporter in adult patients with attention deficit hyperactivity

disorder: effects of methylphenidate as measured by single photon emission computed tomography. Neurosci Lett 2000; 285:107–10.
54. Volkow N, Wang G, Fowler J, et al. Dopamine transporter occupancies in the human brain induced by therapeutic doses of oral methylphenidate. Am J Psychiatry 1998; 155:1325–31.
55. Ratey JJ, Greenberg MS, Bemporad JR, Lindem KJ. Unrecognized attention-deficit hyperactivity disorder in adults presenting for outpatient psychotherapy. J Child Adolesc Psychopharmacol 1992; 2:267–75.
56. McDermott SP, Wilens TE. Cognitive therapy for adults with ADHD. In: Brown T, ed. Subtypes of Attention Deficit Disorders in Children, Adolescents, and Adults. Washington, D.C.: American Psychiatric Press, 2000:569–606.
57. Safren SA, Otto M, Sprich S, Winett C, Wilens T, Biederman J. Cognitive-behavioral therapy for ADHD in medication-treated adults with continued symptoms. Behav Res Ther, 2005; 43:831–42.
58. Wilens T, McDermott S, Biederman J, Abrantes A, Hahesy A, Spencer T. Cognitive therapy in the treatment of adults with ADHD: a systematic chart review of 26 cases. J Cogn Psychother: Int Q 1999; 13:215–26.
59. Wilens T. Drug therapy for adults with attention-deficit hyperactivity disorder. Drugs 2003; 63:2395–411.
60. Wilens T, Spencer T. Pharmacology of amphetamines. In: Tarter R, Ammerman R, Ott P, eds. Handbook of Substance Abuse: Neurobehavioral Pharmacology. New York: Plenum Press, 1998:501–13.
61. Solanto, M. V. Neuropsychopharmacological mechanisms of stimulant drug action in attention-deficit hyperactivity disorder: a review and integration. Behav Brain Res 1998; 94:127–52.
62. Spencer T, Biederman J, Wilens T, et al. Efficacy of a mixed amphetamine salts compound in adults with attention-deficit/hyperactivity disorder. Arch Gen Psychiatry 2001; 58:775–82.
63. Spencer T, Wilens TE, Biederman J, Faraone SV, Ablon S, Lapey K. A double blind, crossover comparison of methylphenidate and placebo in adults with childhood onset attention deficit hyperactivity disorder. Arch Gen Psychiatry 1995; 52:434–43.
64. Wender PH, Reimherr FW, Wood D, Ward M. A controlled study of methylphenidate in the treatment of attention deficit disorder, residual type, in adults. Am J Psychiatry 1985; 142:547–52.
65. Michelson D, Adler L, Spencer T, et al. Atomoxetine in adults with ADHD: two randomized, placebo-controlled studies. Biol Psychiatry 2003; 53:112–20.
66. Wilens T, Biederman J, Prince J, et al. Six-week, double blind, placebo-controlled study of desipramine for adult attention deficit hyperactivity disorder. Am J Psychiatry 1996; 153:1147–53.
67. Wilens T, Prince J, Biederman J, et al. An open study of sustained-release bupropion in adults with ADHD and substance use disorders. Paper Presented at the AACAP, Honolulu, HI, October 2001.

68. Chandler MC. Long-term safety and efficacy of Adderall extended release in children with ADHD. Paper Presented at the Annual Meeting of the American Psychiatric Association, Philadelphia, PA, 2002.
69. Spencer TJ, Biederman J. Efficacy in a 6-month trial of methylphenidate in adults with ADHD. Paper Presented at the Scientific Proceedings of the 49th Annual Meeting: American Academy of Child and Adolescent Psychiatry, San Francisco, CA, October 22–27, 2002.
70. Wilens T, Hammerness P, Biederman J, et al. Blood pressure changes associated with medication treatment of adults with attention-deficit/hyperactivity disorder. J Clin Psychiatry 2005; 66:253–9.
71. Drug Enforcement Administration. Methylphenidate Review Document. Washington, D.C.: Office of Diversion Control, Drug and Chemical Evaluation Section, 1995.
72. Babcock Q, Byrne T. Student perceptions of methylphenidate abuse at a public liberal arts college. J Am Coll Health 2000; 49:143–5.
73. Greenhill LL, Pliszka S, Dulcan MK, et al. Practice parameter for the use of stimulant medications in the treatment of children, adolescents, and adults. J Am Acad Child Adolesc Psychiatry 2002; 41(Suppl. 2):26S–49S.
74. Ratey J, Greenberg M, Lindem K. Combination of treatments for attention deficit disorders in adults. J Nerv Ment Dis 1991; 176:699–701.
75. Markowitz JS, Morrison SD, DeVane CL. Drug interactions with psychostimulants. Int Clin Psychopharmacol 1999; 14:1–18.
76. Bymaster FP, Katner JS, Nelson DL, et al. Atomoxetine increases extracellular levels of norepinephrine and dopamine in prefrontal cortex of rat: a potential mechanism for efficacy in attention deficit/hyperactivity disorder. Neuropsychopharmacology 2002; 27:699–711.
77. Heil SH, Holmes HW, Bickel WK, et al. Comparison of the subjective, physiological, and psychomotor effects of atomoxetine and methylphenidate in light drug users. Drug Alcohol Depend 2002; 67:149–56.
78. Wilens T, Haight BR, Horrigan JP, et al. Bupropion XL in adults with ADHD: a randomized, placebo-controlled study. Biol Psychiatry 2005; 57:793–801.
79. Wilens TE, Spencer TJ, Biederman J, et al. A controlled clinical trial of bupropion for attention deficit hyperactivity disorder in adults. Am J Psychiatry 2001; 158:282–8.
80. Spencer T, Biederman J, Wilens T, Harding M, O'Donnell D, Griffin S. Pharmacotherapy of attention deficit disorder across the life cycle. J Am Acad Child Adolesc Psychiatry, 1996; 35:409–32.
81. Wilens T, Prince J, Spencer T, et al. An open trial of bupropion for the treatment of adults with attention deficit hyperactivity disorder and bipolar disorder. Biol Psychiatry 2003; 54:9–16.
82. Taylor FB. Comparing modafinil to dextroamphetamine in the treatment of adult ADHD. Paper Presented at the 153rd Annual Meeting of the American Psychiatric Association, Chicago, May 12–18, 2000.
83. Cox DJ, Merkel RL, Kovatchev B, Seward R. Effect of stimulant medication on driving performance of young adults with attention-deficit hyperactivity disorder: a preliminary double-blind placebo controlled trial. J Nerv Ment Dis 2000; 188:230–4.

84. Wilens T, Faraone S, Biederman J, Gunawardene S. Does stimulant therapy of ADHD beget later substance abuse: a meta-analytic review of the literature. Pediatrics 2003; 11:179–85.
85. Biederman J, Spencer T, Chrisman AK, Wilens T, Tulloch SJ, Weisler RH. Long-term safety and efficacy of mixed amphetamine salts extended-release for adult ADHD. Paper presented at the American Psychiatry Association 2004. Annual Meeting 2004; New York, NY.
86. Posner ML, Petersen SE. The attention system of the human brain. Annual Review of Neuroscience 1990; 13:25–42.

Section VI: Controversies

26

More Rewards or More Punishment?

Linda J. Pfiffner
Department of Psychiatry, University of California San Francisco, San Francisco, California, U.S.A.

The first inclination adults often have when trying to handle unruly child behavior is to become stricter and to follow the old adage, "spare the rod and spoil the child." Indeed, attention deficit hyperactivity disorder (ADHD) youth are exposed to more punishment and fewer rewards than children without ADHD or other mental health problems. Studies show that teachers and parents tend to rely on punishment to manage the disruptive, impulsive, and noncompliant behavior of ADHD youth and to get through the frequent behavioral and attentional problems surrounding execution of routine activities of daily living (1). The increasing recognition for a genetic or other biological basis of ADHD, suggests that children with ADHD elicit these interaction styles from adults (and other children) rather than the reverse. This may well be a result of a lack of response among children with ADHD to typical contingencies used with children. Unfortunately, the higher rates of punishment and lower rates of rewards typically being used are not serving to "normalize" their behaviors and may even exacerbate their problems. Answers to the questions of how and why ADHD children respond to contingencies are critical for understanding the best contingency mix for improving their behaviors.

THEORETICAL UNDERPINNINGS

Differences in motivational systems have been proposed to underlie the lack of response of ADHD youth to typical contingencies (2; Sonuga-Barke, and Derryberry in this volume). Haenlein and Caul (3) propose that

ADHD is linked to having an elevated reward threshold. In this model, the reward systems for ADHD and normal children are proposed to differ such that children with ADHD require greater amounts of reinforcement to sustain maximal performance than do normal children. Similarly, Douglas and Parry (4,5) suggest that ADHD involves differential sensitivity to rewards. In support of these theories, experimental laboratory data shows that children with ADHD show greater improvement in performance than normal children when continuous, relative to partial reinforcement is provided and perform less well than normal children under a partial reinforcement schedule, but show a similar performance when continuous reinforcement is provided (4,5).

Also consistent with these models, children with ADHD appear to be particularly sensitive to factors affecting reward magnitude and value. Haenlein and Caul (3) note that the amount of effort required to do a task may be one such factor. For easy tasks (presumably more rewarding), the performance of those with and without ADHD was shown to be similar; but on harder tasks (presumably less rewarding) the performance of ADHD youth was shown to be much less than normal children.

Timing of reinforcement is another factor affecting reward magnitude. Numerous studies document that ADHD children have a heightened response to immediate reinforcement and show greater frustration and decrements in performance under conditions of delayed reinforcement (3). Delayed reinforcement is thought to reduce the value of the reward for those with ADHD due to impaired signaling of delayed rewards (6). The "delay aversion hypothesis" (6) refers to a negative emotional reaction to the imposition of delay which results in attempts to avoid or escape the delay. Consistent with the delay aversion hypothesis, children with ADHD show a preference for small, immediate rewards over large, delayed rewards (6,7). Sagvolden et al. (8) suggest that individuals with ADHD have a shorter and steeper delay of reinforcement gradient than those without ADHD whereby the reinforcing effect is greatest when the reward is provided immediately after the response. Interestingly, a recent study found that children were more willing to wait for the larger reward if extra stimulation (looking at a cartoon) was provided during the waiting period (7). Neural evidence for diminished reward anticipation among adolescents with ADHD was recently reported (9).

Another motivational theory posits involvement of the behavioral inhibition system (BIS) in the apparent diminished response to punishment exhibited by ADHD youth. Quay (10) applies Gray's model of emotion and anxiety and theorizes that an underactive BIS underlies the poor response inhibition, motivation, and regulation difficulties of ADHD youth. Quay (10) posits that ADHD children are less avoidant or cautious to cues of punishment or nonreward because of a weak inhibition system. Physiological data such as that reported by Iaboni et al. (11) showing increased skin conductance during extinction trials and increased heart rate habituation to rewards, supports a weak BIS explanation for ADHD. However, other studies are not consistent in finding support for a weak-BIS model (12).

Dysfunctional reward responding as described above has been linked to other aspects of Gray's model (12). The behavioral activation system (BAS) leads to approach behavior when signals of reward are detected or active avoidance to escape punishment (e.g., child avoids teasing peers). As noted above, children with ADHD may be underresponsive to rewards, suggesting a weak BAS. Other findings suggest that children with ADHD may be overresponsive to reward (and hence have an overactive BAS), especially to immediate rewards. This overresponsiveness is proposed to be related to the frequent finding that ADHD children show high levels of impulsive response or difficulty inhibiting responses when cues for rewards are present. Dysregulated BIS and BAS systems may also play a role due to failure of response modulation (13). There is also some evidence for ADHD subtype differences in motivation. Huang-Pollock et al. (14) found that children with ADHD-I tended to give up more easily than those with ADHD-C when rewards became less available on a reward-based variation of the stop-signal paradigm.

Although the focus on this chapter is on motivational factors, poor response inhibition, and attentional problems are not fully accounted for by these factors (15–17), suggesting that other factors perhaps related to arousal or regulatory difficulties play a role as well (see also this volume Sonuga-Barke, pp. 111 and Derryberry, pp. 85). Nevertheless, these motivational theories help guide our understanding of potential mechanisms underlying the atypical response to contingencies observed among children with ADHD.

THE EFFECTS OF MODIFYING CONTINGENCIES

The motivational theories cited above imply that the behavior and performance of children with ADHD should improve by carefully modifying external contingencies for behaviors in the classroom and at home. Although some have argued that external rewards may operate to decrease motivation and therefore be ill-advised, existing data challenges this belief (18). In their meta-analysis of research on intrinsic task interest and creativity, Eisenberger and Cameron (18) reported that tangible rewards for completing tasks or meeting a standard of quality did not impact time spent on the task when the reward was eliminated. In addition, verbal reward increased time on task after the reward's removal and task-liking improved after rewards dependent on performance quality. Reward contingent on creative performance was also shown to increase generalized creativity. The only detrimental effects of reward occurred when reward was provided regardless of performance.

Studies with youth having ADHD support the positive impact of external rewards. Consistent with theories cited above, both experimental and applied studies clearly demonstrate that children with ADHD perform more poorly than controls in the absence of external contingencies. Carlson et al. (19) found that response cost improved accuracy on an arithmetic task relative to reward, but that both rewards and response cost had beneficial effects on motivation (desire to complete the task again) compared to no contingencies; the use of rewards was associated with the highest ratings of wanting to do the task again. The study also revealed that response cost seemed to promote greater intrinsic motivation on a behavioral measure. Neither rewards nor response cost was associated with negative effects on self-reported or observed motivation. In a second study, Carlson and Tamm (20) also found positive effects of both rewards and response cost on performance during high- and low-interest tasks; response cost actually normalized performance. Having a high-interest task also improved performance relative to a low-interest task. Importantly, neither rewards nor response cost reduced motivation, except that during a low-interest task, response cost seemed to reduce task liking.

Applied studies in classroom environments suggest that the value of rewards and punishment depend on how and when they are used. When contingencies consist of primarily praise, the effects are not much different from those without any contingencies (21,22) and are well below those achieved with reprimands alone (22). However, when more potent, individualized incentive systems are used (e.g., stars exchangeable for work breaks, special activities, running errands, stickers, extra recess, special toys, special award tag, posting work, and good note home) and the frequency of positive consequences are increased, on-task behavior and academic accuracy is improved and approximates that achieved when negative consequences are used (23). However, this all-positive approach to classroom management seems to be most effective after children have learned the rules (via negative consequences) and following the gradual removal of the negative consequences (24). Consideration of using such an approach is also dependent on the availability of teacher time and effort, both much higher with the all-positive compared to the combination approach. In addition, the appropriateness of rewards is dependent on the type of behavior they are designed to change. For at least some children, rewards in the form of encouraging comments (keep it up, etc.) contingent upon off-task behavior seem to exacerbate such behavior (25).

In the case of punishment, effectiveness is highly dependent on the specific type of punishment used. Punishment that is "prudent" (e.g., calm, consistent, concrete) is far more effective than imprudent punishment (e.g., loud, emotional, inconsistent) when it comes to on-task behavior and work productivity in the classroom and compliant behavior with parents (22). In fact, imprudent negative consequences appear to be even more deleterious than not using negative consequences at all (22). A number of specific parameters of punishment influence effectiveness. Abramowitz and O'Leary (26) found that immediate reprimands resulted in much lower rates of interactive off-task behavior in the classroom than delayed (by 2 min) reprimands—although differences in noninteractive off-task behavior (e.g., daydreaming) were not detected. Lengthy reprimands have also been shown to be far less effective than brief ones in lowering off-task behaviors in the classroom (27), and consistent reprimands are more effective than inconsistent feedback (sometimes using reprimands sometimes using permissive responses) for reducing inappropriate solicitations (28). Response cost appears to be more effective in decreasing off-task behaviors than reprimands, particularly when delivered consistently (29).

Similar to the experimental studies, reward and cost token programs have been shown to be equally effective in substantially increasing on-task behavior relative to low rates of praise and reprimands only. There was superior maintenance of on-task behavior following fading of response cost relative to reward, especially for the children rated high on hyperactivity and aggression (30), possibly because the fading procedure was more discriminable in the reward than response cost condition. Children with disruptive behavior problems may be particularly sensitive to the fading of rewards due to the motivational theories cited previously.

Other evidence supporting the importance of enhanced positive consequences and prudent negative consequences comes from intervention studies with ADHD. Outcomes from parent training studies with families having a child with ADHD show that parent increases in contingent positive consequences and "good" commands were related to improvements in child compliance (31). In the Multisite Treatment Study of ADHD (MTA Study), children received either combined medication or behavior therapy (BT), only medication, only BT or "treatment as usual" as offered in the community. One of the components of BT was intensive training for parents in the use of more powerful rewards and prudent punishments. The value of this training is clearly seen in the finding that the success of combination treatment for school outcomes (social skills, disruptive behavior) was related to reductions in negative and ineffective parenting practices at home (32,33).

OTHER FACTORS INFLUENCING EFFECTS OF CONTINGENCIES

Medication

Decisions about contingency choices may depend on whether medication is being used. Animal studies show that stimulant medication affects reward centers in the brain and operate to decrease reward thresholds (3,17). A number of studies suggest that this may be true for children with ADHD as well. For example, early studies show enhanced performance with stimulant treatment (ST) on effortful tasks, presumably because the reward value of the task increases with ST (3). More recent studies have found that ST may increase the reward value of reinforcers such as money (34), may dampen inappropriate responding to the arousing and distracting effects of reward and may also increase sensitivity to punishment (35). Along these lines, Abramowitz et al. (36) found that ST reduced the need for the most intense negative consequences (i.e., immediate reprimands) and Fabiano et al. (37) report that low doses of ST increased efficacy of low-intensity behavior modification in the classroom. Reports from the MTA Study show that children in the medication only condition, who by definition did not receive programmed changes in contingencies at school or at home, showed significant improvement relative to the community care control group (38). These findings are consistent with the notion that ST may improve the response to everyday low-intensity contingencies for at least some children.

Comorbid Disorders

The presence of one or more comorbid disorders may also moderate response to contingencies. For example, children with disruptive behavior disorders without anxiety have been reported to have a reward-dominant style, meaning that effects of reward are stronger than the effects of punishment. This style would lead to deficits in avoidance learning when competing rewards and punishments are present. On the other hand, the presence of anxiety has been shown to increase response to cues for punishment and frustrative nonreward, hypothesized to be due to an overly active BIS (39). One implication is that anxious ADHD children may be particularly sensitive to very mild forms of punishment, and more intense punishment may be contraindicated for these children. The MTA findings also show that the effects of behavioral treatment (having a heavy emphasis on contingency management, particularly use of positive consequences) were particularly strong for those with comorbid anxiety (40). Those with a disruptive behavior disorder but without anxiety may be less affected by mild punishment, but very responsive to powerful rewards.

Comorbid oppositional defiant disorder (ODD) and/or CD may also have implications for specific contingency combinations. For example, in the case of impulsive aggressive behavior, prudent punishment is often necessary to stop the behavior immediately, but powerful rewards for self-control at other times would be expected to be important as well. Very little research has been done on how to tailor contingencies for maximal effects across comorbid disorders and behaviors, and the need for such research seems clear.

CLOSING COMMENTS

Relative to normal children, those with ADHD report a preference for less challenging tasks and a greater reliance on external (rather than internal) criteria for success (41). Similarly, parents and teachers report that children with ADHD-C and ADHD-I show motivational deficits including a lack of intrinsic interest in learning, preference for easy work, and a lack of a mastery approach to learning. Booth et al. (41) also report that children with ADHD-I are motivated more by pleasing the teacher and making good grades than by their own internal curiosity or interest. These findings and those cited above strongly support the need for modifying external contingencies to boost the motivation and performance of ADHD youth.

Although the natural tendency is for parents and teachers to decrease their use of rewards and increase their use of punishment to handle the negative behaviors of ADHD youth, the most successful approaches in natural settings appear to involve dense schedules of each, but with a very healthy ratio of powerful rewards to prudent negative consequences, for example, a ratio of at least 5:1 positive to negative comments/consequences (42). Perhaps even more important than the ratio, however, are how and when rewards and negative consequences (punishment) are used. Rewards need to be immediate, frequent (if not continuous when teaching new behavior), of high value and contingent on specific desired behaviors. In addition, reinforcement for competing behaviors should be kept to a minimum. Negative consequences need to be delivered prudently; i.e., immediately, briefly, unemotionally, and backed up with a loss of privilege (response cost) or time-out when necessary. When administered properly, these consequences can produce dramatic improvement in performance without untoward effects on motivation or intrinsic interest in the task.

REFERENCES

1. Johnston C. Parent characteristics and parent–child interactions in families of nonproblem children and ADHD children with higher and lower levels of oppositional-defiant behavior. J Abnorm Child Psychol 1996; 24:85–104.
2. Luman M, Oosterlaan J, Sergeant JA. The impact of reinforcement contingencies on AD/HD: a review and theoretical appraisal. Clin Psychol Rev 2005; 25:183–213.
3. Haenlein M, Caul WF. Attention deficit disorder with hyperactivity: a specific hypothesis of reward dysfunction. J Am Acad Child Adolesc Psychiatry 1986; 26:356–62.

4. Douglas VI, Parry PA. Effect of reward on delayed reaction time task performance of hyperactive children. J Abnorm Child Psychol 1983; 11:313–26.
5. Parry PA, Douglas VI. Effects of reinforcement on concept identification in hyperactive children. J Abnorm Child Psychol 1983; 11:327–40.
6. Sonuga-Barke EJS. Causal models of attention-deficit/hyperactivity disorder: from common simple deficits to multiple developmental pathways. Biol Psychiatry 2005; 57:1231–8.
7. Antrop I, Stock P, Verte S, Wiersema JR, Baeyens D, Roeyers H. ADHD and delay aversion: the influence of non-temporal stimulation on choice for delayed rewards. J Child Psychol Psychiatry 2006; 47:1152–8.
8. Sagvolden T, Aase H, Zeiner P, Berger D. Altered reinforcement mechanisms in attention-deficit/hyperactivity disorder. Behav Brain Res 1998; 94:61–71.
9. Scheres A, Milham MP, Knutson B, Castellanos X. Ventral striatal hyporesponsiveness during reward anticipation in attention-deficit/hyperactivity disorder. Biol Psychiatry 2007; 61:720–4.
10. Quay HC. Inhibition and attention deficit hyperactivity disorder. J Abnorm Child Psychol 1997; 25:7–13.
11. Iaboni F, Douglas VI, Ditto B. Psychophysiological response of ADHD children to reward and extinction. Psychophysiology 1997; 34:116–23.
12. Nigg JT. Is ADHD a disinhibitory disorder? Psychol Bull 2001; 127:571–98.
13. Newman JP, Wallace JF. Diverse pathways to deficient self-regulation: implications for disinhibitory psychopathology in children. Clin Psychol Rev 1993; 13:690–720.
14. Huang-Pollock C, Mikami A, Pfiffner L, McBurnett K. ADHD subtype differences in motivational responsivity but not inhibitory control: evidence from a reward-based variation of the stop signal paradigm. J Clin Child Adolesc Psychol 2007; 36:127–36.
15. Douglas VI, Parry PA. Effects of reward and nonreward on frustration and attention in attention deficit disorder. J Abnorm Child Psychol 1994; 22:281–302.
16. Oosterlaan J, Sergeant JA. Effects of reward and response cost on response inhibition in AD/HD, disruptive, anxious and normal children. J Abnorm Child Psychol 1998; 26:161–74.
17. Solanto MV, Wender EH, Bartell SS. Effects of methylphenidate and behavioral contingencies on sustained attention in attention-deficit/hyperactivity disorder: a test of the reward dysfunction hypothesis. J Child Adolesc Psychopharmacol 1997; 7:123–36.
18. Eisenberger R, Cameron J. Detrimental effects of reward: reality or myth? Am Psychol 1996; 51:1153–66.
19. Carlson CL, Mann M, Alexander DK. Effects of reward and response cost on the performance and motivation of children with ADHD. Cognitive Ther Res 2000; 24:87–98.
20. Carlson CL, Tamm L. Responsiveness of children with attention deficit-hyperactivity disorder to reward and response cost: differential impact on performance and motivation. J Consult Clin Psychol 2000; 68:73–83.
21. Acker MM, O'Leary SG. Effects of reprimands and praise on appropriate behavior in the classroom. J Abnorm Child Psychol 1987; 15:549–58.

22. Rosen LA, O'Leary SG, Joyce SA, Conway G, Pfiffner LJ. The importance of prudent negative consequences for maintaining the appropriate behavior of hyperactive students. J Abnorm Child Psychol 1984; 12:581–604.
23. Pfiffner LJ, Rosen LA, O'Leary SG. The efficacy of an all-positive approach to classroom management. J Appl Behav Anal 1985; 18:257–61.
24. Pfiffner LJ, O'Leary SG. The efficacy of all-positive management as a function of the prior use of negative consequences. J Appl Behav Anal 1987; 20:265–71.
25. Abramowitz AJ, O'Leary SG, Rosen LA. Reducing off-task behavior in the classroom: a comparison of encouragement and reprimands. J Abnorm Child Psychol 1987; 15:153–64.
26. Abramowitz AJ, O'Leary SG. Effectiveness of delayed punishment in an applied setting. Behav Ther 1990; 21:231–40.
27. Abramowitz AJ, O'Leary SG, Futtersak NW. The relative impact of long and short reprimands on children's off-task behavior in the classroom. Behav Ther 1988; 19:243–8.
28. Acker MM, O'Leary SG. Effects of consistent and inconsistent feedback on inappropriate child behavior. Behav Ther 1988; 19:619–24.
29. Pfiffner LJ, O'Leary SG, Rosen LA, Sanderson WC. A comparison of the effects of continuous and intermittent response cost and reprimands in the classroom. J Clin Child Psychol 1985; 14:348–52.
30. Sullivan MA, O'Leary SG. Maintenance following reward and cost token programs. Behav Ther 1990; 21:139–51.
31. Anastopoulos AD, Shelton TL, DuPaul GJ, Guevremont DC. Parent training for attention-deficit hyperactivity disorder: its impact on parent functioning. J Abnorm Child Psychol 1993; 21:581–96.
32. Hinshaw SP, Owens EB, Wells K, et al. Family processes and treatment outcome in the MTA: negative/ineffective parenting practices in relation to multimodal treatment. J Abnorm Child Psychol 2000; 28:555–68.
33. Wells KC, Epstein JN, Hinshaw S, et al. Parenting and family stress treatment outcomes in attention deficit hyperactivity disorder (ADHD): an empirical analysis in the MTA study. J Abnorm Child Psychol 2000; 28: 543–53.
34. Wilkison PC, Kircher JC, McMahon WM, Sloane HN. Effects of methylphenidate on reward strength in boys with attention-deficit hyperactivity disorder. J Am Acad Child Adolesc Psychiatry 1995; 34:897–901.
35. Arnett PA, Fischer M, Newby RF. The effect of Ritalin on response to reward and punishment in children with ADHD. Child Study J 1996; 26:161.
36. Abramowitz AJ, Eckstrand D, O'Leary SG, Dulcan MK. ADHD children's responses to stimulant medication and two intensities of a behavioral intervention. Behav Modif 1992; 16:193–203. [Special Issue: Treatment of children with attention-deficit hyperactivity disorder (ADHD)].
37. Fabiano G, Pelham Jr. W, Gnagy E, et al. The single and combined effects of multiple intensities of behavior modification and methylphenidate for children with ADHD in a classroom setting. Sch Psychol Rev 2007; 36:195–214.

38. MTA. A 14-month randomized clinical trial of treatment strategies for attention-deficit/hyperactivity disorder. Arch Gen Psychiatry 1999; 56: 1073–86.
39. O'Brien BS, Frick PJ. Reward dominance: associations with anxiety, conduct problems, and psychopathy in children. J Abnorm Child Psychol 1996; 24: 223–40.
40. Jensen PS, Hinshaw SP, Kraemer HC, et al. ADHD comorbidity findings from the MTA study: comparing comorbid subgroups. J Am Acad Child Adolesc Psychiatry 2001; 40:147–58.
41. Booth J, Carlson CL, Shin MC, W. Parent, teacher, and self-rated motivational styles in eh ADHD subtypes. ADHD Report 2001; 9:8–11.
42. Pelham WE. Evidence-based Psychosocial Treatment for ADHD Children and Adolescents. Buffalo, NY: Center for Children and Families, Department of Psychology, State University of New York at Buffalo, 2004.

27

Against the Grain: A Proposal for a Psychosocial First Approach to Treating ADHD—the Buffalo Treatment Algorithm

William E. Pelham, Jr.

Center for Children and Families, State University of New York at Buffalo, Buffalo, New York, U.S.A.

Attention deficit hyperactivity disorder (ADHD) is a prevalent and chronic mental health disorder associated with adverse outcomes through the life span. These include severe disruptions in relationships with parents, teachers, peers and siblings during childhood, academic problems throughout the school years, delinquency in adolescents, and substance use difficulties in adulthood (1). With a prevalence rate of 2% to 9% (2,3), it is one of the most common problems encountered in mental health, primary care, and educational settings. Further, the prevalence of ADHD is consistent with this rate throughout the rest of the world (4).

Because of its adverse outcomes and prevalence, ADHD is a costly problem for society. It is estimated that the annual per child cost of illness (COI) of ADHD in the United States in 2005 is more than US $14,000—more than US $40 billion annually—and that this number is likely underestimated by 50% due to lack of available figures (5). Of this total, estimates for pharmacological treatment with a long-acting stimulant (currently used in over 80% of cases) are US $1440 per year (not including physician's costs); other health care costs associated with ADHD (e.g., emergency room visits due to accidents) average US $1000 annually per child. Much larger amounts are spent annually by schools, juvenile justice systems, and, though limited data are available, families. These costs approximate those of major depression and stroke in the United States (5). Thus, ADHD is a major public health problem in the United States and worldwide.

There are currently three evidence-based treatments for ADHD: (1) behavior modification, (2) stimulant medication, and (3) their combination (2). Stimulant medication, behavioral treatment, and multimodal treatment all have well-established proof of efficacy in short-term studies—hundreds of studies of stimulants (6), 175 studies of behavioral treatments, and 25 studies of combined interventions (7,8). The acute effects of the two modalities are quite substantial and generally comparable, with moderate to large effect sizes across a range of measures, including symptoms of ADHD (e.g., as rated by parents and teachers), classroom behavior and seatwork productivity, compliance with adult requests, and interactions with peers (9). The impact of medication is generally larger on symptom scales, while behavioral treatments have larger effects on functional measures (8,9). Current guidelines call for medication to be administered across settings and days of the week. Behavioral treatments with solid evidence include those provided to parents (parent training), in schools (behavioral classroom management), and to ADHD children themselves for problems with peers (8).

Despite the large evidence base and comparable effects for the two treatments, most medical professionals believe that medication is more effective than behavioral treatments. Indeed, leading ADHD researchers have argued that the effectiveness of medication means that most ADHD children do not need behavioral treatments (10–13). Prominent psychiatric and advocacy groups who have published guidelines in the past 5 years have advocated that stimulant medications be the first-line and often the only treatment provided to ADHD children (3,14–17). In contrast, we are aware of only a single guideline that has suggested that behavioral interventions be employed first-line (9) and only one that states that either treatment could be so employed (2). As a result of this emphasis on medication, the great majority of identified ADHD children receive pharmacotherapy, which is widely available and commonly funded by insurance carriers. Current estimates are that stimulants are taken by 5% to 7% of the elementary-aged U.S. population—70% to 90% of identified ADHD children (3), and prescription rates are even increasing exponentially for preschoolers (18). A recent report (19) showed that utilization of ADHD medications increased by 49% from 2000 to 2003. The extensive pharmaceutical industry marketing to consumers and physicians no doubt contributes to this increase. Further, FDA approval of six new formulations of medications for ADHD in the past 5 years will increase these trends for the near future. This dramatic increase in use has led to growing concern among the media and the lay public about whether medication should be so widely used. Much of the controversy surrounding this issue results from a lack of information regarding whether all of these children need to be medicated.

Given that there are three evidence-based treatments for ADHD, a central question that faces every practitioner and family of ADHD children following identification and diagnosis is the following: Which of the treatments should a given child receive and in what sequence? Clearly physician practice is to begin treatment with medication and rely on medication alone. Parents' and teachers' preferences are to begin treatment with behavior therapy and only add medication if necessary. The most prominent parent advocacy group for ADHD children has argued that all children should receive multimodal treatments, with both modalities started simultaneously (www.CHADD.org). Given the availability of behavior modification and the fact that many parents prefer it to medication, a pertinent question is whether children who begin treatment with behavior therapy need medication—that is, whether medication use (or dosage) would decrease if behavioral treatments were begun first. Similarly, for parents who do not mind using medication alone with their child, medication alone might be the less costly treatment, and certainly involves less effort than does medication on the part of parents and teachers. If parents prefer to combine the two modalities, the use, dosage, and cost of behavioral treatments might be minimized if children were started on medication first and only subsequently received behavior therapy. Which of these strategies yields greater benefit for ADHD children in the short term? Which is likely to lead to the best long-term outcomes?

Despite all of the guidelines recommending medication as first-line treatment, the extant research literature has evaluated whether the treatments work in the short term when implemented independently or simultaneously. There have just begun to be studies of the appropriate sequence of treatments for a given patient that would provide guidance to address some of the questions raised above. The decision regarding with which treatment to begin in a given case must currently be based on factors other than the extant literature. We believe that a risk:benefit assessment of the two main evidence-based treatments that is provided clearly to parents is the primary consideration that should be used to develop treatment strategies for a given patient. What is known about the relative risks (and benefits) of the two evidence-based treatments?

RISKS AND BENEFITS OF THE INTERVENTIONS

Pharmacotherapy

Despite their widespread use and acute benefits, stimulant medications have limitations when used as the sole form of intervention for ADHD. For example, not all ADHD children show positive responses to stimulant drugs—70% to 80% are responders—and less than half show sufficient improvement for their behavior to fall within the normal range on teacher rating scales (20,21). Further and most important, there is a uniform lack of evidence that the drugs improve ADHD children's long-term prognosis, either in development of antisocial behaviors or in academic achievement

(22,23). Forty years of research have failed to show that medication provided as the sole intervention alters the abysmal long-term outcomes that characterize most ADHD children.

Furthermore, the stimulants are associated with risks of serious side effects, in addition to the well-known acute side effects (e.g., appetite suppression, motor tics, insomnia), (1) reductions in growth (12), (2) cardiac effects as recently cited in the FDA safety advisory panel's recommendation that stimulants receive a black box warning, as well as the FDAs decision to add warning language to all stimulants and to direct the development of parental warnings (54), and (3) possible increased risk of later substance use/abuse (24–26).

While some of these concerns may be minimized by employing very low doses, the trend among psychatrists is in the opposite direction. In general, studies have shown that increasing stimulant dose beyond a low-to-moderate level increases side effects at a faster rate than improvement (27,28). However, current influential practice guidelines argue for titrating dose to a level just below that at which side effects are obtained and no further room for improvement is available (2,3,10,11). However, this dosing strategy results in escalating doses—25% increase annually—to maintain effectiveness (29) and is associated with reductions in growth of 1 cm per year over 2–4 years (12). This trend is clearly toward using higher doses, prolonging active dosing well into the evening hours [e.g., with the long-acting stimulants that comprise the majority of the stimulant market, medicating 7 days per week, and toward continuing medication treatment for many years (3,14)]. A typical ADHD child who takes one of the newer long-acting formulations of methylphenidate (MPH; e.g., Concerta) and is medicated daily for a decade will consume nearly 150,000 mg of MPH over his childhood/adolescent years. Such a medication regimen has been widely recommended in recent years by ADHD experts (6,16). That dose is 15 to 30 times higher than the typical lifetime doses that were consumed in the medication regimen that was common in the 1980s and early 1990s, when the norm was short-acting stimulants for school hours only for a year or two (30). The safety and efficacy of such a high-dose, long-term stimulant regimen has never been investigated (24).

In short, although it has clear and often large acute beneficial effects on ADHD symptoms, stimulant medication is not without risks, which are largely unknown in the long run. What do we know about the risks and benefits of behavioral treatments?

Behavioral Interventions

As noted above, a large body of research has shown that behavioral treatments are acutely effective for children with ADHD (8,31). Furthermore, behavioral treatments specifically address the problems in functioning that predict and mediate long-term outcomes and therefore lead to long-term improvement if remediated (e.g., parenting skills, peer relationships, and academic functioning) that medication alone does not address (22,32,33). Furthermore, behavioral treatments have major impacts on these domains—typically larger than medication (8). Although there are not yet long-term studies as these findings suggest that behavior therapy should result in improvements in long-term outcomes for ADHD children. Finally, behavioral interventions do not have adverse side effects. Behavioral parent training and classroom management programs have no known side effects. Although some have suggested that group-based peer interventions have iatrogenic effects, systematic evaluations of this putative effect have not supported this speculation (34,35). Thus, behavioral interventions have no known side effects. Furthermore, parents strongly prefer nonmedication treatment to medication treatment for their children (36). In the multimodal treatment for ADHD (MTA), strong parent satisfaction with treatment was doubled from one-third to two-thirds of families when a behavioral component was present (38). Not surprisingly, family attitudes toward treatment are predictive of long-term treatment adherence (38), which is essential when dealing with chronic diseases such as ADHD.

Unfortunately, most children with ADHD in the United States receive psychosocial treatments that are not evidence-based in community mental health settings (39,40). These frequently used and often commonly reimbursed treatments include individual psychotherapy, play therapy, generic counseling, neurotherapy or biofeedback, sensory integration therapy, and occupational therapy. However, none of these interventions have any scientific support (8,9,16,39,40). In other words, they do not work. The result is that insurers and governmental entities that underwrite community-based treatments both locally and nationally are faced with paying for costly treatments (e.g., individual counseling for the child) that are not proven to be effective but use valuable resources (e.g., therapist time) and therefore ultimately contribute to the economic burden of mental healthcare in United States.

Thus, in contrast to a medication-first or usual clinic care model for treating ADHD, some professionals have begun to argue that a "do-no-harm" or "safety-first" approach, which characterizes most of pediatric care, should be applied to ADHD (9). Such an approach would prioritize evidence-based psychosocial (i.e., behavioral) treatments as a first-line treatment with medication as a second-line, adjunctive treatment. What might be the benefits of such an approach?

BENEFITS OF A BEHAVIORAL-FIRST TREATMENT APPROACH

The major potential benefits of a behavioral-first approach involve reducing the need for medication and thus the number of medicated children and reducing the dose of medication that will be necessary if a behavioral intervention is insufficient and adjunctive medication is needed. We will briefly illustrate these outcomes with results from several recent studies.

In the MTA study, children in the combined treatment group (behavior therapy plus medication) were receiving endpoint doses that were 20% less than those in the medication only groups (10,11). The reason for the difference is that medication had to be increased over the intervention year in the medication group in order to maintain efficacy (29). Although this was an impressive reduction in medication dosage, design factors in the MTA study limited the reduction in dose that could be obtained in this group. For example, reductions in dose were prohibited unless driven by side effects, that is, a child could not have his or her dose reduced if the therapist thought that it was unnecessarily high. Previous studies had suggested that dose could be reduced by as much as 50% in a combined versus medication alone group (41) but this was not systematically attempted in the MTA.

To examine this question, we recently conducted a study to find out whether concurrent behavioral treatment could produce even larger reductions than the MTA and earlier research, in the dose of medication that is needed if behavioral treatments are implemented. In that study, comparative and combined impacts of different doses of behavioral intervention (none, low, and high) and MPH (pl, 0.15, 0.3, and 0.6 mg/kg per dose t.i.d.) were evaluated in a summer program setting (42,43). The low behavioral "dose" involved rules, consistent staff praise and feedback, daily "when...then" contingencies, and a daily report card (DRC) with weekly rewards; the enhanced or high behavioral "dose" involved the same low dose variables plus a point system and daily rewards. All of the above were removed in the control, no-treatment condition. Results showed that the higher dose of behavioral intervention was more effective than the lower dose in both classroom and recreational settings on multiple measures of functioning (Fig. 1 for results on classroom rule violations). The same was true for medication. Unexpectedly and in contrast to medication, the behavioral intervention function appeared to be quadratic rather than linear—lower behavioral doses were closer to higher behavioral doses than to no treatment, implying that the higher dose may not have been necessary for many children. The low behavioral dose was comparable to the moderate dose of MPH, while the enhanced behavior modification condition was comparable to the high doses of medication. As Figure 1 illustrates and as in previous studies (41), effects of MPH beyond the lowest dose were minimal in the presence of behavior modification.

What is novel about this study is that the dose of MPH on which effects were maximized, 0.15 mg/kg per dose, was half that employed in earlier studies (44). This result suggests that if appropriate behavioral interventions are employed, then the dose of MPH necessary as an adjunct might be reduced by as much as 75%—in this study from an average dose of 20 to 5 mg/dose. At this low dosage level in this study, there were no side

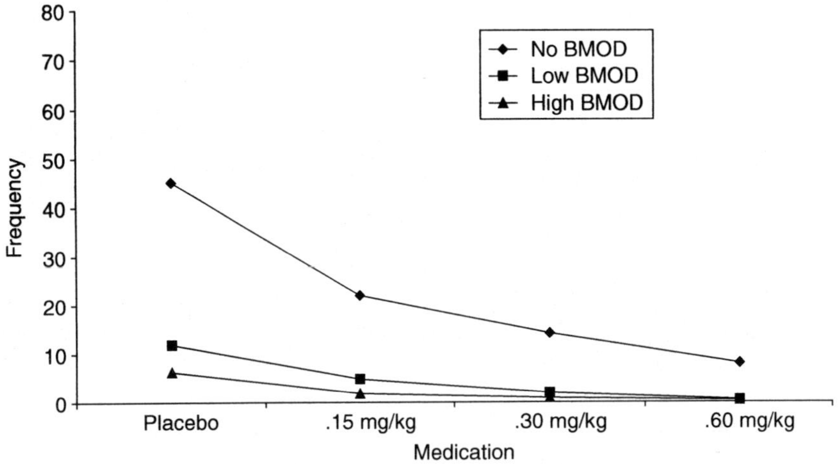

Figure 1 Rule violations in the classroom as a function of treatment condition.

effects, including no tics, no increase in heart rate and blood pressure, no appetite suppression, and no insomnia (45).

These findings are interesting but are limited, as is the MTA by the fact that the two modalities were provided concurrently rather than sequentially. As low as the dose that maximum benefit was, it is possible and even likely that some children functioned so well with the behavioral treatment alone that they did not need adjunctive medication. After all, the difference between the placebo and low dose conditions in Fig. 1 is rather small. We thus decided to ask the question of whether medication was needed at all in these children had behavioral interventions been initiated first?

The children were enrolled in a follow-up study in which they returned to their regular schools at the beginning of the school year without medication (46). All parents had received nine sessions of weekly large group parent training during the summer study. At the beginning of the school year, they were randomly assigned to receive behavioral intervention as follow-up (the opportunity to attend monthly large group parent booster sessions) or to receive nothing as follow-up. A DRC was implemented by a consultant in the classrooms of the children who were assigned to the behavioral follow-up condition. Regular evaluations were conducted to examine functioning in school, at home, and the need for adjunctive medication. If medication was needed according to the regular evaluations, it was provided either at home or at school or both, as indicated.

For analysis, subjects were divided into those who had begun their treatment with behavioral intervention (e.g., had not been medicated prior to the study), and those who had been previously medicated. By the end of the school year, more than 90% of the children who had not been previously medicated and whose parents received parent training and behavioral follow-up remained medication-free in the home setting, and two-thirds of those were also medication-free at school. These rates were reduced dramatically if children had been previously medicated or if parents were not receiving follow-up behavioral interventions. Only 35% and 15% of parents of children who had been previously medicated (i.e., had received medication prior to the behavioral treatment) and who did not receive follow-up were successful in keeping their children off medication at home and school, respectively.

This follow-up study thus suggests that the majority of ADHD children can be maintained with good functioning at school and especially at home if their treatment is begun with a clinical level of behavioral intervention (standard behavioral parent training and a school DRC). There are limitations to this conclusion that include the fact that the children were all exposed to medication and to a summer treatment program in the context of the summer study, but the findings are provocative.

The findings of one additional study, the MTA study, are relevant to this discussion. Seventy-five percent of the children assigned to the behavioral treatment only group (equivalent to the high dose behavior modification group described above) in the MTA study "survived" the treatment year without medication, with that figure rising to 85% for children who had not been previously medicated (10,11). Further, more than 80% of those children remained medication-free 1 or 2 years later (12,13). Thus, although the MTA was not planned as a sequencing study, its results can be interpreted as supporting our contention that the vast majority of ADHD children can be well treated and maintained without medication if a comprehensive behavioral intervention is provided as first-line treatment.

Considered together, the MTA study and our studies shed light on the dosage of behavioral intervention that might be necessary to avoid medication. The amount of parent training provided in our studies—a standard set of 9 large group (16 families) weekly sessions with monthly large booster group sessions available—was far less than that provided in the MTA study [35 planned sessions divided into weekly small group (6 families) and monthly individual sessions]. However, the results in terms of preventing need for medication at home were similar, 85% versus 90%. In addition to the results shown in Fig. 1, this comparison suggests that for many families of ADHD children, a standard course of group parent training may be sufficient to produce functioning that parents consider adequate to avoid using medication. In other words, many if not most of the parents in the MTA study may not have needed the intensive parenting intervention that they received.

Regarding school intervention, our follow-up behavioral treatment involved only two brief contacts with the child's teacher to establish a home-based DRC, compared to 20 weekly teacher contacts, 5 parent–teacher meetings, and a 9-week half-time aide in the MTA study. Eighty-five percent of the previously unmedicated MTA children with this intensive intervention were maintained without medication versus 60% of our previously unmedicated children with a much less intensive intervention (vs. 35% of our previously unmedicated children with no follow-up intervention). This comparison suggests four conclusions: (1) that parent training alone may apparently be sufficient to enable some parents to maintain their children without medication at school; (2) that a consultant-facilitated, teacher-implemented DRC can nearly double that number; (3) that a far more intensive behavioral intervention might be needed and effective for an additional 25% of the children; and (4) that the remaining 15% may need adjunctive medication at school.

Altogether, these studies suggest that most ADHD children can be treated effectively with a relatively simple behavioral intervention and will not need adjunctive medication or intensive behavioral interventions. Conceivably, such an approach to treatment might reduce the number of ADHD children in the US receiving psychoactive medication from more than 4% to no more than 1%. This outcome would be well received by families of ADHD children. An important question is what impact will this have on the societal cost of ADHD? While it is widely believed that medication is less expensive than psychosocial treatment, an evidence-based but low-intensity behavioral treatment (e.g., 12 group parent training sessions plus a consultant to visit the child's teacher to establish a DRC) may be implemented for a cost (approximately US $1500) that is less than that the annual cost of today's long-acting stimulant preparations [about US $1800 per year, assuming quarterly physician contact (5)]. Furthermore, because of the lack of long-term gains, medication must be continued indefinitely once it has begun, whereas effective behavioral treatments have been shown to produce longer term maintenance of treatment gains (12,13). A liberal estimate of the cost of the intensive behavioral or combined treatment provided in the MTA was US $6000 to US $8000 (13)—about equally divided among the parent training, school intervention, and summer treatment program. This was considerably more than the cost of medication in the MTA study, but as our discussion above shows, the majority of ADHD children do not need either adjunctive medication or behavioral treatment of this intensity. Thus, provision of a low dose of behavioral intervention as the starting treatment for ADHD children may be more cost-effective than medication alone and can avoid the expensive, intensive treatments provided in the MTA study if they are not needed for a given child.

IMPLICATIONS FOR TREATMENT

What can be concluded about how clinicians should be implementing treatment with ADHD children? We believe that the literature and a

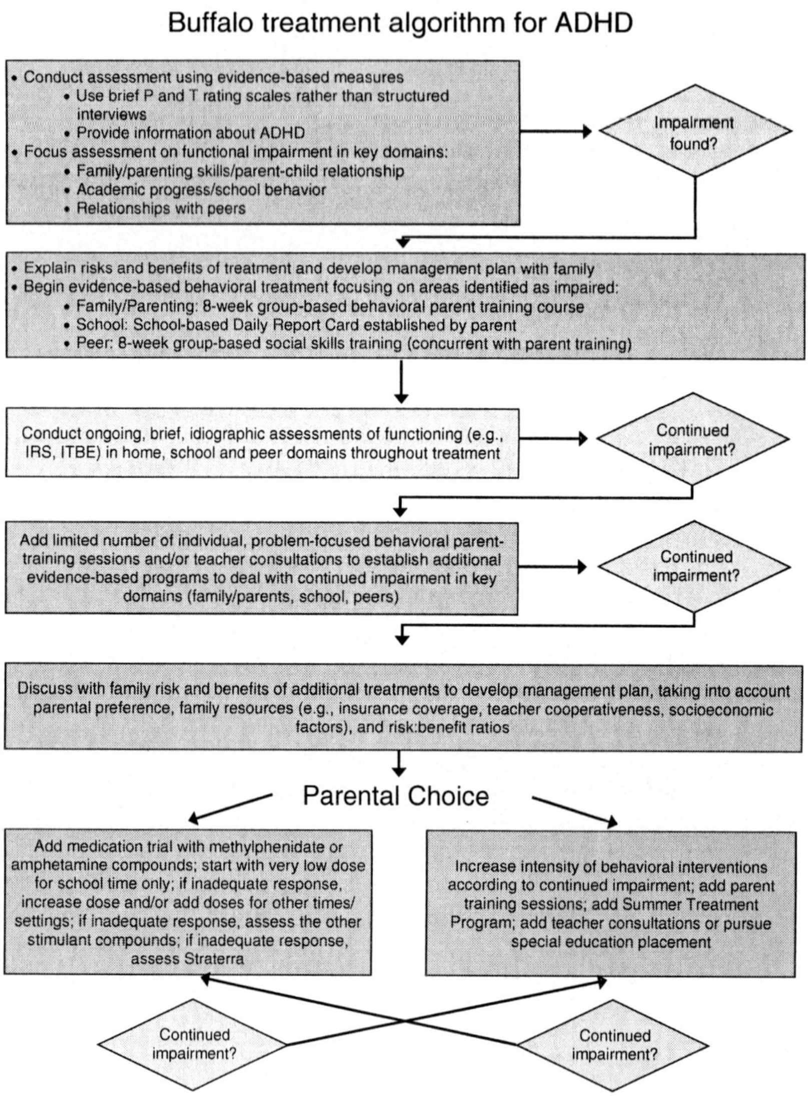

Figure 2 Buffalo treatment algorithm for ADHD.

risk: benefit assessment suggest the treatment algorithm that we present in Fig. 2, the Buffalo treatment algorithm. First, evidence-based treatment should begin with an evidence-based assessment that is focused on functional outcomes rather than DSM symptoms. Because there is little evidence that psychiatric comorbidities make a difference in treatment planning or outcome, the diagnostic process should be conducted as efficiently as possible. Thus, rating scales rather than systematic structured clinical interviews should be employed so that relatively more professional time can be devoted to treatment development than to diagnosis. Functional analyses should be conducted to select target behaviors and identify the antecedent and consequent variables that influence them and will be utilized in treatment, and these should be ongoing using simple, inexpensive instruments (47; instruments downloadable at http://ccf.buffalo.edu) as new targets are identified and addressed (48). When such assessments reveal dysfunction in peer, classroom, and family domains, as will typically but not always be the case, a management plan should be discussed with the family explaining what treatments could be initiated. Based on the literature on parent preferences, our assumption is that the vast majority of parents will elect to begin intervention with the clinical behavioral approach shown in the algorithm. If selected by parents, children with ADHD should have school-, home-, and peer-based behavioral treatments initiated, as indicated, with the management plan developed with the family.

Given the importance of cost of services in a public health model, we propose (1) that initial behavioral treatment be relatively simple and inexpensive, (2) that need for additional behavioral components treatment be based on ongoing assessments (see above) in domains of impairment, and (3) that the treatment be adaptively determined based on need. Thus, a standard course of any one of the evidence-based group behavioral parent training (BPTs) (49–52; Webster-Stratton, www.incredibleyears.com) should be implemented initially. A limited number of individual sessions (53) could be used after the parenting group, if indicated by ongoing brief assessments. A DRC should be concurrently implemented with parent training. Because the effectiveness of DRCs has been ubiquitously documented in the studies with ADHD and because they are relatively simple interventions, a DRC would clearly be a first-line classroom program. A standardized packet for developing and implementing a school-based DRC that has been used in multiple studies can be downloaded at http://ccf.buffalo.edu. DRC implementation can be a topic in parent training groups, and parents can take the lead in initiating this with their child's teacher. As with individual parenting sessions, more intensive classroom programs can be implemented subsequently with a limited number of contacts as necessary. In a clinic setting, this would typically involve having a consultant work with the classroom teacher directly or through a school psychologist or counselor, assisting in the development and implementation of behavioral programs in the child's classroom. When initial assessment identifies problems in peer relations, an evidence-based peer intervention should be included. There is limited evidence for social skills training but some evidence that provided concurrently with parent training weekly groups can be helpful (54).

If such a behavioral intervention has been insufficient, then one of two alternatives for increasing treatment intensity should be presented to the family—adjunctive or increased dose of stimulant medication (depending on whether it has already been utilized) or enhanced and more complex behavioral interventions (e.g., enhanced individualized parent training, a summer treatment program for peer or academic problems) and/or more restrictive educational placement. Based on parent preferences, resources, and a discussion of risk:benefit tradeoffs, families should be counseled to select one of these alternatives. If the chosen alternative is insufficient, the other would become the only remaining option based on the current literature regarding intervention for children with ADHD (i.e., second-line medications show little evidence of efficacy and other psychosocial approaches to treatment also lack an evidence base).

ADHD is a chronic disorder (2). As in the case of other chronic disease states it is inappropriate to think that a brief, time-limited treatment regimen, whether behavioral, pharmacological, or combined, will be a sufficient and effective intervention for a child with ADHD. For most children with ADHD and their families, sustained treatment that is palatable for the family and that promotes engagement and adherence to the selected regimen for protracted periods of time will be required. It is our firm belief that the treatment approach outlined in the Buffalo treatment algorithm that begins with behavioral interventions best meets these goals. By minimizing medication use and dose, this approach reduces risk of adverse effects–both known short-term side effects and unknown long-term adverse events. By emphasizing treatment components that impact on the key domains that mediate long-term outcomes—parenting, school functioning, and peer relations—this approach has the best chance of maximizing the long-term adaptive outcomes of children with ADHD and their families. By minimizing adverse effects, maximizing adaptive outcomes, and cost-effectiveness, the approach we have outlined should also reduce the societal costs of ADHD.

ACKNOWLEDGMENTS

During the preparation of this manuscript, Dr Pelham was supported in part by grants from the National Institute of Mental Health (NIMH; MH62946-01A1, MH069614-01A2, MH053554-11A1, MH069434-01A2, MH065899-02, and MH078051-01A1), National Institute on Alcohol Abuse and Alcoholism (AA11873-06), National Institute on Drug Abuse (DA12414-01A2), and the Department of Education, Institute of Educational Sciences (IES; R305L0300065A, R324J06024, R324B06045). The author would also like to thank the many collaborators and staff that have been involved in the projects mentioned herein.

Correspondence concerning this chapter should be addressed to William E. Pelham, Jr., State University of New York at Buffalo, Center for Children and Families, 106 Diefendorf Hall, 3435 Main Street, Building 20, Buffalo, New York 14214. Email: pelham@ascu.buffalo.edu.

REFERENCES

1. Barkley RA. Attention Deficit Hyperactivity Disorder: A Handbook for Diagnosis and Treatment. New York: The Guilford Press, 2006.
2. American Academy of Pediatrics. Clinical practice guideline: treatment of the school-aged child with attention-deficit/hyperactivity disorder. Pediatrics 2001; 108:1033–44.
3. American Academy of Child & Adolescent Psychiatry. Practice parameter for the use of stimulant medications in the treatment of children, adolescents, and adults. J Am Acad Child Adolesc Psychiatry 2002; 41:26S–49.
4. Polanczyk G, Silva de Lima M, Horta BL, Biederman J, Rohde LA. The worldwide prevalence of ADHD: a systematic review and metaregression analysis. Am J Psychiatry 2007; 164:942–8.
5. Pelham WE, Foster EM, Robb JA. The economic impact of attention-deficit/hyperactivity disorder in children and adolescents. Ambul Pediatr 2007; 7 (Suppl.):121–31.
6. Greenhill LL, Ford RE. Childhood attention-deficit/hyperactivity disorder: pharmacological treatments. In: Nathan PE, Gorman JM, eds. A Guide to Treatments that Work. 2nd ed. New York: Oxford University Press, 2002: 25–55.
7. Fabiano GA, Pelham WE, Coles EK, Gnagy EM, Chronis AM, O'Connor B. (under review). A meta-analysis of behavioral and combined treatments for ADHD.
8. Pelham WE, Fabiano GA. (in press). Evidence-based psychosocial treatment for attention-deficit/hyperactivity disorder: an update. J Clin Child Adolesc Psychol.
9. APA Working Group on Psychoactive Medications for Children and Adolescents. Report of the Working Group on Psychoactive Medications for Children and Adolescents. Psychopharmacological, Psychosocial, and Combined Interventions for Childhood Disorders: Evidence Base, Contextual Factors, and Future Directions. Washington, D.C.: American Psychological Association, 2006.
10. MTA Cooperative Group. 14-month randomized clinical trial of treatment strategies for Attention Deficit Hyperactivity Disorder. Arch Gen Psychiatry 1999; 56:1073–86.
11. MTA Cooperative Group. Moderators and mediators of treatment response for children with attention-deficit/hyperactivity disorder: the multimodal treatment study of children with ADHD. Arch Gen Psychiatry 1999; 56:1088–96.
12. MTA Cooperative Group. National Institute of Mental Health Multimodal Treatment Study of ADHD Follow-up: 24-month outcomes of treatment strategies for attention-deficit/hyperactivity disorder. Pediatrics 2004; 113:754–61.
13. Jensen PS, Arnold LE, Swanson J, et al. Follow-up of the NIMH MTA study at 36 months after randomization. J Am Acad Child Adolesc Psychiatry 2007; 46:989–1007.

14. American Academy of Child and Adolescent Psychiatry. Practice parameters for the assessment and treatment of children and adolescents with attention-deficit/hyperactivity disorder. J Am Acad Child Adolesc Psychiatry 2007; 46: 894–921.
15. Greenhill LL, Pliszka S, Dulcan MK, et al. Practice parameter for the use of stimulant medications in the treatment of children, adolescents, and adults. J Am Acad Child Adolesc Psychiatry 2002; 41(Suppl. 2):26S–49.
16. Hinshaw SP, Klein RG, Abikoff H. Childhood attention deficit hyperactivity disorder: nonpharmacological and combination treatments. In: Nathan PE, Gorman JM, eds. A Guide to Treatments that Work. 2nd ed. New York: Oxford University Press, 2002:3–23.
17. Pliszka SR, Matthews TL, Braslow KJ, Watson MA. Comparative effects of methylphenidate and mixed salts amphetamine on height and weight in children with attention-deficit/hyperactivity disorder. J Am Acad Child Adolesc Psychol 2006; 45:520–6.
18. Zito JM, Safer DJ, dosReis S, Gardner JF, Boles M, Lynch F. Trends in the prescribing of psychotropic medications to preschoolers. J Am Med Assoc 2000; 283:1025–30.
19. Medco Health Solutions. Drug Trend Report. San Diego, CA: Medco Health Solutions, Inc, 2004.
20. Swanson JM, Cantwell D, Lerner M, McBurnett K, Hanna G. Effects of stimulant medication on learning in children with ADHD. J Learn Disabil 1991; 24:219–30.
21. Swanson JM, Kraemer HC, Hinshaw SP, et al. Clinical relevance of the primary findings of the MTA: success rates based on severity of ADHD and ODD symptoms at the end of treatment. J Am Acad Child Adolesc Psychiatry 2001; 40:168–79.
22. Loe IM, Feldman HM. Academic and educational outcomes of children with ADHD: literature review and proposal for future research. Ambul Pediatr 2007; 7 (Suppl. 1):82–90.
23. NIH Consensus Conference. Diagnosis and Treatment of Attention Deficit Hyperactivity Disorder. NIH Consensus Statement 1998, Nov. 16–18; 16:1–37.
24. Volkow ND, Insel TR. What are the long-term effects of methylphenidate treatment? Biol Psychiatry 2003; 54:1307–9.
25. Lambert NL, McLeod M, Schenk S. Subjective responses to initial experience with cocaine: an exploration of the incentive-sensitization theory of drug abuse. Addiction 2006; 101:713–25.
26. Pelham WE, Molina BSG, Gnagy EM, Meichenbaum DL, Greenhouse JB. (under review). The impact of childhood stimulant medication on later substance use.
27. Evans SW, Pelham WE, Smith BH, et al. Dose-response effects of methylphenidate on ecologically valid measures of academic performance and classroom behavior in adolescents with ADHD. Exp Clin Psychopharmacol 2001; 9:163–75.
28. Smith BH, Pelham WE, Evans S, et al. Dosage effects of methylphenidate on the social behavior of adolescents diagnosed with attention deficit hyperactivity disorder. Exp Clin Psychopharmacol 1998; 6:1–18.

29. Vitiello B, Severe JB, Greenhill LL, et al. Methylphenidate dosage for children with ADHD over time under controlled conditions: lessons from the MTA. J Am Acad Child Adolesc Psychiatry 2001; 40:188–96.
30. Greenhill L, Osman BP, eds. Ritalin: Theory and Patient Management. New York: MaryAnn Liebert, Inc, 1991.
31. Pelham WE, Wheeler T, Chronis A. Empirically supported psychosocial treatments for attention deficit hyperactivity disorder. J Clin Child Psychol 1998; 27:190–205.
32. Cunningham CE. A family-centered approach to planning and measuring the outcome of interventions for children with attention-deficit/hyperactivity disorder. Ambul Pediatr 2007; 7 (Suppl.):60–72.
33. Hoza B. Peer functioning in children with ADHD. Ambul Pediatr 2007; 7 (Suppl.):101–6.
34. Mager W, Milich R, Harris MJ, Howard A. Intervention groups for adolescents with conduct problems: is aggregation harmful or helpful? J Abnorm Child Psychol 2006; 33:349–62.
35. Weiss B, Caron A, Ball S, Tapp J, Johnson M, Weisz JR. Iatrogenic effects of group treatment for antisocial youth. J Consul Clin Psychol 2005; 73:1036–44.
36. Power TJ, Hess LE, Bennett DS. The acceptability of interventions for attention-deficit hyperactivity disorder among elementary and middle school teachers. Dev Behav Pediatr 1995; 16:238–43.
37. Pelham WE, Erhardt D, Gnagy EM, et al. (under review). Parent and teacher evaluation of treatment in the MTA: consumer satisfaction, perceived effectiveness, and demands of treatment.
38. Weiss B, Catron T, Harris V, Phung TM. The effectiveness of traditional psychotherapy. J Consult Clin Psychol 1999; 67:82–94.
39. Weisz JR, Jensen-Doss A, Hawley KM. Evidence-based youth psychotherapies versus usual clinical care: a meta-analysis of direct comparisons. Am Psychol 2006; 61:671–89.
40. Carlson CL, Pelham WE, Milich R, Dixon MJ. Single and combined effects of methylphenidate and behavior therapy on the classroom performance of children with attention-deficit hyperactivity disorder. J Abnorm Child Psychol 1992; 20:213–32.
41. Fabiano GA, Pelham WE, Gnagy EM, et al. The single and combined effects of multiple intensities of behavior modification and multiple intensities of methylphenidate in a classroom setting. School Psychol Rev 2007; 36:195–216.
42. Pelham WE, Burrows-MacLean L, Gnagy EM, et al. (under review). A between groups study of behavioral, pharmacological and combined treatment for children with ADHD.
43. Pelham WE, Burrows-MacLean L, Gnagy EM, et al. Transdermal methylphenidate, behavioral, and combined treatment for children with ADHD. Exp Clin Psychopharmacol 2005; 13:111–26.
44. Pelham WE, Burrows-MacLean L, Gnagy EM, et al. (under review). A dose-ranging crossover study of behavioral, pharmacological, and combined treatment in a recreational setting for children with ADHD.

45. Coles EK, Pelham WE, Gnagy EM, et al. A controlled evaluation of behavioral treatment with children with ADHD attending a summer treatment program. J Emotion Behav Disorder 2005; 13:99–112.
46. Fabiano GA, Pelham WE, Waschbusch D, et al. A practical impairment measure: psychometric properties of the Impairment Rating Scale in samples of children with attention-deficit/hyperactivity disorder and two school-based samples. J Clin Child Adolesc Psychol 2006; 35:369–85.
47. Mash EJ. Treatment of child and family disturbance: a cognitive-behavioral systems perspective. In: Mash EJ, Barkley RA, eds. Treatment of Childhood Disorders. 3rd ed. New York: The Guilford Press, 2006:3–62.
48. Barkley RA. Defiant Children: A Clinician's Manual for Parent Training. New York: The Guilford Press, 1987.
49. Cunningham CE, Bremner R, Secord-Gilbert M. The community parent education (COPE) program: a school-based family systems oriented course for parents of children with disruptive behavior disorders. Chedoke-McMaster Hospitals and McMaster University, 1998.
50. McMahon RJ, Forehand RL. Helping the Noncompliant Child: Family Based Treatment for Oppositional Behavior. 2nd ed. New York: Guilford Press, 2003.
51. Sanders MR, Markie-Dadds C, Turner KMT. Practitioner's Kit for Standard Triple P. Brisbane, Queensland, Australia: Families International, 1998 (http://www.pfsc.uq.edue.au/02_ppp/ppp.html).
52. Hembree TL, McNeil CB. Parent-Child Interaction Therapy. New York: Plenum Press, 1995.
53. Pfiffner LJ, McBurnett K. Social skills training with parent generalization: treatment effects for children with attention deficit disorder. J Consult Clin Psychol 1997; 65:749–57.
54. U.S. Food and Drug Administration, 2006.

28

Stimulants in ADHD: Effects on Weight and Height

Glen R. Elliott

The Children's Health Council, Palo Alto, and University of California San Francisco, San Francisco, California, U.S.A.

INTRODUCTION

Issues about growth patterns in individuals with attention deficit hyperactivity disorder (ADHD) have long been of interest to families and professionals. By far the greatest attention has been paid to the possible effects of stimulants on height and weight, since these medications typically are used to treat ADHD in children during a significant interval of the growth development. Current evidence indicates that, on average, persistent use of stimulants does result in decreased rates of growth for both height and weight, especially during the first several years when used in prepubertal children. The magnitude of the effect seems to be related to total medication exposure. Less clear is whether stopping the medication either with "drug holidays" or completely while a child is still growing permits for "growth rebound." This latter issue relates, in part, to unresolved questions about whether ADHD itself may be associated with changes in growth patterns.

As thoroughly documented in other chapters of this volume, ADHD has been a well-recognized disorder for many years. It is perhaps not a coincidence that stimulants have been widely accepted as an effective treatment for ADHD for many of those years, dating back to at least the early 1960s (1). Although other medication and nonmedication interventions also have clear benefits for ADHD, stimulants remain the gold standard for medicating individuals with this disorder (2). Since 1990, use of stimulants for this purpose has expanded markedly in multiple ways: more individuals are receiving higher doses for more days of the week, more weeks of the year, and more years (3). This expanded use of stimulants has had many contributing factors, two important ones being relatively high efficacy rates and acceptable side effect profile.

Although potential effects of growth, specifically height and weight, may initially seem only peripherally interesting as a medication side effect, clinicians quickly learn otherwise. Most parents are intensely interested in the eating habits of the children; so, a notable decrease in appetite, let alone loss of weight or even a failure to gain weight typically is a cause for concern. Similarly, at least in the United States, being tall is a valued trait especially for males and increasingly for females. Therefore, information about medication effects on either weight or height is of understandable interest.

Concerns about possible effects especially on height are not new. For example, Safer et al. (4) proposed that stimulants slowed physical growth rates. However, by the late 1970s and into the late 1990s, the general consensus was that effects on growth were of minor concern (5,6). In fact, some research suggested that, even if stimulants did have a short-term effect of growth suppression, this effect was negated by growth rebound once stimulants were discontinued (7).

This sanguine view of the impact of stimulants on growth has been shaken in the past few years by a number of studies that indicate that the growth-suppressive effects of stimulants are more persistent than earlier studies suggested. As discussed below, the magnitude of those effects and their importance in clinical management remain to be determined.

It may seem surprising that, with stimulants having been widely used for decades, there would be any remaining uncertainties about their effects on weight and height. However, it is important to keep in mind the changes that have occurred in stimulant use (cf. 3). Up through the mid-1990s, the most common way of administering stimulants was as an immediate-release, short-acting form once or twice a day just on school days; usually, stimulant use stopped sometime around the onset of puberty. Now, children routinely take stimulant preparations that work for 8 to 12 hr a day or longer, often 7 days a week, all year long. In addition, they may start taking stimulants at a younger age and are apt to continue taking them throughout adolescence, that is, during their entire growth phase.

STIMULANT EFFECTS OF WEIGHT

The acute effect of stimulants on appetite is not controversial: most individuals who take stimulant experience a notable suppression of appetite that typically lasts for several hours with short-acting preparations. Usually, the effect is most notable with medication-naïve individuals, but the effect often persists and may be severe enough to be perceived by patients or their parents as an unacceptable side effect. More commonly, however, the acute appetite-suppressing properties of stimulants change the pattern of eating during the day, with most caloric intake occurring in the morning and late afternoon or evening. Less well-studied are possible effects on the types of calories consumed, with parents sometimes reporting that children crave certain types of foods, for example, carbohydrates, when they are hungry.

One potential effect of appetite suppression is decreased overall caloric intake, with resulting slowing of weight gain or even actual weight loss. In one of the few controlled studies of using stimulants to treat ADHD over a prolonged period, the Multimodal Treatment of ADHD (MTA) found that, over 14 months of treatment, subjects with ADHD who received stimulants daily, gained on average 1.2 kg/year less than those who did not receive stimulants (8). By 36 months, the difference in weight between these two groups was 2.7 kg (9). Similarly, a recent study of the use of stimulants in preschoolers with ADHD found a slowing in weight gain at 1 year (10).

However, not all studies have shown such sustained differences in weight as a result of stimulant use. For example, Kraemer et al. (11) followed a sample of children with ADHD, treated with stimulants as children, into adulthood and found no statistically significant effects on weight compared to unmedicated family members or community controls. Spencer et al. (12) have proposed that an apparent initial effect on weight might actually reflect an ADHD-related delay in maturation. However, their methodology used a cross-sectional evaluation. The longitudinal results from the MTA (9) failed to support such a hypothesis.

Pragmatically, clinicians should warn parents and children that use of stimulants may have an effect on appetite, especially early on. Parents need to know that children often will have little to no interest in lunch and that the best times for encouraging them to eat a healthy meal will be at breakfast and then later in the day. Occasionally, especially with higher doses of long-acting formulations of stimulants, appetite does not return till late evening. Under such circumstances, it may be appropriate to arrange for the child to have a healthy meal shortly before bedtime; it is essential that parents be warned not to allow any guilt they may feel, about having caused their child's poor appetite, to result in their letting the child indulge at such times in poorly balanced snacks of low nutritional value.

If appetite suppression is severe and persistent and results in weight loss or even just a failure to gain weight at the expected pace, it may be necessary to consider using another medication. Sometimes switching to a different preparation or to a different stimulant is sufficient. Other times, it may best to utilize a nonstimulant medication.

STIMULANT EFFECTS OF HEIGHT

As noted earlier, the effect of stimulants on height has been more controversial than that on weight. Early studies suggested that stimulants decelerated height growth rates (4). However, later reports suggested that early effects on height were either transient or reversed once stimulants were stopped (7,13). Further, studies done in the late 1980s that followed samples of patients into adulthood (11,14) found no differences in ultimate height as a function of exposure to stimulants during childhood. As mentioned earlier, Spencer et al. (12) proposed that the apparent observed effect of stimulants might simply reflect a maturational lag that co-occurs with ADHD.

More recent studies of growth, however, again raised concerns about possible immediate effects of stimulants on growth, although the results are inconsistent. In independent studies of children in the United States (15) or Australia (16) researchers found evidence of growth reduction in children taking stimulants; these chart-reviews found no evidence of growth rebound over the 3 years studied. However, two other chart-review studies found no such reduction in growth (17,18).

The MTA, mentioned earlier, is one of the few studies that combine random treatment assignment with long-term follow-up. At the time the study was designed (19), effects on height and weight were thought to have been settled and were not a major focus of the research plan. However, measures of both were included at regular intervals. The first assessment of the impact of treatment on height revealed that, compared to those who received no medications, subjects who received stimulants during the 14 months of active treatment grew an average of 1cm/year more slowly (8). This effect was sustained at 3 years, the most recent data reported (9), with a 3 cm difference between the groups. An intermediate group with exposure to stimulants that was more intermittent resulted in intermediate rates of growth.

The MTA results (8,9) also raise questions about the hypothesis of maturational delay. The researchers found that, if anything, unmedicated children with ADHD grew at a faster rate than did normal controls. In fact, they proposed that one possible explanation for reports of growth rebound in other studies was that the children with ADHD resumed their more rapid pattern of growth once off medications. Among their subjects, they found no evidence for rebound or for maturational delay.

The mechanism by which stimulants might affect growth remains unknown, but it almost certainly is independent of their effects on appetite and caloric intake (20). Whatever the cause, the MTA data seem to suggest that the effect of stimulants on height is incremental and directly related to persistent exposure to stimulants.

CLINICAL IMPLICATIONS

Clinically, the available data suggest that clinicians need to inform families of the potential effects of stimulants on weight and height. Regular measurement of both in standardized fashion should be a routine part of care, with use of growth charts to monitor how the child is doing over time. It is quite likely that the effects are not uniform, with some children potentially having profound growth reduction and others having little to none. In the latter cases, no studies have suggested any possibility of a "sleeper effect": if a child shows no deviation from his or her growth curve potential, no unanticipated abrupt loss of height or weight will occur later.

On the other hand, if children show marked reductions in acquisition of either height or weight over time, then it behooves the clinician to bring such side effects to the attention of the family and help them consider options. Here, research is relatively silent. Clinical experience suggests that switching from one stimulant to another may result in a different side effect profile. Alternatively, several new nonstimulant medications are now available. Most of these are still so new that scant information exists about their possible long-term effects on growth, but they at least offer a potentially viable alternative. In the end, the family and clinician will, as usual, have to balance perceived benefit with potential risks in deciding on the most appropriate clinical course.

REFERENCES

1. Conners CK, Eisenberg L. The effects of methylphenidate on symptomatology and learning in disturbed children. Am J Psychiatry 1963; 120:458–64.
2. American Academy of Child and Adolescent Psychiatry. Practice parameter for the use of stimulant medications in the treatment of children, adolescents, and adults. J Am Acad Child Adolesc Psychiatry 2002; 41S:26S–49S.
3. Olfson M, Marcus SC, Weissman MM, Jensen PS. National trends in the use of psychotropic medications by children. J Am Acad Child Adolesc Psychiatry 2002; 41:514–21.
4. Safer D, Allen R, Barr E. Depression of growth in hyperactive children on stimulant drugs. N Engl J Med 1972; 287:217–20.
5. Roche AF, Lipman RS, Overall JE, Hung W. The effects of stimulant medication on the growth of hyperkinetic children. Pediatrics 1979; 63: 847–50.
6. NIH Consensus Committee. Diagnosis and treatment of attention deficit hyperactivity disorder (ADHD). NIH Consensus Statement 1998; 16:1–37.
7. Safer DJ, Allen RP, Barr E. Growth rebound after termination of stimulant drugs. J Pediatrics 1975; 86:113–6.
8. MTA Cooperative Group. National Institute of Mental Health multimodal treatment study of ADHD follow-up: changes in effectiveness and growth after the end of treatment. Pediatrics 2004; 113:762–9.
9. Swanson JM, Elliott GR, Greenhill LL, Wigal T, Arnold LE, Vitiello B, et al. for the MTA Collaborative Group. Effects of stimulant medication on growth rates across 3 years in the MTA follow-up. J Am Acad Child Adolesc Psychiatry 2007; 46:1015–27.

10. Swanson JM, Greenhill LL, Wigal T, Kollins S, Nguyen A, Davies M, for the PATS Study Group. Stimulant-related growth suppression in preschool children with ADHD. J Am Acad Child Adolesc Psychiatry 2006; 45:1304–13.
11. Kramer JR, Loney J, Ponto LB, Roberts MA, Grossman S. Predictors of adult height and weight in boys treated with methylphenidate for childhood behavior problems. J Am Acad Child Adolesc Psychiatry 2000; 39:517–24.
12. Spencer T, Biederman J, Harding M, O'Donnell D, Faraone SV, Wiles TE. Growth deficits in ADHD children revisited: evidence for disorder-associated growth delays? J Am Acad Child Adolesc Psychiatry 1996; 35:1460–9.
13. Satterfield JH, Cantwell DP, Schell A, Blaschke T. Growth of hyperactive children with methylphenidate. Arch Gen Psychiatry 1979; 36:212–7.
14. Klein R, Mannuzza S. Hyperactive boys almost grown up. III. Methylphenidate effects on ultimate height. Arch Gen Psychiatry 1988; 45: 1131–4.
15. Lisska MC, Rivkees SA. Daily methylphenidate use slows the growth of children in a community sample. J Pediatr Endocrin Metabol 2003; 16:711–8.
16. Poulton A, Cowell CT. Slowing of growth in height and weight on stimulants: a characteristic pattern. J Paediatr Child Health 2003; 39:180–5.
17. Pliszka S, Matthews TL, Braslow KJ, Watson MA. Comparative effects of methylphenidate and mixed salts amphetamine on height and weight in children with attention deficit hyperactivity disorder (ADHD). J Am Acad Child Adolesc Psychiatry 2006; 45:520–5.
18. Spencer T, Faraone SV, Biederman J, Lerner M, Cooper KM, Zimmerman B, on behalf of the Concerta Study Group. Does prolonged therapy with a long-acting stimulant suppress growth in children with ADHD? J Am Acad Child Adolesc Psychiatry 2006; 45:527–37.
19. Arnold LE, Abikoff HB, Cantwell DP, Conners CK, Elliott GR, Greenhill LL. NIMH collaborative multimodal treatment study of children with ADHD (MTA): design challenges and choices. Arch Gen Psychiatry 1997; 54:865–70.
20. Greenhill LL, Osman BB, eds. Ritalin: Theory and Practice. 2nd ed. New York: Mary Ann Liebert, 2000:443.

29

Why Controversy Over ADHD Won't "Go Away"

Lawrence Diller

Private Practice, Walnut Creek, and University of California San Francisco, San Francisco, California, U.S.A.

Several years ago I noted a pediatrician's frustration with the persistence of criticism over the attention deficit hyperactivity disorder (ADHD) diagnosis and the use of prescription stimulant drugs like Ritalin in the United States. He complained, what with the thousands of studies supporting the validity of the ADHD diagnosis and the effectiveness and safety of the stimulant drugs, why critics, like me, continue to raise concerns. Enough already, was his conclusion; let's move on to other important concerns of our times where real questions remain unanswered. At least with ADHD and Ritalin, according to this pediatrician, the important questions have been settled.

Indeed, controversy over stimulant drugs for children's performance and behavior problems has been present since Bradley's first report of the effects of benzedrine in hyperactive children in 1937 (1). Despite nearly 70 years of use and the plethora of research associated with these drugs and ADHD, some of the original ethical concerns about these medications continue to resonate despite the pediatrician's lamentation. The explosive growth of the ADHD diagnosis and the use of stimulants beginning in the early 1990s, initially in school-age children and then spreading to teenagers and adults, have only heightened concerns about the long-term effectiveness and safety of these medications. And if one is of a questioning nature (who in this case is also a physician who has routinely prescribed stimulant drugs for over a quarter century), this more recent, wide use of the ADHD diagnosis and stimulant drugs, raises even broader questions about our society's values and beliefs about children.

The most fundamental assumptions of any belief system are invariably also the most challengeable. The medical model is most commonly invoked as the scientific and ideological underpinnings upon which ADHD diagnosis and use of stimulant drugs rest. That framework emphasizes biological process that are genetic and biochemical in nature. Even most ardent proponents of the medical model do not deny some importance attributed to experience when it comes to behavior. However, "nurture" is not routinely invoked with mainstream ADHD research, presentations, or professional publications.

Yet even the devastating effects of a thoroughly well-described genetic condition like phenylketonuria (PKU) deficiency can be avoided by making changes in the environment (avoiding foods that contain phenylalanine). Such a child can otherwise lead a completely normal life.

I often mused over the meaning of the heritability of ADHD. It's contribution to the variance of the syndrome is said to be as high as 0.8 or similar to the genetic contribution towards adult height. Such data have been used politically and emotionally to justify ADHD as a genetically based disorder that has nothing to do with parenting.

But I wonder whether the full penetrance or expression of an ADHD set of heritable personality characteristics (as an aside I believe qualities of persistence and intensity to be far more problematic in the raising of children than impulsivity, but practically speaking all are often lumped together as ADHD) would appear if, say between the ages of 24 and 60 months, the child and family received the kind of intensive, in-home behavior modification programs offered at a similar age to children with another biological-based problem, that of autis (2).

While complete remission of autistic signs occurs in only 10% to 20% of those children who received such interventions, nearly 80% become compliant, an outcome worth noting when contemplating a similar intensive psychosocial regimen for ADHD. Many of these autistic children are also inattentive and hyperactive but if they respond to a "no" then medication is not likely to be necessary in their management.

The parenting/interventions of applied behavioral analysis (ABA) are fairly rigorous (the equivalent of kiddie boot camp, according to some). It may not be for the faint hearted parent who is committed to a more cognitive conflict avoidance type of parenting that has gained predominance culturally in our country. Indeed, while the reasons are legion for the explosive growth in the past 15 years of the ADHD diagnosis and stimulant use in our country, one contributing factor might be the ADHD temperament profile, which has always been part of the spectrum of human behavior (at least since the Ice Ages), in combination with our current parenting styles in America. The genetics of ADHD—is not to be ignored—but may not be the complete explanation for behavior expressed in the current epidemic.

Stimulant medication works to improve the behavior and performance of children with ADHD—there are no questions about that at all. And 70 years experience suggests, despite recent negative publicity and the lack of long-term (more than 2 years) randomized studies, that stimulants are also quite safe (at least in the under teen population—see below). But the effect that stimulant drugs have on improved focus and concentration and decreased impulsivity is true for everyone, not just ADHD children, or adults for that matter (3). This too we have known through studies for 25 years but it is also confirmed by the current widespread illegal use of prescription stimulants by teens and young adults.

However, that stimulants work and are relatively safe do not make them the equivalent to addressing the needs of children at their schools and home with nondrug interventions. But nearly all the scientific literature operates within the constraints and limitations of the medical model which ignores ethical considerations. Consider the following circumstances.

Critics of critics like me invoke well-run studies like the Multimodal Treatment Study of Children with Attention Deficit Hyperactivity Disorder (MTA) or Klein series which purport to prove that psychosocial treatments neither work as well as stimulant drugs in addressing the symptoms of ADHD, nor do they really add much to improvements achieved by stimulant drugs alone. It does not matter that both sets of studies can be (and have been) deconstructed to make a better case for psychosocial interventions for ADHD.

But to go beyond the analyses of these studies, surely the qualities of impulsivity, inattention, and hyperactivity fall within a bell-shaped dimensional model for all children. When considering ADHD in gross terms one looks at the left side of the curve (Fig. 1) at those with the most extreme and clear problem behaviors. They will be few in number compared to those children with a mild or borderline condition for ADHD.

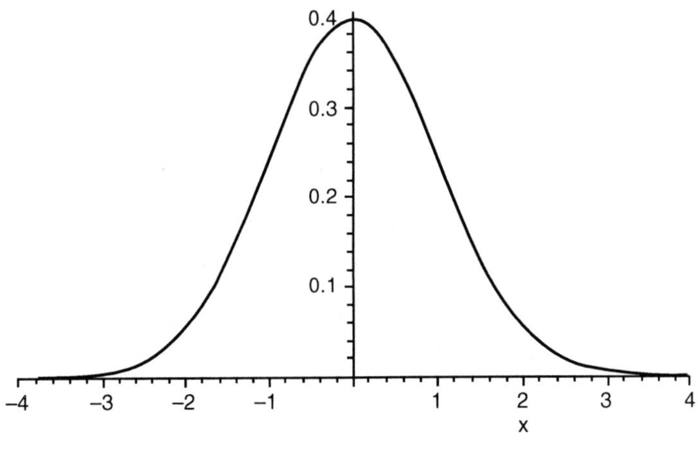

Figure 1 Bell-shaped dimensional model for ADHD.

University studies undoubtedly screen children more rigorously for ADHD diagnosis compared to community standards. Children within MTA and Klein were far more likely to have serious ADHD compared to those diagnosed in the community and treated with stimulant medication (4,5). The Great Smokey Mountain Study offers clues to how medication is actually used on the community level (6). A medication rate of 5% in this population of 4000 children seemed reasonably appropriate given many other studies of ADHD prevalence and medication rates.

Researchers found that 75% of the children who met ADHD criteria were receiving stimulants. However, over half the children being prescribed stimulant medication in this sample did not meet threshold criteria for ADHD or were being treated for a variety of other behavioral and performance issues. The authors did not even address the relative impairment of the medicated children, which ultimately should be the determining factor for treatment, but limited themselves to using the current judgment criteria of our day which was a count of DSM-based symptoms for ADHD.

Other surveys of ADHD prevalence and medication use demonstrate wide variability based on geographic region, ethnicity, and income level—which support the kind of treatment picture we get from the Great Smokey Mountain Study. What we are left with is a very wide set of children being treated with stimulants in our country compared to those carefully screened well-diagnosed children of the MTA and Klein series. It is within the community diagnosed set of children that ethical questions of equivalency of means of treatment can be especially raised.

Just because one kind of treatment works equally well compared to another does not make them morally equivalent (7). Certainly in cases with extreme ADHD, drugs are both indicated and are most likely quite necessary, no matter what environment, or what other nondrug interventions might be available to those children. But for the vast bulk of children in the community being treated with stimulant drugs the same caveat does not apply.

Pelham and others have shown quite clearly that behavioral interventions will reduce ADHD behavior and lower the dose of, or the need for, psychostimulant drugs (8). Just because Ritalin works does not make it the same as offering parents and teachers effective behavioral tools for intervening with impulsive or inattentive behavior. Since children are being treated with stimulants for a variety of behavioral and school performance issues in the real world, making certain educational and learning needs are being addressed in the classroom, with special educational interventions, is ethically required.

I offer a Swiftian "modest proposal" in order to make this lack of moral equivalency clearer. With an estimated 3 million children currently taking stimulant medication in our country, and classroom size averaging about 29 children per class, I propose we increase the number of children on medication to 5 million and in the process we could probably increase classroom size to 40 children per class and save our communities a great deal of money in teachers' salaries. Are there any takers to my offer? Most politicians and community leaders would reject such an offer as completely unethical—that medication is not the equivalent of giving children proper or enough attention. Yet to a degree that already happens in our country today in many communities and areas.

Critics of the critic often respond with medical analogies. But "Would you deny insulin to a diabetic child?" or just simply try to change the environment. The charge is disingenuous. There is a small group of ADHD children (relative to those treated in the United States) who are like insulin-dependent diabetic children. They would need their Ritalin regardless of family, community, or culture. But they represent a minority (my guess is one-eighth to one-tenth of whom we treat medically today). Ironically the diabetes metaphor for ADHD can be used to justify psychosocial interventions. Type II diabetes is clearly a medical problem and is probably a better analogy for ADHD than Type I. Type II diabetes does respond to insulin or oral hypoglycemic agents, but the first interventions recommended are typically environment related—diet and exercise. Only after they fail (and they often do) are medical interventions employed (as should be the case with ADHD—yet official recommendations are for drugs as the first-line treatment).

America's love affair with legal and illegal stimulant drugs raises many questions about the nature of our society. One wonders whether the fact that the United States uses 80% of the world's legal stimulant production is a sign of our advanced thinking on these problems, or some perverse fixation we have on performance at any cost (9). More recently I have come to the conclusion that our obsession with performance drug use in children is an ironic response to our over concern about our children's self-esteem and self-image. However, the cultural implications of this speculation go beyond this essay and the reader is referred to essays in "The Last Normal Child" (10).

My final area of concern has to do with growing signs and evidence of prescription stimulant misuse and abuse particularly in teenagers and young adults. America has experienced three waves of doctor prescribed stimulant abuse since World War II and we are currently deeply into our fourth. The last prescription stimulant abuse epidemic occurred in the 1970s when doctors routinely prescribed amphetamine for weight loss primarily in women. Many patients became addicted to the drug. In the end society judged (through congressional hearings and individual state laws prohibiting doctors from prescribing stimulants for weight control) that the benefits of these drugs for weight loss far outweighed the risks involved.

As I mentioned, stimulants have an enviable safety record in children. In the past our society (also true in Europe and Japan) has concluded that stimulant drugs are potentially dangerous to adults—the main reason that

Ritalin, Concerta, and Adderall are all Schedule II controlled substances in the United States. Beginning in the mid-1990s the diagnosis of ADHD in teens and adults burgeoned, as did the use of prescription stimulants. Recent surveys by Medco have prescription rates doubling in this age group between 2000 and 2003 (11). Centers for Disease Control (CDC) estimates of adult prescription stimulants use is at 1.5 million in 2002 but is likely to be much higher now.

Anecdotal reports of widespread availability of prescription stimulants on high school and college campuses abound. Up to one quarter of college students at certain campuses admit to the illegal use of prescription stimulants (12). In early 2006 a study of data collected in 2002 first reported on the number of individuals over the age of 12 who had illegally used prescription stimulants (13). Twenty-one million people overall admitted to illegal use at least once. Three million used only prescription stimulants. Seventy-five thousand between the ages of 12 and 25 admit to a level of use which meets DSM criteria for addiction and abuse. This number represents about 1 in 10 young persons who admitted to casual use.

This data analysis for the first time gives physicians and the general community a handle on the scope of prescription stimulant abuse. The information was from a 2002 survey. Undoubtedly, the number of seriously affected individuals four years later is higher. My own experience prescribing to college students over the last five years has been regularly problematic. I have been less concerned about over use by these individuals. Rather, their use appears sporadic and intermittent until exam time when binging is likely. Despite vigorous efforts on my part to have a regular connection with these patients (via telephone, email, in person appointments, etc.), such use does not treat ADHD effectively and potentially permits and/or exacerbates an ADHD lifestyle of procrastination with intense catch-up activity under high anxiety. I suspect, but cannot be certain, that some of my patients share or sell their medication. The widespread illegal use of these drugs has to be coming from some legitimate source.

Even in more responsible adult patients, tolerance—that need for increasing dosages in order to maintain effectiveness or length of action—appears to develop in about one-quarter of the patients I have treated for 5 years or longer. There is nothing in the medical literature as of September 2007 on this phenomenon in ADHD adult patients. Tolerance is rarely if ever seen in children (even younger teens). But tolerance was absolutely a problem for the women of the 1970s who took stimulant medication for weight control. The Santayana conclusion—those who do not study history are condemned to repeat it—comes to mind.

The answers to my concerns about legitimate prescription stimulant use for ADHD in adults as of this writing are not forthcoming. In part there is no monetary incentive on the short term to study any drug beyond the drug approval period of several months. The history of stimulant use in this country screams out concern but has been overwhelmed by short-term studies and the anecdotal reports of success promoted by drug companies to physicians and patients alike.

We may be entering a period shortly when a backlash against stimulant drugs develops once news of abuse hits the front pages of the newspaper and are discussed in the halls of Congress. Even without this major specter of a fourth wave of stimulant abuse hovering, ethical concerns will continue about the balance between the use of stimulants and nondrug interventions for children who misbehave or under perform in our country. I'm afraid these worries will not go away; nor should they.

REFERENCES

1. Bradley C. The behavior of children receiving Benzedrine. Am J Psychiatry 1937; 94:577–85.
2. Cohen H, Amerine-Dickens M, Smith T. Early intensive behavioral treatment: replication of the UCLA model in a community setting. J Dev Behav Pediatr 2006; 27:S145–55.
3. Rapoport JL, Buchsbaum MS, Weingartner H, et al. Dextroamphetamine: its cognitive and behavioral effects in normal and hyperactive boys and normal men. Arch Gen Psychiatry 1980; 49:728–38.
4. Special Section: ADHD, comorbidity and treatment outcomes in the MTA study. J Am Acad Child Adolesc Psychiatry 2001; 40:134–96.
5. Abikoff H, Hechtman L, Klein RG, et al. Symptomatic improvement in children with ADHD treated with long-term methylphenidate and multi-modal psychosocial treatment. J Am Acad Child Adolesc Psychiatry 2004; 43:802–11.
6. Angold A, Erkanli A, Egger HL, Costello EJ. Stimulant treatment for children: a community perspective. J Am Acad Child Adolesc Psychiatry 2000; 39: 975–984.
7. Parens E. Is better always good? Hastings Center Report, Special Supplement (Jan–Feb) 1998:S1–17.
8. Chako A, Pelham WE, Gnagy EM, et al. Stimulant medication effects in a summer treatment program among young children with attention-deficit hyperactivity disorder. J Am Acad Child Adolesc Psychiatry 2005; 44:249–257.
9. UN International Narcotics Control Board. Report of the UN International Narcotics Control Board. New York: UN Publications, 2000.
10. Diller LH. The Last Normal Child: essays on the intersection of kids, culture and psychiatric drugs. Westport CT: Praeger Publishers, 2006.
11. Harris G. Use of attention-deficit drugs is found to soar among adults. New York Times, September 2005; 15, p. A14.
12. McCabe SE, Knight JR, Teter CJ, Wechsler H. Non-medical use of prescription stimulants among U.S. college students: prevalence and correlates from a national survey. Addiction 2005; 99:96–106.
13. Kroutil LA, Van Brunt DL, Herman-Stahl MA, et al. Non-medical use of prescription stimulants in the United States. Drug Alcohol Depend 2006; 84: 135–43.

Section VII: Consensus

30

The American Academy of Pediatrics ADHD Practice Guidelines: A Critique

Thomas A. Blondis
University of Chicago School of Medicine, Chicago, Illinois, U.S.A.

Kerry A. Brown
La Rabida Children's Hospital, Chicago, Illinois, U.S.A.

In 1996 the Committee on Quality Improvement of the American Academy of Pediatrics (1) selected a subcommittee composed of pediatricians, four developmental and behavioral pediatricians, one neurodevelopmental disabilities pediatrician, and one pediatric neurologist. Joining the committee and participating as liaison representatives was one representative from each of the following organizations: the American Psychiatric Association, the Child Neurology Society, the American Academy of Family Physicians, and the Society for Pediatric Psychology. The aim of this subcommittee was to develop practice guidelines for general pediatricians to provide competent (1) diagnosis of attention deficit hyperactivity disorder (ADHD) of 6- to 12-year-olds, and (2) treatment and management of 6- to 12-year-old children who are diagnosed with ADHD (2–6).

The subcommittee collaborated with the Agency for Healthcare Research and Quality to develop the evidence-based literature on the topic of the diagnosis of ADHD. For the treatment guidelines segment the committee partnered with the Agency for Healthcare Research and the evidence-based practice center at McMaster University, Ontario, Canada, to develop the evidence-based literature in the areas of treatment and management of ADHD. A "Clinical Practice Guideline" was produced for the diagnosis of ADHD, and a subsequent "Clinical Practice Guideline" was produced for the treatment of the school-aged child with ADHD (5).

The Committee on Quality Improvement of the AAP undertook this project due to ADHD being "the most common neurobehavioral disorder" of childhood. It is estimated that between 4% and 12% of school-aged children or as many as 3.8 million children, most of them boys, have ADHD. The AAP recognizes that ADHD is among the most prevalent chronic health conditions affecting school-aged children. The National Institute of Health's Consensus Statement (7) found ADHD to be a major public health problem in the United States. Also of concern were the increasing public interest in ADHD and the debate in magazines, newspapers, television, and the internet concerning the diagnostic and treatment strategies (8).

DIAGNOSIS

The diagnostic portion of the AAP practice plan begins by affirming the behavioral requirements for ADHD in its three forms [predominantly inattentive type (PIT), predominantly hyperactive-impulsive type (PHT), and combined type (CT)] as defined in the *Diagnostic and Statistical Manual of Mental Disorders*, Fourth Edition (DSM-IV) (9). The practice guidelines clearly delineate the core IA symptoms along with the core HI symptoms from the DSM-IV. It maintains that ADHD is the most common neurobehavioral disorder of childhood. Additionally, since a wide variety of other psychological and developmental disorders (e.g., oppositional defiant disorder, conduct disorder, depression, Tourette's, anxiety disorder, and learning disorders) frequently coexist in children with ADHD, the importance of a thorough assessment is emphasized. The National Institutes of Health in their Consensus Statement (7) affirmed the core behaviors in DSM-IV to be optimum symptoms at that time.

Diagnostic Recommendation # 1

"In a child 6 to 12 years old who exhibits inattention, hyperactivity, impulsivity, academic underachievement, or behavior problems, primary care clinicians should initiate an evaluation for ADHD (Strength of evidence: good; strength of recommendation: strong)."

Pediatricians are often the first medical professionals that parents bring their child to when they are concerned about the child's ability to attend and/or behave appropriately. As aforementioned, since ADHD is comorbid with a number of other disorders, it is pertinent that the primary care physician (PCP) evaluate the ADHD patient for associated mental health conditions. Unfortunately, there is a scarcity of both developmental/behavioral pediatricians and child psychiatrists. Therefore, screening parents of patients during routine visits may assist in early recognition that a child may need to receive a thorough ADHD evaluation. Following the new practice guidelines, the PCP should be able to evaluate straightforward cases of ADHD.

Diagnostic Recommendation # 2

"The diagnosis of ADHD requires that a child meet DSM-IV criteria (strength of evidence: good; strength of recommendation: strong)."

The diagnosis must be based on the 18 DSM-IV symptoms that occur in two separate scales. This includes nine symptoms on the IA scale and nine symptoms on the HI scale. The physician needs to recognize the criteria for the three subtypes:

- ADHD-PIT (exhibiting at least 6/9 IA behaviors)
- ADHD-PHT (exhibiting at least 6/9 HI behaviors)
- ADHD-CT (exhibiting at least 6/9 HI behaviors AND at least 6/9 IA behaviors)

Symptoms must have been present before 7 years of age, have persisted for at least 6 months, and occur in two or more settings (i.e., home and school). Furthermore, these symptoms must be accompanied by a significant functional impairment in at least one of the following areas:

- Academic failure
- Occupational failure
- Social failure

Finally, the physician or psychologist must determine that these failures are not due to another mental health or neurological disorder.

The AAP subcommittee adapted four other recommendations for the diagnostic practice guidelines.

Diagnostic Recommendation # 3

"The assessment of ADHD requires evidence directly obtained from parents or caregivers regarding the core symptoms of ADHD in various settings, the age of onset, duration of symptoms, and degree of functional impairment (strength of evidence: good; strength of recommendation: strong)."

Diagnostic Recommendation # 4

"The assessment of ADHD requires evidence directly obtained from the classroom teacher (or other school professional) regarding the core symptoms of ADHD, the duration of symptoms, the degree of functional impairment, and coexisting conditions... (strength of evidence: good; strength of recommendation: strong)."

Diagnostic Recommendation # 5

"Evaluation of the child with ADHD should include assessment for coexisting conditions (strength of evidence: strong; strength of recommendation: strong)."

Diagnostic Recommendation # 6

"Other diagnostic tests are not routinely indicated to establish the diagnosis of ADHD (strength of evidence: strong; strength of recommendation: strong)."

The PCP who has the experience and the time to evaluate comorbidity should be able to manage generalized anxiety disorder, disruptive behavioral disorders, and dysthymia. The PCP with the help of the child's school district or a private child psychologist should be able to help determine if the child has a learning disability. However, more complex comorbidity such as possible bipolar disorder should be referred to a child psychiatrist.

A meta-analysis of published data on the reliability, sensitivity, and selectivity of behavioral questionnaire scales was performed by the National Initiative for Children's Healthcare Quality (NICHQ) group. The results demonstrated that broadband scales' sensitivity for ADHD was less than would be required to support a diagnosis. For example, broadband scales analyzed were the CBCL/4–18 Parent Form and the CBCL/TRF, Total Problem Scale (Achenbach, 1991), and the DSMD-Total Scale (Devereaux Scales of Mental Disorders; 10) all of which failed to yield a specific diagnosis for ADHD. These results are published in "Diagnosis of Attention Deficit/Hyperactivity Disorder" (3).

Results from the Green et al. (3) study, however, reached significantly different conclusions in their analysis of ADHD-specific short-band questionnaires. The Conners Parent Rating Scale—1997 Revised Version: Long Form, ADHD Index Scale (CPRS-R:L-ADHD Index) for 6- to 17-year-old males and females had an effect size of 3:1 and 95% confidence limits of 2.5, 3.7. The Conners Teacher Rating Scale—1997 Revised Version: Long Form, ADHD Index Scale (CTRS-R:L-ADHD Index) for 6- to 17-year-old males and females had an effect size of 3:3 and 95% confidence limits of 2.8, 3.8. Finally, Barkley's School Situations Questionnaire-Original Version, Number of Problem Setting Scale (SSQ-O-1) (Breen 1989) for 6- to 11-year-old females had an effect size of 1.3 and 95% confidence limits of 0.5, 2.2, and the SSQ-O-1, Mean Severity Scale had an effect size of 2.0 and 95% confidence limits of 1.0, 2.9. In conclusion, short-band questionnaires appear to more validly assess ADHD due to its sensitivity to ADHD symptomology.

The subcommittee dealt with comorbidity, but failed to address mimic disorders. If the practice guidelines contained a description of each mimic disorder, the focus of the guidelines would be diminished and the length could decrease the number of PCPs who take the time to read the guidelines.

However, these multiple disorders that could be mistaken for ADHD should be added to the toolkit. The PCP needs to be reminded of sickness and other conditions that often include the ADHD core symptoms (11,12).

TREATMENT

The first point the committee established was that since ADHD is a chronic condition, treatment must be managed like all other chronic medical conditions (e.g., diabetes, asthma, sickle cell). The subcommittee, partnered by the Agency for Healthcare Research and Quality and the Evidence-Based Practice Center at McMaster University (5), developed treatment recommendations for the school-aged ADHD child between the ages of 6 and 11 years. The recommendations also integrated important findings from the MTA study (13,14). The key recommendations include:

1. Primary care clinicians should establish a treatment program that recognizes ADHD as a chronic condition (strength of evidence: good; strength of recommendation: strong).
2. The treating clinician, parents, and the child, in collaboration with school personnel, should specify appropriate target outcomes to guide management (strength of evidence: good; strength of recommendation: strong).
3. The clinician should recommend stimulant medication (strength of evidence: good) and/or behavioral therapy (strength of evidence: fair), as appropriate to improve target outcomes in children with ADHD (strength of recommendation: strong).
   For children on stimulants, if one stimulant does not work at the highest feasible dose, the clinician should recommend another.
4. When the selected management for a child with ADHD has not met target outcomes, clinicians should evaluate the original diagnosis, use of all appropriate treatments, adherence to the treatment plan, and presence of coexisting conditions (strength of evidence: weak; strength of recommendation: strong).
5. The clinician should periodically provide a systematic follow-up for the child with ADHD. Monitoring should be directed to target outcomes and adverse effects by obtaining specific information from parents, teachers, and the child (strength of evidence: fair; strength of recommendation: strong).

William E. Pelham, Ph.D., a professor at SUNY-Buffalo and a consultant to the guidelines committee, reported that one of the most crucial functions of the guidelines is its emphasis on the chronic nature of ADHD and the necessity for the treatment plan to reflect this chronicity. In addition, Dr. Pelham notes another important strength of the guidelines including its focus on difficulties of daily life, rather than just the clinical symptomatology of ADHD. Finally, its recognition of the vast research findings that medication and behavioral therapy are the two most empirically validated treatments is another important strength of the guidelines (15,16).

Another benefit of the guidelines is that it can provide additional opportunities for the fields of pediatrics and psychology to collaborate. Specifically, now that PCPs are being encouraged to utilize behavioral treatment in conjunction with medication in the treatment of ADHD, psychologists play a crucial role. Some psychologists receive specialized training regarding assessing/evaluating ADHD, providing school consultations with teachers of ADHD students, and providing useful behavioral interventions for children with ADHD (individual therapy, parent training, social skills groups) (6,17).

On the other hand, the guidelines also have weaknesses. Some believe that the guidelines are both vague and unrealistic. Specifically, they argue that the guidelines fail to provide specific information to help clinicians determine the appropriate treatment approach for specific, individual patients. Additionally, the guidelines seem to be less helpful in treating children with comorbid mental health conditions.

The treatment guidelines will hopefully add Atomoxetine as an ADHD drug in the near future. Atomoxetine was not yet available at the time of publication. Eli Lilly carried out a 5-year placebo versus Atomoxetine investigation that clearly demonstrated that ADHD patients on Atomoxetine are significantly more attentive and less hyperactive. Safety issues were closely investigated and there were no significant negative cardiovascular side effects. A further study demonstrated Atomoxetine to be as effective as short-acting methylphenidate when both are compared to a placebo (18,19).

THE AAP ADHD TOOLKIT

The "Caring for Children with ADHD: a Resource Toolkit for Clinicians" was codeveloped by the AAP and the NICHQ and published in 2002 (20). The goal of this toolkit was to simplify and organize the process by putting all of the most effective tools for diagnosing and treating ADHD in one place. It mirrors the AAP guidelines and is designed to streamline the practice guidelines for pediatricians.

This toolkit includes:

- An introduction
- Diagnostic materials
    - Introduction explaining the diagnostic process
    - NICHQ ADHD primary care evaluation form
    - Scoring instructions for the NICHQ Assessment Scales

- NICHQ Vanderbilt Assessment Scale-PARENT Information
- Cover letter for teachers
- NICHQ Vanderbilt Assessment Scale-TEACHER information

A drawback to the toolkit is that the NICHQ Vanderbilt Assessment Scale-PARENT and TEACHER Information was not a part of the meta-analysis that Green et al. (3) conducted for the AAP Subcommittee on ADHD. Additionally, scoring fails to consider different norms for gender or age changes deeming the results for middle school-aged children less specific than scales that include gender and age norms. This is particularly problematic because at the National Institute of Health Consensus Conference, the panel of scientists agreed that current measures of ADHD are flawed because they do not take into account the ADHD child's age. For example, the norms for CPRS-R and the CTRS-R both reflect the decline of hyperactivity symptoms over the age span. This leads to the concern that boys over the age of nine years may be misclassified as ADHD-IA (PIT) (7). Therefore, the consensus concludes that clinicians and investigators must take into account age in tools that are developed for ADHD diagnosis, and the toolkit currently ignores this factor. With the exception of this tool, the NICHQ toolkit is generally based on evidence-based research and at this time can be considered a solid working device for the PCP who adheres to the practice guidelines.

Several regions of the country have begun to establish networks making the diagnosis and treatment of ADHD more feasible for the PCP (21,22). Leslie et al. (23) published results of a two and half year attempt to implement the AAP diagnostic guidelines. Money from a national grant paid for an ADHD Coordinator, who received, scored, and summarized packets of questionnaires sent by seven pediatric practices. Seven "research naïve" primary care offices in the San Diego area were recruited to participate. The pediatricians and their office staff were trained in the San Diego Attention-Deficit/Hyperactivity Disorder Project (SANDAP) protocol that was based upon the AAP practice guidelines and utilized the NICHQ Toolkit. More than 40% of the subjects demonstrated discrepant results on the Vanderbilt scales, with only the parent or teacher endorsing sufficient symptoms to meet DSM-IV criteria for ADHD. Significant barriers plague the primary care providers. One such barrier is that providers do not have the mechanisms for implementing the ADHD diagnostic guidelines. Also, without the study, ADHD coordinators, physicians' offices, and in some cases care providers would have to take the time to score questionnaires and summarize this data. At this time private primary care providers cannot take the amount of time that is required to diagnose and manage ADHD utilizing the AAP practice guidelines.

If primary care providers are to treat ADHD and ADHD associated mental health conditions, third-party payers will have to pay for the time that it takes to do a competent job. Currently, there is no incentive for the loss of revenue that implementation of the AAP diagnostic and treatment plans will bring about. This requires significantly more time that the 10-minute office visit PCPs are reimbursed for by third-party payers.

REFERENCES

1. American Academy of Pediatrics. The Classification of Child and Adolescent Mental Diagnoses in Primary Care: Diagnostic and Statistical Manual for Primary Care (DSM-PC) Child and Adolescent Version. Elk Grove Village, IL: American Academy of Pediatrics, 1996.
2. Academy of Pediatrics, Committee on Quality Improvement and Subcommittee on Attention-Deficit/Hyperactivity Disorder. Diagnosis and evaluation of the child with attention-deficit/hyperactivity disorder. Pediatrics 2000; 105: 1158–70.
3. Green M, Wong M, Atkins D, Taylor J, Feinlieb M. Diagnosis of Attention-Deficit/Hyperactivity Disorder. Technical Review # 3a. Rockville, MD: Agency for Health Care Policy and Research, 1999.
4. American Academy of Pediatrics, Committee on Quality Improvement and Subcommittee on Attention-Deficit/Hyperactivity Disorder. Clinical practice guideline: treatment of school-aged child with attention-deficit/hyperactivity disorder. Pediatrics 2001; 108:1033–44.
5. Jadad AR, Boyle M, Cunningham C, et al. Treatment of Attention Deficit/Hyperactivity Disorder. Evidence Report/Technology and Quality, 1999. (AHRZ publication no. 00–E005.)
6. Brown RT, Freeman WS, Perrin JM, et al. Prevalence and assessment of Attention-Deficit/Hyperactivity Disorder in primary care settings. Pediatrics 2001; 107:e43–60.
7. National Institutes of Health. Diagnosis and Treatment of Attention-Deficit/Hyperactivity Disorder. NIH Consensus Statement 16(2). Washington, D.C.: U.S. Government Printing Office, 1998.
8. Gibbs N. Latest on Ritalin. Time 1998; 152:86–96.
9. American Psychiatric Association. Diagnostic and Statistical Manual for Mental Disorders, 4th ed. Washington, D.C.: American Psychiatric Association, 1994.
10. Naglieri JA, LeBuffe PA, Pfeiffer SI. Manuel for the Devereaux Scales of Mental Disorders. San Antonio, TX: Psychological Services, 1994.
11. Accardo TA, Blondis TA, Whitman BY, Stein M, eds. Attention Deficit Disorders and Hyperactivity in Children and Adults. New York: Marcel Dekker, 2000.
12. Castellanos FX, Giedd JN, Elia J, et al. Controlled stimulant treatment of ADHD and comorbid Tourette's syndrome: effects of stimulant and dose. J Am Acad Child Adolesc Psychiatry 1997; 36:589–96.
13. Jensen P, Arnold L, Richters J, et al. 14-month randomized clinical trial of treatment strategies for attention deficit hyperactivity disorder. Arch Gen Psychiatry 1999; 56:1073–86.

14. Swanson JM, Kraemer HC, Hinshaw SP, et al. Clinical relevance of primary symptoms of the MTA: success rates based on severity of symptoms at the end of treatment. J Am Acad Child Adolesc Psychiatry 2001; 40:147–5817.
15. Pelham WE Jr, Wheeler T, Chronis A. Empirically supported psychosocial treatments for attention deficit hyperactivity disorder. J Clinical Child Psychology 1998; 27:190–205.
16. Smith D. Guidance in treating ADHD. Monitor Psychol January 2002:34–5.
17. Leslie LK, Weckerly J, Landsverk J, Hough RL, Hurlburt M, Wood PA. Racial/ethnic differences in the use of psychotropic medication in high-risk children and adolescents. J Am Acad Child Adolesc Psychiatry 2003; 42: 1433–42.
18. Kratochvil CJ, Heiligenstein JH, Dittmann R, et al. Atomoxetine and methylphenidate treatment in children with ADHD: a prospective, randomized, open-label trial. Journal of the American Academy of Children and Adolescent Psychiatry 2002; 41:776–84.
19. Michelson D, Faries D, Wernicke J, et al. Atomoxetine in the treatment of children and adolescents with attention-deficit/hyperactivity disorder: a randomized, placebo-controlled, dose-response study. Pediatrics 2001; 108:E83.
20. American Academy of Pediatrics, National Initiative for Children's Healthcare Quality. Caring for Children with ADHD: A Resource Toolkit for Clinicians. Chicago: Centers for the Education and Research on Therapeutics, 2002.
21. Leslie LK. Improving care for ADHD in primary care pediatrics; caring for children in child welfare; developmental screening and enhancement project; impact of screening and triage for developmental problems on service use by children in child welfare; children's care connection (CASRC); www.casrc.org/People/Internal_Investigators/leslie.htm, 2004
22. Olfson M, Gameroff MJ, Marcus SC, Jensen PS. National trends in the treatment of attention deficit hyperactivity disorder. Am J Psychiatry 2003; 1600:1071–7.
23. Leslie LK, Weckerly J, Plemmons D, Landsverk J, Eastman S. Implementing the American Academy of Pediatrics Attention-Deficit/Hyperactivity Disorder diagnostic guidelines in primary care settings. Pediatrics 2004; 114:129–40.
24. Adenbach TM. Integrative guide for the 1991 CBCL/4–18, YSR, and TRF profiles. Berlington, VT: University of Vermont, Department of Psychiatry, 1991.
25. Breen MJ, Alteper TS, Factor Structures of the Home Situations Questionnaire and the School Situations Questionnaire. Journal of Pediatric Psychology 1991; 16(1):59–67.

31

Educational Policy

Perry A. Zirkel and George J. DuPaul
College of Education, Lehigh University, Bethlehem, Pennsylvania, U.S.A.

Children with attention deficit hyperactivity disorder (ADHD) experience significant academic and/or social difficulties in school settings (1). Approximately 90% of students with this disorder underachieve academically and about 30% have specific learning disabilities (2). Given these pervasive and chronic difficulties, school services (e.g., special education) may be necessary to enhance the academic and social functioning of students with ADHD. Over the past decade, the nature of school services available to children with this disorder has been shaped by educational policy related to education for students with disabilities. Educational policy starts with legislation but also includes what is largely neglected in the limited relevant literature (3), published interpretations by the administering agency.

Whether the clinician refers to ADHD as a "disability," the child's legal entitlement to accommodations or services in elementary or secondary school will depend on whether the child meets the criteria for "disability" under either the Individuals with Disabilities Education Act (IDEA) or Section 504 of the Rehabilitation Act (§ 504). The third pertinent federal law, the Americans with Disabilities Act (ADA), has the same definition as does § 504; its only additional relevance here is that it applies to private schools that do not receive federal financial assistance.

In this chapter, we will provide (1) an overview of the disability definitions and related information for the IDEA and § 504, (2) a chronological, stage-by-stage summary of the relevant policy interpretations under each of these overlapping statutory frameworks, and (3) a brief discussion of the clinical implications of educational policy related to identification and diagnosis.

IDEA AND § 504

The IDEA legislation dates back to 1975. It was basically a funding act, providing federal funds to school districts along with a set of detailed state and local requirements. Congress has amended the Act several times. The Office of Special Education Programs (OSEP) is the agency, which is part of the federal Department of Education that administers the Act, including the issuance of policy interpretations (4). In contrast, § 504 is a civil rights act—in parallel to Title VI for race and national origin and Title IX for gender—that succinctly prohibits organizations receiving federal financial assistance from discrimination based on disability. It is older than the IDEA, dating back to 1973, but its regulations were not issued until 1978. § 504 has remained largely unchanged, except for amendments in 1990, upon passage of its sister statute, the ADA, which changed the term "handicap" to "disability" and made revisions in terms of substance abuse. The agency charged with administering § 504 and the ADA in relation to schools, including the issuance of policy interpretations, is the Office for Civil Rights (OCR), which is another part of the federal Department of Education (5).

The IDEA regulations (6) define "child with a disability" in terms of two essential elements: (i) meeting the criteria of one or more of 13 specified categories, such as "other health impairment" (OHI) or "specific learning disability" (SLD); and (ii) needing, "by reason thereof," special education. Available in the form of a practical checklist (7), the IDEA criteria for OHI are (i) a chronic or acute health condition that results in (ii) limited strength, vitality, or alertness, having (iii) an adverse effect on the child's educational performance that (iv) necessitates special education (with or without related services).

In contrast, the amended § 504 legislation (8) defines "individual with a disability" in terms of three essential elements: (i) a physical or mental impairment, (ii) that substantially limits, (iii) a major life activity. The courts have clarified the meaning and measurement of these elements. For example, they have held that the measurement of "substantially limits" is with reference to other students in the general population and with, not without, the mitigating effects of medication (9). In relation to students with ADHD, the major developments in terms of the application of the IDEA's and § 504's statutory eligibility definitions have largely been, first, the regulations, and second, interpreting the ambiguities and filling in the gaps, OSEPs and OCRs policy interpretations of these respective laws. Courts generally defer to regulations and, to a lesser extent, to the policy interpretations that supplement them (10). In contrast, very few published court decisions have focused on the eligibility of ADHD students under the IDEA (11) or under § 504 (12,13). Moreover, the guidance that they provide, particularly those under the IDEA, has been limited, except that these decisions continue to reinforce the case-by-case "it depends" answer rather than the automatic "yes" or "no" answer (14,15). These policy interpretations may be grouped into succeeding stages under the IDEA and § 504, respectively.

IDEA: STAGES OF POLICY INTERPRETATIONS

The policy interpretations under the IDEA are relatively frequent. They fit into four succeeding stages of policy evolution.

Stage 1

The first major policy change relating to students with ADHD was the Joint Policy Memorandum (16), jointly issued by the OSEP, the OCR, and the Office of Elementary and Secondary Education. This Memorandum, issued in the wake of a notice of inquiry soliciting public comment on the education of children with ADHD mandated by the 1990 Amendments of the IDEA, concluded that no change was necessary in the IDEA definition of disability. The explanation was that children with ADHD could qualify as OHI or under the other specified categories, such as SLD or emotional disturbance (ED), under the IDEA where they needed special education and related services. This policy interpretation further explained that when such children did not meet the IDEA requirements, they "may fit" (p. 118) under the broader definition of disability under § 504 depending on the severity of their condition. This alternative is discussed in the subsequent part of this chapter.

Stage 2

The second stage was an assortment of policy interpretations in the early and later 1990s, including another joint endeavor (17) that reiterated and supplemented the Joint Memorandum. One line of the policy letters during this period clarified when the IDEA eligibility evaluation must be conducted for a child who has or may have ADHD. Specifically, the OSEP has repeated that district's have an affirmative "child find" obligation to evaluate, without undue delay, all children who have or are suspected of having a disability under the IDEA (18). Parents may request such an evaluation at any time, but the district's obligation is only triggered if—based on the parents' request and/or other information—the district has reason to suspect that the child is eligible under the two-part test of eligibility under the IDEA (19,20).

Another line of the policy letters during this period addressed the roles of educators, including school psychologists, and physicians in the diagnosis of ADHD. First, the OSEP clarified and reiterated that a district may not refuse to evaluate a child for possible IDEA eligibility for the reason that the child has a medical diagnosis of ADHD (19,21). Second and more importantly, a physician is not necessary under the IDEA for the diagnosis of ADHD (17,21). Rather, when a district conducts an evaluation of OHI as a result of ADHD, the multidisciplinary team must include "an individual who is knowledgeable about the possible adverse effects of ADD on a child's educational performance" (21, p. 964). Third, if state law or the local policy/practice opts to require a physician for this purpose, which is within their discretion (17,22), a physician's diagnosis of ADHD is not sufficient to establish IDEA eligibility (22); rather, the district must ensure that this diagnosis is at no cost to the parents (17,21) and that "any necessary evaluation by other professionals are also conducted and considered as part of the eligibility determination process" (21, p. 965).

Stage 3

The third stage was the express recognition in the 1999 IDEA regulations, in the wake of the 1997 IDEA Amendments, that ADHD was one of the chronic or acute health conditions in the definition of OHI and that the "limited alertness" in the same definition may be met by the "heightened alertness to environmental stimuli" attributable to ADHD. On one hand, this recognition effectively added more legal force to the possible eligibility of ADHD students under the IDEA, taking the form of a regulation rather than just policy interpretations. On the other hand, all that this recognition did was fulfill two of the essential elements of OHI. The IDEA evaluation process, including the impartial second and binding opinion of a hearing and/or review officer and, if appealed, one or more levels of the judiciary, must conclude not only that the child has ADHD but also that the child's ADHD meets the remaining criteria of adverse effect on educational performance and the need for special education.

Stage 4

In a final, postregulations stage, the OSEP has issued two further policy interpretations in response to the continuing inquiries of interested individuals and organizations in ADHD issues under the IDEA. Both revisit the issue of the respective roles of physicians and educators. In the first letter, the OSEP confirmed its long-standing position that the IDEA does not require a medical diagnosis of ADHD for purposes of OHI eligibility, allowing the district instead "to use qualified personnel other than a licensed physician to conduct the [eligibility determination] as long as all of the protections in evaluation procedures under IDEA are met" (23, p. 151). More interestingly, the second policy letter responds to the increasing concern about educators pressing parents to secure medication for their children with ADHD. Specifically, the OSEP endorsed the position of Rhode Island's department of education that districts may not condition educational services upon the parents' consent to medicate the child (24). Second and perhaps less obvious, the OSEP announced what it characterized as part of "its long-standing policy" that "[a]t parents' request and with their consent, educators may provide input about a student's behavior that may aid medical professional in making a diagnosis, but it not the role of educators to attempt to medically diagnose or recommend medical treatment for students with ADD or ADHD" (23, p. 794). The two distinctions that are noteworthy in this policy statement are (i) the qualifier of a "medical" diagnosis and treatment, as compared to the IDEA, or a primarily educational, determination of eligibility or services; and (ii) the more subtle and arguably new qualifier of educators only providing such information "at the parents' request and with their consent" (23, p. 794).

SECTION 504 (AND THE ADA): STAGES OF POLICY INTERPRETATION

Although some districts use § 504 as, in effect, a consolation prize for students, including those with ADHD, who do not attain or whose parents oppose eligibility under the IDEA, the corresponding policy statements have been less frequent from the OCR. They appear to fit into two successive stages.

Stage 1

First, the Joint Memorandum (16) pointed out that "the protections of Section 504 extend to some children who do not fall within the disability categories specified in [the IDEA]" (p. 117) and, more specifically, reciting the three-part definition of disability under § 504, concluded that "depending on the severity of their condition, children with ADD *may* fit within that definition" (p. 118). Additionally, the memorandum traced the related § 504 requirements, including the obligation to evaluate the child "if parents believe that their child is handicapped by ADD" (p. 118); the parent's right to contest an adverse decision via a due process hearing; and the child's right, in the wake of a favorable eligibility determination, to appropriate education in the least restrictive environment. Finally, the memorandum stated that state and local education agencies "should" take necessary steps "to train regular education teachers and other personnel to develop their awareness about ADD and its manifestations and the adaptations that can be implemented in regular education program to address the instruction needs of these children" (p. 118). The specified examples of such adaptations included the use of behavior management techniques, modified test delivery, and tailored homework assignments. On the other hand, the memorandum also specified examples of more restrictive steps or strategies, including reduced class size, one-on-one tutorials, and classroom aides.

Stage 2

In the absence of any change in the regulations, the remaining stage has been the entire period after the Joint Memorandum, marked by three policy interpretations and a limited assortment of other pertinent legal developments. In the first policy interpretation, the OCR first qualified its statement in the

Joint Memorandum about triggering a district's duty to evaluate in terms of § 504 eligibility. More specifically, in tandem with the IDEA, the OCR clarified that the standard that triggers an evaluation for § 504 eligibility is "reason to believe," not parental suspicion or demand (25). The difference from the IDEA, however, is that this reasonable suspicion standard applies to a wider definition of "disability" and "appropriate education." This same policy interpretation also includes reiterations or clarifications that (i) children with ADHD are not automatically protected under § 504; (ii) districts may not refuse to evaluate a child with ADHD solely because the child did meet the eligibility criteria under the IDEA; (iii) districts may use the same or a different process from that of the IDEA for § 504 evaluation; and (iv) districts may use the same or different procedures from those under the IDEA for impartial due process hearings (25).

Soon thereafter, in a second policy interpretation, the OCR repeated even more emphatically that under § 504, for students with ADHD or other physical or mental impairments "there is no absolute right to an evaluation on demand" (26, p. 1128). Rather, based on the same "suspected disability" standard, applied to a broader criteria of physical or mental impairment that substantially limits a major life activity and needs special or regular education, the district is obligated to either evaluate the child or, if it refuses on the basis of no purportedly reasonable basis to do so, provide notice to the parents of their right to an impartial due process hearing to challenge that refusal (26). Second, in the same policy letter the OCR confirmed that the IDEA-eligible children are typically double-covered, which is also entitled to protection under § 504. Finally, pointing out that "appropriate education" under the § 504 regulations, is defined more broadly than it is under the IDEA as consisting of "special or regular education and related services," the OCR included these additional examples of students with ADHD covered by this entitlement:

- a student with ADHD who meets the three-part definition of disability under § 504 and who needs "what the district considers to be adjustments in the regular classroom (e.g., providing a structured learning environment, simplifying instruction about in-class and homework assignments, using behavioral management techniques, modifying test delivery, using audio-visual equipment)"
- a student with ADHD who meets the three-part definition of disability under § 504 and who needs "regular administration of medication to attend regular class" (26, p. 1128).

However, the double-covered case and the two additional examples require some cautionary warnings in light of more recent relevant legal developments. First, in relation to the double-covered child with ADHD, the OCR more recently issued the more general clarification that it is the district's decision whether to provide special education under the IDEA individualized educational program and that if the district elects to do so and the parent insists instead on a § 504 plan, "the parent would essentially be rejecting" what they were entitled to under § 504 (27, p. 296). Second, although the entitlement of "appropriate education" is undeniably broader, because it attaches related services to regular education as an alternative to special education, the courts in more recent years have applied the definition of eligibility, particularly the criterion of substantial limitation, rather restrictively (9,12) and, in any event, § 504 is an "unfunded mandate," that is, it is triggered by the receipt of federal financial assistance but provides no funding itself. Third, it may be, based on recent case law, that some students with ADHD who require regular administration of medication and who have the requisite parental consent and medical prescription may not meet the definition of disability under § 504 in the first place (9).

Finally, in the second joint policy interpretation (15), the OCR reiterated that whether a child's ADHD is an impairment that substantially limits a major life activity must be determined on an individual basis. With regard to the overlapping definitions of disability, the OCR commented: "While it is possible that a child with ADD might be covered by Section 504, but might not be eligible for services under [the IDEA], the reverse—that the child is eligible for services under [the IDEA], but not covered by Section 504—is difficult to imagine" (p. 76). Based on the recent Supreme Court decisions about mitigating measures, such as medication (9), the reverse today is more possible to imagine—specifically, in the case where 1) the parents agree to medication for their child with ADHD, 2) the district obtains baseline data showing that with the medication the ADHD does not substantially limit learning, 3) the parents then decide to discontinue the medication, and 4) the ADHD, without the mitigating effects of the medication, so adversely affects the child's educational performance as to necessitate special education. On the other hand, for a child not covered by the IDEA, the determination must be careful and individualized, not absolute or stereotyped, particularly in light of the courts' imprecision in further defining and specifically applying the three elements of the definition of disability under § 504 (13).

The Williams letter (17) also clarified with respect to children suspected of having ADHD the OCRs more general position (28) that, "like the IDEA" (p. 77), § 504 does not require a school district to conduct a medical diagnosis, but that if the district determines that one is necessary in addition to or instead of alternative assessment methods, the district must ensure that it is at no cost to the parents.

CLINICAL IMPLICATIONS

The express requirements and policy interpretations of the IDEA and § 504 directly influence the process of identifying students with ADHD who may require special education services and/or general education accommodations. Zirkel (7) has designed a checklist for determining the legal eligibility for special education services in accordance with the regulations enumerated above. Using this checklist as a guide, several steps should be followed in determining whether a specific child will require special education services for ADHD (for more detailed procedures, see Ref. 1).

The first step in the eligibility process is to conduct the IDEA evaluation of ADHD and related difficulties (1). Does the child meet the criteria for one of the IDEA classification categories and, as a result thereof, need special education services? The multidisciplinary team needs to pay special but not exclusive attention to the OHI category. Specifically, if the child is found to meet the criteria for ADHD, then, by definition, the child has a chronic condition that significantly limits alertness, thus satisfying two components of the "other health impaired" eligibility criteria. Two OHI criteria remain.

Next, does the child's ADHD-related behavior in the classroom significantly limit his or her educational performance? The team can determine a child's educational functioning by using academic performance data, such as norm-referenced achievement tests or, more preferably, curriculum-based measurement (29).

Finally, does the child need special education services because of his or her ADHD? This ambiguous criterion could be interpreted in a variety of ways. One way to reach a relatively objective decision regarding this criterion is through evaluating the efficacy of regular classroom interventions (30). Baseline data should be collected on a number of target behaviors prior to implementing a specific intervention (including medication). After implementing the recommended treatment(s), the clinician collects data on the same variables to assess behavioral change. If significant improvement in child functioning does not occur, the clinician can follow one of three possible courses of action. First, changes could be made to the intervention program in the general education classroom. Alternatively, the child could receive some form of special education programming. A third alternative would be to make changes in general education interventions and provide special education programming. The efficacy of both general and special education interventions should be evaluated on a continuous basis to determine when changes in programming and/or placement are necessary.

A similar data-based decision-making process should be followed to identify those students who may require accommodation in general education instruction under § 504. A clinician must first determine whether the child is suffering from "a physical or mental impairment which substantially limits one or more*major life activities" (5) including learning. Thus, a multimethod assessment procedure (2,31) can be used to determine whether a child has ADHD (i.e., a mental impairment) and whether the symptoms of this disorder lead to substantial impairment in educational performance.

In particular, this assessment must include reliable and valid measures of academic functioning and should establish a connection between ADHD symptoms and decrements in educational performance. It is important to note that the framework is used for determining whether ADHD symptoms substantially limit learning in the "average" student in the general population, and, for those children who are medicated, the determination is made with medication, not without it (9).

CONCLUSION

Federal legal policymaking concerning eligibility of ADHD in elementary and secondary education has proceeded on two fronts during the same period—the IDEA and § 504. The primary action has been on the IDEA front, and it has proceeded through several stages marked by refinements rather than reversals in policy. The end results include (1) the recognition, on the elevated level of regulations, that ADHD may qualify under the OHI category; (2) the continuing recognition, in various policy letters, that ADHD may also qualify for other categories, such as SLD, but that the determination will be on an individual basis in terms of the remaining criteria, including the need for special education; (3) the refined recognition, in the second stage of policy letters, that the district's evaluation duty is triggered when it has reason to suspect that a child's ADHD is of sufficient severity to qualify under one of the IDEA categories, and (4) the recent recognition, in the final stage of policy letters, that the IDEA does not require a physician's diagnosis for determination of OHI eligibility and that educators may give their input but may not interfere with the parents' and physicians' roles regarding the medical diagnosis of ADHD for purposes of medication and other such treatment.

The activity under § 504 and, since 1990, its sister statute the ADA, has been less frequent but largely parallel within the context of a broader definition of "disability" and "appropriate education." At the first stage, the Joint Memorandum (16) formalized the recognition that a child with ADHD may meet the three-part definition of disability. During the more recent stage, the OCR clarified that (1) the same "reason to suspect," rather than parental demand per se, is the triggering standard for an eligibility evaluation, (2) the interpretation regarding medical diagnoses also parallels that under the IDEA, and (3) § 504 provides a parallel, albeit more streamlined, notice requirement for procedural safeguards, centering on the parents' right to proceed to a due process hearing.

Finally, clinicians must follow a data-based decision-making model in determining the eligibility of individual students with ADHD for special education services or accommodations to instruction in general education classrooms. Practitioners should use psychometrically sound assessment measures that include multiple sources and methods to evaluate whether guidelines under the IDEA and/or § 504 are met.

REFERENCES

1. DuPaul GJ, Stoner G. ADHD in the Schools: Assessment and Intervention Strategies. 2nd ed. New York: Guilford, 2003.
2. Barkley RA. Attention-deficit/Hyperactivity Disorder: A Handbook for Diagnosis and Treatment. 2nd ed. New York: Guilford, 1998.
3. Latham PS, Latham PH. Attention Deficit Disorder and the Law. 2nd ed. Washington, D.C.: JKL Communications, 1997.
4. Yell M. The Law and Special Education. Upper Saddle River, NJ: Prentice-Hall, 2006.
5. Zirkel P. Section 504, the ADA and the Schools. Horsham, PA: LRP Publications, 2004.
6. IDEA regulations, 34 C.F.R. § 300.8 (2007).
7. Zirkel P. A checklist for determining legal eligibility of ADD/ADHD students. The Special Educator 1992; 8:93–7.
8. § 504 legislation, 29 U.S.C. § 705(20) (2007).
9. Zirkel P. Conducting legally defensible §504/ADA eligibility determinations. Educ L Rep (West) 2003; 176:1–11.
10. Zirkel P. Do OSEP policy letters have legal weight? Educ L Rep (West) 2002; 171:391–6.
11. Kozak v. Hampton Twp. Sch. Dist., 655 A.2d 641 (Pa. Commw. Ct. 1995).
12. Bercovitch v. Baldwin Sch., 133 F.3d 141 (1st Cir. 1998).
13. T.J.W. v. Dothan City Bd. of Educ., 26 IDELR 999 (M.D. Ala. 1997).
14. Alvin Indep. Sch. Dist. v. A.D., 46 IDELR ¶221 (S.D. Tex. 2006).
15. West Chester Area Sch. Dist. v. Chad C., 194 F. Supp. 2d 417 (E.D. Pa. 2002).
16. Joint Policy Memorandum, 18 IDELR 116 (OSEP/OCR/OESE 1991).
17. Williams, Letter to, 21 IDELR 73 (OSEP/OCR 1994).
18. Thomason, Letter to, 18 IDELR 536 (OSEP 1991).
19. Sisisky, Letter to, 21 IDELR 995 (OSEP 1994).
20. Williams, Letter to, 20 IDELR 1210 (OSEP 1993).
21. Parker, Letter to, 18 IDELR 963 (OSEP 1991).
22. Gallagher, Letter to, 24 IDELR 177 (OSEP 1996).
23. Anonymous, Letter to, 34 IDELR ¶35 (OSEP 2000).
24. Hoekstra, Letter to, 34 IDELR ¶204 (OSEP 2000).
25. OCR Memorandum, 19 IDELR 876 (OCR 1993).
26. Mentink, Letter to, 19 IDELR 1127 (OCR 1993).
27. McKethan, Letter to, 25 IDELR 295 (OCR 1996).
28. Veir, Letter to, 20 IDELR 864 (OCR 1993).
29. Shinn MR, ed. Advanced Applications of Curriculum-based Measurement. New York: Guilford, 1998.
30. Gresham FM. Conceptualizing behavior disorders in terms of resistance to intervention. Sch Psychol Rev 1991; 20:23–36.
31. Anastopoulos AD, Shelton TL. Assessing Attention-deficit/Hyperactivity Disorder. New York: Kluwer Academic/Plenum, 2001.

Section VIII: New Directions

32

Sluggish Cognitive Tempo: The Promise and Problems of Measuring Syndromes in the Attention Spectrum

Keith McBurnett

Department of Psychiatry, University of California San Francisco, San Francisco, California, U.S.A.

Sluggish cognitive tempo (SCT) is a term used to describe a syndrome of excessive daydreaming, sluggishness, drowsiness, and forgetfulness, hypothesized to accompany some cases of the inattentive type of attention deficit hyperactivity disorder (ADHD). The term SCT was introduced by Lahey et al. (1). Items describing "daydreams" and "seems sluggish or drowsy" were included in rating scales, e.g., Revised Behavior Problem Checklist (2) and Child Behavior Checklist (3), which were widely used in research in the 1980s. These symptoms were observed to be elevated in children with DSM-III attention deficit disorder without hyperactivity (ADD-WO) (4–6). These symptoms were present in data sets because of their inclusion in behavior rating scales used by these researchers. In those years, no concerted efforts were made toward gathering a more complete set of descriptors, or in more fully delineating SCT beyond those two items. The shift away from recognition of an inattentive type of ADHD in DSM-III-R hindered progress in studying the construct. A renaissance of interest in SCT began around the time of DSM-IVs introduction and has slowly continued, although progress continues to be limited by the lack of a psychometrically sound and generally accepted measure of SCT.

Daydreaming

Research in the 1960s from Jerome Singer's group (7,8) demonstrated that individual differences in daydreaming could be experimentally manipulated, and furthermore that high frequency daydreamers exhibit marginally poorer vigilance in signal detection that sharply deteriorates over time, compared to low frequency daydreamers. This attention decrement was associated with an increase in self-reported daydreaming. Although individuals who frequently daydream are impaired from the viewpoint of sustained attention, it is not known whether children who appear to be daydreaming are actively engaged in processing off-task information (in which case, daydreaming may be associated with divergent rather than convergent thinking, with potential benefits in creativity and problem solving) or with episodic lapses in awareness (e.g., microsleep).

HYPOACTIVITY

Research in the 1970s from Roscoe Dykman's laboratory demonstrated that individual differences in activity level extended from hyperactivity to normoactivity to hypoactivity. Dykman et al. (1970) (24), divided children with learning disabilities (ages 8–11) on the basis of parent and teacher reports into hyperactive, normoactive, and hypoactive groups and tested them along with controls on a variety of conditioning and reaction time tasks. Although all clinical groups tended to perform worse than controls, the hypoactive group consistently displayed longer response latencies across experimental paradigms. Participant matching using chronological and mental ages did not eliminate these disparities. Follow-up data when the children were in their midteens suggests that hypoactivity is a stable characteristic. Behavioral ratings at follow-up found the percentage of participants who were "extremely slow moving" was 0% for the hyperactive and control groups, 20% for the normoactive group, and 65% for the hypoactive group. Some findings suggested that deviation from normal activity levels in either direction is pathognomonic. Neurological abnormalities and soft signs were observed in all three clinical groups at baseline but only in the hyperactive and hypoactive groups at follow-up. Social adjustment at follow-up differed little between normoactives and controls. Hyperactives had more conflicts with family and authorities, whereas hypoactives had more difficulties with self-esteem, social withdrawal, and internalizing symptoms.

PRIMARY DISORDER OF VIGILANCE

Weinberg and Brumback (9) reported six cases that exhibited what they called a primary disorder of vigilance (PVD), and they offered diagnostic criteria for classifying cases with PVD. These criteria included difficulty sustaining alertness and arousal, daydreaming, difficulty focusing attention, losing one's place in activities and conversation, slow/delayed/incomplete tasks, susceptibility to boredom, fidgeting and other behaviors to improve alertness, and a "caring, compassionate, affectionate, kind temperament" (9, p. 721). The most detailed case report is what we consider to be the prototypical representation of SCT: teacher reports were "slow moving, a dawdler, a procrastinator, not competitive, immature, a daydreamer with poor attention, easily distracted, lazy and wanting to avoid work, kind, affectionate, compassionate, sensitive, a very good child who was never a behavior problem" (p. 721). The authors acknowledged an overlap of PVD and ADHD but argued in favor of considering PVD to be distinct in its unique cognitive impairments. Of considerable interest are their observations that (1) half of the reported cases were accompanied by clinical depression; (2) PVD impairment increases over the course of the life span; and (3) methylphenidate resulted in "excellent response" in all six cases. Among the diagnostic criteria for PVD was a requirement that the PVD symptom complex precede the onset of other disorders (including depression, narcolepsy, medication use, alcohol/drug abuse, hypothyroidism), which can cause secondary hypovigilance.

SCT IN DSM-III

DSM has always structured ADHD categories such that there were no cognitive symptoms that were unique to an inattentive type of attention disorder. Thus, DSM-III distinguished types solely on the basis of whether hyperactivity was present. Studies using DSM-III categories reported that the cognitive deficits in ADD-WO sometimes differed from those in ADD with hyperactivity (ADD-H). The chief difference was that some children with ADD-WO exhibited slow retrieval and information processing, low levels of alertness, and mild problems with memory/orientation (4–6). Clinically, there were reports of peers' calling these children "space cadets," a pejorative term that reflects their being briefly but frequently nonresponsive ("spacing out") during periods of daydreaming or wandering attention. In a review of studies of DSM-III defined cases (i.e., ADHD with and without hyperactivity), Barkley et al. (10) reported that both types share deficits on tests of frontal lobe functions, but that additional problems in perceptual-motor speed and processing may be specific to the ADD-WO group. In their review, Goodyear and Hynd (11) suggest that several neurocognitive deficits, including dysfunction of automatized information processing and slow cognitive speed, may be specific to ADD-WO.

Interestingly, the pattern of comorbidities seen with hyperactive and hypoactive learning disabled (LD) children (see above) was also observed in DSM-III. ADD-H was associated with oppositional and conduct problems, and ADD-WO was associated with social withdrawal and internalizing symptoms (12,13).

SCT IN DSM-IV

DSM-III-R did not distinguish types at all, thus curtailing research into that aspect of ADHD. When DSM-IV was being developed, two SCT items ("often daydreams" and "is often sluggish or drowsy") were included in the Field Trials for Attention and Disruptive Behavior Disorders. As symptoms, SCT items were found to have excellent positive predictive power (PPP) for the Inattention group of symptoms, meaning that their presence was highly associated with the presence of the remaining symptoms of Inattention. However, they demonstrated poor negative predictive power (NPP), meaning that when an SCT symptom was not endorsed, it did not provide much information about whether inattention symptoms were generally absent. This lowered the overall utility of the SCT items as symptoms of Inattention. In other analyses, the SCT items were found to be mainly associated with ADHD-I and not with the other types. The DSM-IV child work group chose not to include the tested items ("often daydreams" and "is often sluggish or drowsy") as DSM-IV Inattention symptoms, largely because of the group's intention to adhere to a set of cognitive symptoms that were common to both ADHD-I and ADHD-C (B.B. Lahey, personal communication).

Nevertheless, evidence has accrued suggesting that the two major DSM-IV types do not share the same neurocognitive dysfunction. At least three studies have found higher rates of SCT symptoms in ADHD-I (14–16). Klorman et al. (17) found executive function deficits only for the ADHD-C group. Houghton et al. (18) found greater deficits in perseveration and response inhibition among the ADHD-C group. Bauermeister et al. (14) found deficits for ADHD-I on a factor measuring vigilance and persistence of effort. Studies by Weiler et al. (19) and Lockwood et al. (20) report slow information processing speed, possibly reflective of low arousal, in children with ADHD-I.

EXTERNAL VALIDITY

The presence of SCT appears to indicate difficulties beyond those that can be accounted for by ADHD. Carlson et al. (21) found that among children with ADHD-I, those with more severe SCT symptoms exhibited more unhappiness, anxiety/depression, withdrawn behavior, and social dysfunction. Mikami et al. (22) conducted an analog Internet chat room experiment with children with ADHD and normal controls. Even after controlling for DSM-IV diagnostic group, computer skill, IQ, and reading achievement, SCT symptoms predicted fewer total verbal responses; less perception of subtle social cues; less memory for the conversation, and a smaller proportion of hostile responses.

MEASUREMENT DIFFICULTIES

Progress in studying SCT is hampered by the absence of a good way to measure it. The measures of SCT that have been employed nearly equals the number of studies in this area: McBurnett et al. (16) used three items from the DSM-IV Field Trials symptom pool; Huang-Pollock et al. (25) used two of these but a different third item; Todd et al. (26) used two items similar to those used by McBurnett et al. in 2001; Bauermeister et al. used five items from the Teacher Rating Form and four from the Child Behavior Checklist; and Hartman et al. (15) used five items, including two used by McBurnett et al. (16). The lack of a consistent approach introduces ambiguity when comparing studies, and it is likely to be daunting to new investigators looking to expand this literature. Moreover, the paucity of SCT items hinders the investigation of latent structure (28). A final concern is that the symptoms of SCT are nonspecific and are likely to be secondary to other problems, particularly mood and anxiety problems.

FUTURE DIRECTIONS

Efforts are currently underway to assemble a large pool of items that may indicate an internally consistent latent construct resembling SCT. McBurnett and Pfiffner (27) developed a semistructured interview, the Kiddie-SCT (K-SCT) interview, which uses a format similar to that of the Schedule for Affective Disorders and Schizophrenia for School-Age Children (K-SADS) (23). The instrument uses a stem-contingent format, in which clinicians first decide whether the item is present or absent for a given case. If present, follow-up questions are then asked which assess the duration and variability of the item, and its relationship to any anxiety or mood problems. The clinician then uses this information to decide whether the item is primary (relatively stable and characteristic of the individual) or secondary (highly variable and tending to resolve when emotional disturbance, anxiety, fatigue, etc. are not prominent). The hope is that primary symptom candidates can be reliably identified, and that latent structural analyses can be used to demarcate the relationship of SCT items to those of Inattention in ADHD.

REFERENCES

1. Lahey BB, Stempniak M, Robinson E, Tyroler MJ. Hyperactivity and learning disabilities as independent dimensions of child behavior problems. J Abnorm Psychol 1978; 87:330–40.
2. Quay HC, Peterson DR. Manual for the Revised Behavior Problem Checklist. Coral Gables, FL: Authors, 1987.
3. Achenbach TM. Manual for the Child Behavior Checklist/4-18 and 1991 Profile. Burlington, VT: Department of Psychiatry, University of Vermont, 1991.

4. Barkley RA, DuPaul GJ, McMurray MB. Comprehensive evaluation of Attention Deficit Disorder with and without Hyperactivity as defined by research criteria. J Consult Clin Psychol 1990; 58:775–89.
5. Lahey BB, Schaughency EA, Frame CL, Strauss CC. Teacher ratings of attention problems in children experimentally classified as exhibiting Attention Deficit Disorder with and without Hyperactivity. J Am Acad Child Psychiatry 1985; 24:613–6.
6. Lahey BB, Schaughency EA, Hynd GW, Carlson CL, Piacentini JC. Attention Deficit Disorder with and without Hyperactivity: comparison of behavioral characteristics of clinic-referred children. J Am Acad Child Adolesc Psychiatry 26:718–23.
7. Antrobus JS, Coleman R, Singer JL. Signal-detection performance by subjects differing in predisposition to daydreaming. J Consult Psychol 1967; 31:487–91.
8. Singer JL. Daydreaming. New York: Random House, 1967.
9. Weinberg WA, Brumback RA. Primary disorder of vigilance: a novel explanation of inattentiveness, daydreaming, boredom, restlessness, and sleepiness. J Pediatr 1990; 116:720–5.
10. Barkley RA, Grodzinsky G, DuPaul GJ. Frontal lobe functions in attention deficit disorder with and without hyperactivity: a review and research report. J Abnorm Child Psychol 1992; 20:163–88.
11. Goodyear P, Hynd GW. Attention-deficit Disorder with (ADD/H) and without (ADD/WO) Hyperactivity: behavioral and neuropsychological differentiation. J Clin Child Psychol 1992; 21:273–305.
12. Lahey BB, Carlson CL, Frick PJ. Attention-deficit disorder without hyperactivity. In: Widiger TA, Frances AJ, Pincus HA, Ross R, First MB, Davis W, eds. DSM-IV Sourcebook, Vol 3. Washington, D.C.: American Psychiatric Press, 1997:163–88.
13. McBurnett K. Attention-Deficit/Hyperactivity Disorder: review of diagnostic issues. In: Widiger TA, Frances AJ, Pincus HA, Ross R, First M, Davis W, eds. DSM-IV Sourcebook, Vol 3. Washington, D.C.: American Psychiatric Association, 1997:111–44.
14. Bauermeister JJ, Matos M, Reina G, et al. Comparison of the DSM-IV combined and inattentive types of ADHD in a school-based sample of Latino/Hispanic children. J Child Psychol Psychiatry 2005; 46:166–79.
15. Hartman CA, Willcutt EG, Rhee SH, Pennington BF. The relation between sluggish cognitive tempo and DSM-IV ADHD. PubMed 2004; 32:491–503.
16. McBurnett K, Pfiffner LJ, Frick PJ. Symptom properties as a function of ADHD type: an argument for continued study of sluggish cognitive tempo. J Abnorm Child Psychol 2001; 29:207–13.
17. Klorman R, Hazel-Fernandez LA, Shaywitz SE, et al. Executive functioning deficits in attention-deficit/hyperactivity disorder are independent of oppositional defiant or reading disorder. J Am Acad Child Adolesc Psychiatry 1999; 38:1148–55.
18. Houghton S, Douglas G, West J, et al. Differential patterns of executive function in children with attention-deficit hyperactivity disorder according to gender and subtype. J Child Neurol 1999; 14:801–5.

19. Weiler MD, Bernstein JH, Bellinger DC, Waber DP. Processing speed in children with attention deficit/hyperactivity disorder, inattentive type. Neuropsychol Dev Cogn Sect C Child Neuropsychol 2000; 6:218–34.
20. Lockwood KA, Marcotte AC, Stern C. Differentiation of attention-deficit/hyperactivity disorder subtypes: application of a neuropsychological model of attention. J Clin Exp Neuropsychol 2001; 23:317–30.
21. Carlson CL, Booth JE, Shin M, Canu WH. Parent-, teacher-, and self-rated motivational styles in ADHD subtypes. J Learn Disabil 2002; 35:104–13.
22. Mikami AY, Huang-Pollock C, Pfiffner L, McBurnett K, Hangai D. Social skills differences among Attention-Deficit/Hyperactivity Disorder types in a chat room assessment task. J Abnorm Child Psychol 2007; 35:509–21.
23. Kaufman J, Birmaher B, Brent D, et al. Schedule for affective disorders and schizophrenia for school-age children-present and lifetime version (K-SADS-PL): initial reliability and validity data. J Am Acad Child Adolesc Psychiatry 1997; 36:980–8.
24. Dykman RA, Walls RC, Suzuki T, Ackerman PT, Peters JE. Children with learning disabilities: conditioning, differentiation, and the effect of distraction. Am J Orthopsychiatry 1970; 40:766–82.
25. Huang-Pollock CL, Mikami AY, Piffiner L, McBurnett K. ADHD subtype differences in motivational responsivity but not Inhibitory control: evidence from a reward-based variation of the stop signal paradigm. J Clin Child Adolesc Psychol 2007; 36:127–36.
26. Todd RD, Rasmussen ER, Wood C, Levy F, Hay DA. Should sluggish cognitive tempo symptoms be included in the diagnosis of attention-deficit/hyperactivity disorder? J Am Acad Child Adolesc Psychiatry 2004; 43:588–97.
27. McBurnett K, Pfiffner L. Sluggish cognitive tempo module to supplement K-SADS interviews. University of California, San Francisco 2006.
28. Devellis RF. Scale Development: Theory and Applications. 2nd Edition. New York: Sage, 2003.

33

ADHD Pharmacogenomics: Past, Present, and Future

James J. McGough
Division of Child and Adolescent Psychiatry, UCLA Semel Institute for Neuroscience and Human Behavior and UCLA Child and Adolescent Psychopharmacology Program and ADHD Clinic, Los Angeles, California, U.S.A.

Mark A. Stein
Department of Psychiatry, and HALP Clinic and ADHD Research Center, University of Illinois at Chicago, Chicago, Illinois, U.S.A.

INTRODUCTION

Clinicians who choose to prescribe a particular medication based on a family history of positive results are practicing a simple form of pharmacogenetics. Pharmacogenetics is the study of genetic variability in medication response (1). Pharmacogenetics had its formal beginnings in the 1950s when clinicians noted increased patterns of adverse reactions within certain families or ethnic groups. One example pertinent to psychiatry was the discovery that some patients receiving electroconvulsive therapy developed prolonged muscular paralysis after administration of succinylcholine due to a mutation within the gene coding for the enzyme succinylcholine esterase (2). Other early pharmacogenetic findings included attribution of peripheral neuropathy to slow acetylation of isoniazid in patients with tuberculosis, and hemolysis to glucose-6-phosphate deficiency in African-American males treated for malaria (1). The molecular genetic causes for these inherited differences were subsequently elucidated in the 1980s (3).

In contrast to pharmacogenetics, pharmacogenomics refers more specifically to the study of variations in genes and gene products and their relationship to medication response (4). Studies in pharmacogenomics have become much more practical with technological advances in gene sequencing and complete mapping of the human genome. Obvious foci of pharmacogenomic investigations include drug metabolic pathways and drug targets, such as transporters and receptors (5). Although there remain many challenges, several established pharmacogenetic findings are likely to significantly impact mental health treatment.

At present, the most widely appreciated pharmacogenetic finding is that polymorphisms at the gene for hepatic cytochrome P450 2D6 (CYP2D6) isozymes lead to slow metabolism of many psychotropic medications in 5% to 10% of Caucasians and 0% to 19% of African-Americans (6) (see later discussion of atomoxetine). Polymorphisms are defined as variations in a single allele that occur in more than 1% of the population (7). Other recent association studies have demonstrated relationships between polymorphisms in the serotonin transporter (SERT) and response to antidepressant therapy (8), as well as associations between polymorphisms at several dopamine and serotonin receptors and increased likelihood for positive response or risk of side effects in clozapine treatment of schizophrenia (9).

Linkage studies, utilizing haplotype mapping, are also being conducted in attention-deficit/hyperactivity disorder (ADHD), and have potential relevance to pharmacogenomic study (10). A haplotype is a combination of alleles that are found together on the same chromosome. With increased identification of single-nucleotide polymorphisms (SNPs), tagging of common haplotypes can economically identify regions of interest which more fully represent common genetic variation in association with drug response (51). Consequently, pharmacogenomic studies might examine relationships between drug response and candidate polymorphisms and haplotypes.

ADHD has an estimated heritability in the range of 80% and is theorized to arise from the interaction of multiple genes and environmental factors (11). Molecular genetic findings for ADHD are among the most highly replicated of any psychiatric disorder (12). However, the majority of studies have utilized broad phenotype definitions of ADHD (52). Therefore, given the heterogeneity of ADHD samples as currently defined by DSM criteria, it is not surprising that only a small percentage of the variance in ADHD is accounted for by specific genes (13). Candidate gene investigations in ADHD have largely been guided by the recognition that stimulant medications have their putative targets of activity on catecholaminergic and serotonergic pathways (12,14). Candidate genes associated with increased risk for ADHD include the dopamine transporter (DAT1), the dopamine receptors (DRD2, DRD4, and DRD5), the serotonin receptor (5HT1B), dopa-β-hydroxylase (DBH), synaptosomal-associated protein (SNAP-25), catechol-*O*-methyltransferase (COMT), and others.

While knowledge about the presumed mechanisms of activity of ADHD medications initially informed searches for polymorphisms related to increased risk for the disorder, it is also reasonable to assume that these same polymorphisms might predict medication outcomes. Although stimulant medications have a large effect on ADHD symptoms in short- and intermediate-term studies (e.g. the MTA study done in 1999), long-term prognosis has not been demonstrated to change significantly. Moreover, the high prevalence of ADHD, its significant heritability, variability in drug response, and the need to individually titrate doses, creates a compelling case for pharmacogenomic investigations of treatment response. In addition, the cost of failed treatment trials is significant as many families choose not to pursue pharmacotherapy for ADHD if the child does not respond to the first medication trial or displays significant side effects. The promise of ADHD pharmacogenomics is far reaching, and includes the potential to develop individualized medication regimens that improve symptom response, decrease risk of side effects, improve long-term tolerability, and thus contribute to long-term treatment compliance and improved effectiveness and general functioning. Pharmacogenomic studies of ADHD may also add to our understanding of the pathophysiology of the disorder, as the moderating effects of polymorphisms are increasingly utilized in psychopathology research.

PRELIMINARY STUDIES

Several preliminary reports indeed suggest that candidate genes related to catecholamines, such as dopamine or norepinephrine, predict response to ADHD medications. However, the nature, direction, and magnitude of these associations remain unclear. These early pharmacogenomic studies have utilized modest samples sizes and, not surprisingly, have yielded inconsistent results. The majority are limited to investigations of methylphenidate response, include retrospective reports and both open-label and placebo-controlled clinical trials, and emphasize ADHD symptom reduction as the primary outcome measure. Nonetheless, these early trials attest to the feasibility of pharmacogenomic studies of ADHD and provide a foundation for future research investigation.

Dopamine Transporter (DAT1)

DAT1 is located on chromosome 5. The gene contains a variable number tandem repeat (VNTR) of a 48-bp sequence within its 3′-untranslated region. Common allelic polymorphisms result from different VNTRs. Cook et al. (15) first described an association between the 10-repeat (480 bp) DAT1 polymorphism and ADHD. This association has been replicated in some (16,17), but not all studies (18) and explains a small percentage of the variance in ADHD symptoms (12).

Several reasons underlie interest in DAT1 as a candidate gene for ADHD treatment response. First, as noted previously, numerous studies suggest an association between variants at DAT1 and increased risk for categorically defined ADHD. More recently, Cornish et al. (19) reported an association between dimensional measures of ADHD symptoms, response inhibition, and the 10/10 DAT1 genotype in a sample of non-referred children. Second, methylphenidate, and to some extent amphetamine, specifically targets and blocks the dopamine transporter (20,21). This results in an increase in extracellular dopamine in dopamine-rich brain regions, which project to the striatum, nucleus accumbens, prefrontal cortex, and hypothalamus. These brain regions are frequently implicated in the pathophysiology of ADHD (22). Third, several neuroimaging studies reveal increased dopamine transporter densities in striatal regions of adults with ADHD, giving rise to the hypothesis that blockade of the transporter in ADHD patients might correct underlying brain pathophysiology (23). Moreover, Durston et al. (24) recently demonstrated that DAT1 influences caudate volume.

In the first pharmacogenomic investigation of ADHD, Winsberg and Comings (25) reported that 86% of "poor" responders to methylphenidate (defined as less than a 50% reduction in ADHD symptoms on parent ratings) were homozygous for the 10-repeat allele (10/10) in a sample of 30 African-American children with ADHD. Roman et al. (26) and Cheon et al. (27) utilizing similar methodology described similar findings in Brazilian and Chinese samples respectively. In these studies, approximately 30–50% of the homozygous youth (10/10) responded positively to methylphenidate (MPH) as compared to a response rate of 70–100% in the predominantly 10/9 genotype groups.

It should be noted that the 10/10 and 10/9 genotypes are the two most common genotypes of DAT1. The Winsberg and Colleagues studies prematurely assumed that the 9-repeat allele was dominant. Two other studies that did not make this assumption found improved response to methylphenidate in patients heterozygous or homozygous for the 10-repeat allele. Based on retrospective recall of medication outcomes, Kirley and colleagues (13) reported that "very good" responders were more likely to have at least one copy of the 10-repeat allele, and that a linear relationship existed between number of 10-repeat alleles and degree of positive response. Similarly, Stein and colleagues (28) found that the presence of one or two 10-repeat alleles was associated with increased response rates in patients receiving 36 or 54 mg doses of OROS-methylphenidate as compared to those without a copy of the 10-repeat allele, who did not display a linear dose–response curve. Those individuals with the less common, 9/9 genotype of DAT1 not only displayed a different dose–response curve, they displayed more stimulant side effects and the majority remained impaired during MPH treatment. In contrast, methylphenidate treatment was associated with mild to minimal impairment in 80% of those with either the 10/9 or 10/10 genotype (Fig. 1).

The Stein et al. study (28) was the first pharmacogenomic study of ADHD to analyze the 9/9 group separately. Subsequent reanalysis of the Kirley study (13) also found a poor stimulant response rate (25%) for those

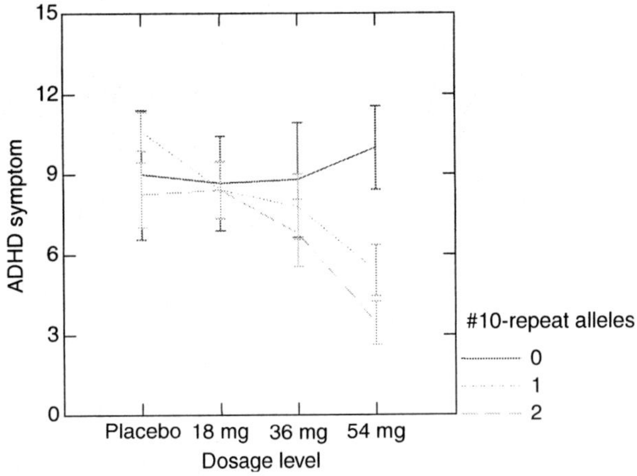

Figure 1 Total ADHD parent rating scale IV scores (with standard errors) by dosage level and by genotype. *Source*: From Ref. 28.

with the 9/9 genotype as compared to a robust positive response rate (65%) for those with one or two 10-repeat alleles.

Interestingly, a similar effect of the 9/9 genotype on amphetamine response was reported by Lott and colleagues (29). In this study, healthy college students homozygous for the 9-repeat allele were less sensitive to amphetamine effects in terms of subjective ratings and diastolic blood pressure. For example, individuals with the 9/9 genotype were less sensitive to the subjective effects of amphetamine as suggested by ratings of feels drug (Fig. 2).

Thus, three studies indicate that when the 9/9 is examined separately or not combined with the 9/10 genotype, there appears to be a clear difference in stimulant response. Although the statistical significance of the effect of the 9/9 genotype on methylphenidate response is robust, replication is necessary for the results to be more conclusive and to determine any clinical significance of this finding.

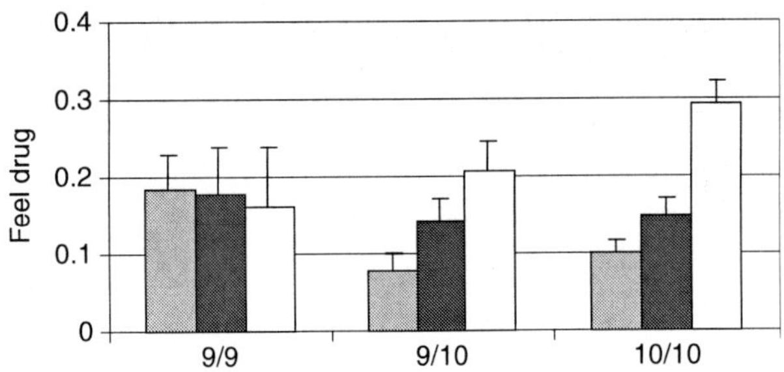

Figure 2 Visual analog scale of ratings of feels drug. *Source*: From Ref. 29.

Several studies are ongoing with the goal of determining clinical predictors of nonresponse, specific adverse events associated with DAT1 genotypes and other candidate genes, and neuropsychological or neurophysiological endophenotypes (30,31). In a National Institute of Mental Health (NIMH) sponsored study, Dr Jeffrey Newcorn, Dr Mark Stein and colleagues are testing whether those with the 9/9 genotype respond to nonstimulant treatment (e.g., atomoxetine). Additionally, Dr Chandan Vaidya and colleagues at Georgetown University are examining the relationship between DAT1 genotypes and striatal activity utilizing functional magnetic resonance imaging (fMRI).

Dopamine Receptors (DRD2, DRD4, DRD5)

DRD2, DRD4, and DRD5 are presumed targets of postsynaptic catecholaminergic activity. DRD2 is located on chromosome 11 and is involved in central reward-mediating mesocorticolimbic pathways. DRD2 has been implicated in risk for alcoholism and nicotine addiction. DRD4 is also located on chromosome 11. The 7-repeat (48 bp) VNTR polymorphism found in the coding region of DRD4 exhibits odd ratios for increased ADHD risk ranging from 1.4 to 1.9 in numerous studies (32). DRD5 is located on chromosome 4. The 148-bp allele of DRD5 has a pooled odds ratio of 1.24 for ADHD risk in meta-analysis, although the association is mostly confined to the inattentive and combined subtypes (12).

In vitro studies of the DRD4 7-repeat suggest that this allelic variant is functionally less responsive to dopamine effects (33,34). Consistent with this, one study demonstrated that patients with at least a single copy of the 7-repeat required higher doses of methylphenidate for optimal symptom reduction (35). In contrast, Winsberg and Comings (25) failed to demonstrate any relationship between DRD4, DRD2, and treatment outcomes.

Salee et al. (36) reported that ADHD children with at least one DRD4 4-repeat allele showed a trend toward improved response to the nonstimulant atomoxetine, in contrast to methylphenidate response, which was unaffected by DRD4 genotype. Furthermore, improvement on the ADHD-Rating Scale hyperactivity subscale was maximized by the absence of the 7-repeat allele. The results of this study suggest an interaction between atomoxetine and DRD4 genotype, supporting a role of the dopamine D4 receptor in ADHD, and also suggest possible relevance of pharmacogenomic factors associated with atomoxetine treatment.

Norepinephrine Transporter (NET) Protein 1

NET is located on chromosome 16 and has been implicated in susceptibility for orthostatic hypotension. NET is a likely candidate for studies of medication outcome as the NET is also targeted and blocked by methylphenidate. NET blockade is also the presumed mechanism of activity for atomoxetine (37).

Bobb et al. (38) reported an association between NET and ADHD. In addition, one study in Han Chinese evaluated the relationship between the G1278A polymorphism at NET and medication response (39). These investigators found that individuals homozygous for the less common A/A genotype had decreased symptom reductions compared with the G/A or AA groups. The authors noted that, since the G1278A allele has no known functional activity, the allele might be in linkage disequilibrium with another allele responsible for outcome differences.

Cytochrome P450 2D6 (CYP2D6)

Atomoxetine metabolism is regulated by the CYP2D6 enzyme system. In one of the first examples of pharmacogenomics applied during ADHD drug development, the effects of CYP2D6 polymorphisms were evaluated for atomoxetine. Whereas most individuals are extensive metabolizers (EMs), approximately 7% of the U.S. population are poor metabolizers (PMs) (40). Atomoxetine has a plasma half-life of approximately 5 hr in EMs. In PMs, atomoxetine has a longer plasma half-life of approximately 22 hr (Eli Lilly, personal communication, July 2005). In a review of several studies, PMs displayed greater symptom improvement than EMs and were more likely to continue treatment (41). Not surprisingly, decreased appetite and insomnia were reported more frequently in PMs taking any dose of atomoxetine. PMs also displayed a greater increase in pulse and diastolic blood pressure compared with EMs, while EMs gained more weight than PMs. Thus, both efficacy and adverse events to atomoxetine appear to be moderated by the CYP2D6 enzyme system.

GENOME-WIDE INVESTIGATIONS

An alternative to candidate gene studies is the whole genome or genome-wide scan approach. Several genome-wide scans have importance for ADHD risk (12). A genome-wide scan makes no a priori assumptions regarding the potential functional significance of particular genes, but examines the entire genome to identify possible regions of functional importance. A similar approach has been proposed to identify regions in the genome with implications for ADHD treatment outcomes. In one study, investigators used quantitative trait analysis to test for linkage with methylphenidate response in a genome-wide scan (42). The authors found regions of moderate significance on chromosome 7, with additional regions on chromosomes 3, 5, and 9. With the development of high-density SNP genotyping arrays, whole-genome association studies are now technically (if not financially) feasible for study of pharmacogenetic response (or study of etiology).

CLINICAL RELEVANCE

Although stimulant medications are regarded as effective first-line ADHD therapies, the majority of treatment studies are short-duration trials with long-term efficacy being much more modest (43). In a 5-year prospective study, 50% of children did not continue methylphenidate into the second year, and many who remained in treatment reported clinically meaningful side effects (44). Moreover, in two open-label studies of both methylphenidate and amphetamine, fewer than 60% of previously stabilized patients remained on medication after 12 months of treatment (45,46). At 14 months follow-up in the ADHD Multimodal Treatment Study (MTA), only 56% of patients assigned to intensive medication management continued to meet criteria as excellent responders (47). In one community study, 49% of children who were receiving stimulant medications met full symptomatic criteria for ADHD (48). In most longitudinal studies of ADHD, although ADHD symptoms tend to decline with age, impairment tends to persist or worsen. Thus, impairment as well as ADHD symptoms should be studied as outcome measures in pharmacogenomic investigations (28).

ADHD pharmacogenomics might ultimately lead to individualized medication prescriptions based on a patient's own genomic information. More individually tailored ADHD treatments could conceivably lead to improved tolerability, enhanced symptom reduction, and associated improvements in patient compliance. Alternatively, pharmacogenomics might identify patients at increased risk for certain side effects, allowing physicians to minimize exposing individuals at risk of adverse events. Pharmacogenomics might also play a role in the development of new ADHD medications.

FUTURE DIRECTIONS

There is growing international interest in ADHD pharmacogenomics. Future studies will consider an expanded range of treatment outcomes, including variability in tolerability and side effects, symptom change, pharmacokinetics, and metabolic pathways (49). These studies are likely to consider individual variation in responses to multiple medications, such as amphetamine, atomoxetine, guanfacine, buproprion, and other compounds deemed selectively useful in treating ADHD and related disorders, symptoms, or dimensions. Research is apt to consider a broader set of candidate genes, with samples large enough to examine gene–gene and gene–environment interactions.

Larger controlled clinical trials will require multisite collaborative networks of clinicians and researchers working with the support of government agencies and the pharmaceutical industry. In this regard, there is much to be learned from other illnesses, such as cancer, in developing infrastructures to promote pharmacogenomic studies of ADHD. Such collaborations will increase the speed of findings, reduce research costs considerably, and also increase the rate at which findings are translated into clinical practice. Consideration of pharmacogenetics early in drug development might promote identification of new drug targets as well as subsets of patients likely to respond to a specific treatment. Conversely, subjects with increased risk of side effects could be excluded from clinical trials, allowing others to benefit from medications that might have otherwise been rejected during early development.

The goal of ADHD pharmacogenomics is to be able to individualize medication based on a patient's own genomic information. More individually tailored ADHD treatments could conceivably lead to improved tolerability, enhanced symptom reduction, and associated improvements in patient compliance. Alternatively, pharmacogenomics might identify patients at increased risk for certain side effects, allowing physicians to minimize exposing individuals at risk of adverse events. Advances in pharmacogenetics may also lead to increased understanding of ADHD pathophysiology, which may also have implications for diagnosis and treatment. Finally, pharmacogenomic studies might also play a role in the development of new ADHD medications with more specific drug targets.

SUMMARY

Pharmacogenomic studies of ADHD are in a relatively early stage, but hold considerable promise for improving treatment of this disorder. Several studies suggest differences in stimulant response between individuals with DAT1 genotypes. Children with the much less common 9/9 genotype do not benefit from usual clinical methylphenidate doses and might be less sensitive to stimulant effects. Larger samples are needed to clarify inconsistent findings and to determine the magnitude of pharmacogenetic effects in different samples. There are also promising leads with other candidate polymorphisms, such as NET and the CY2D6 enzyme system and atomoxetine.

Pharmacogenetic and pharmacogenomic studies have progressed from small samples looking at single genes and ADHD symptom reductions, to larger studies looking at a broader phenotype of clinically relevant stimulant response and various neurophysiological and neuropsychological endophenotypes (30). As noted by Cook (50), replication of positive findings with adequately powered samples and determination of the positive and negative predictive value are the next steps.

Being able to predict which individuals are likely to respond positively or which individuals do not tolerate a particular medication or class of medications would alter the trial and error approach to stimulant treatment of ADHD. Ultimately, it is hoped that further understanding of the genetic variability in ADHD treatment response may shed light on both genetic and nongenetic factors which contribute to the outcome.

ACKNOWLEDGMENTS

This study was supported by NIMH grants K23MH01966 to Dr McGough and K24MHO1823 and R01 MH70564-01A to Dr Stein. The authors wish to thank Edwin Cook Jr., MD for his comments on an earlier version of this manuscript.

REFERENCES

1. Weber WW. Pharmacogenetics. New York: Oxford Press, 1997.
2. Kalow W. Pharmacogenetics: Heredity and the Response to Drugs. Philadelphia: W.B. Saunders, 1962.
3. Evans WE, Relling MV. Pharmacogenomics: translating functional genomics into rational therapeutics. Science 1999; 286:487–91.
4. Meyer UA. Pharmacogenetics and adverse drug reactions. Lancet 2000; 356: 1667–71.
5. Masellis M, Basile V, Muglia P, Ozdemir V, Macciardi FM, Kennedy JL. Psychiatric pharmacogenetics: personalizing psychostimulant therapy in attention-deficit/hyperactivity disorder. Behav Brain Res 2002; 130:85–90.
6. Xie H-G, Kim RB, Wood AJ, Stein CM. Molecular basis of ethnic differences in drug disposition and response. Annu Rev Pharmacol Toxicol 2001; 41: 815–50.
7. Meyer UA. Genotype or phenotype: the definition of a pharmacogenetic polymorphism. Pharmacogenetics 1991; 1:66–7.
8. Murphy DL, Lerner A, Rudnick G, Lesch KP. Serotonin transporter: gene, genetic disorders, and pharmacogenetics. Mol Interv 2004; 4:109–23.
9. Wilffert B, Zaal R, Brouwers JR. Pharmacogenetics as a tool in the therapy of schizophrenia. Pharm World Sci 2005; 27:20–30.
10. Sklar P. Principles of haplotype mapping and potential applications to attention-deficit hyperactivity disorder. Biol Psychiatry 2005; 57:1357–66.
11. Faraone SV, Doyle AE. The nature and heritability of attention-deficit/hyperactivity disorder. Child Adolesc Psychiatr Clin N Am 2001; 10:299–316.
12. Faraone SV, Perlis R, Doyle AE, et al. Molecular genetics of attention-deficit/hyperactivity disorder. Biol Psychiatry 2005; 57:1313–23.
13. Kirley A, Lowe N, Hawi A, et al. Association of the 480 bp DAT1 allele with methylphenidate response in a sample of Irish children with ADHD. Am J Med Genetics 2003; 121B:50–4.
14. Ogdie MN, Macphie IL, Minassian SL, et al. A genome-wide scan for attention-deficit/hyperactivity disorder: suggestive linkage on 17p11. Am J Hum Genet 2003; 72:1268–79.
15. Cook EH, Stein MA, Krasowski MD, Cox NJ, Oikon DM, Kieffer JE. Association of attention-deficit disorder and the dopamine transporter gene. Am J Hum Genet 1995; 56:993–8.

16. Gill M, Daly G, Heron S, Haw Z, Fitzgerald M. Confirmation of association between attention deficit hyperactivity disorder and a dopamine transporter polymorphism. Mol Psychiatry 1997; 2:311–3.
17. Waldman ID, Rowe DC, Abramowitz A, Kozel ST, Mohr JH, Sherman SL. Association and linkage of the dopamine transporter gene and attention deficit hyperactivity disorder in children. Am J Hum Genetics 1998; 63:1767–76.
18. Todd RD, Jong YJ, Lobos EA, Reich W, Heath AC, Neuman RJ. No association of the dopamine transporter gene 3′ VNTR polymorphism with ADHD subtypes in a population sample of twins. Am J Med Genetics 2001; 105:745–8.
19. Cornish KM, Manly T, Savage R, et al. Association of the dopamine transporter (DAT1) 10/10-repeat genotype with ADHD symptoms and response inhibition in a general population sample. Mol Psychiatry 2005; 10: 686–98.
20. Melega WP, Williams AC, Schmitz DA, DiStefano EW, Cho AK. Pharmacokinetic and pharmacodynamic analysis of the actions of D-amphetamine and D-methamphetamine on the dopamine terminal. J Pharmacol Exp Ther 1995; 274:90–6.
21. Volkow ND, Wang G, Fowler JS, et al. Evidence that methylphenidate enhances the saliency of a mathematical task by increasing dopamine in the human brain. Am J Psychiatry 2004; 161:1173–80.
22. Swanson J, Castellanos FX, Murias M, LaHoste G, Kennedy J. Cognitive neuroscience of attention deficit hyperactivity disorder and hyperkinetic disorder. Curr Opin Neurobiol 1998; 8:263–71.
23. Spencer TJ, Biederman J, Madras BK, et al. In vivo neuroreceptor imaging in attention-deficit/hyperactivity disorder: a focus on the dopamine transporter. Biol Psychiatry 2005; 57:1293–300.
24. Durston S, Fossella JA, Casey BJ, et al. Differential effects of Drd4 and DAT1 genotype on fronto-striatal gray matter volumes in a sample of subjects with attention deficit hyperactivity disorder, their unaffected siblings, and controls. Mol Psychiatry 2005; 10:678–85.
25. Winsberg BG, Comings DE. Association of the dopamine transporter gene (DAT1) with poor methylphenidate response. J Am Acad Child Adolesc Psychiatry 1999; 38:1474–7.
26. Roman T, Szobot C, Martine S, Biederman J, Rohde LA, Hutz MH. Dopamine transporter gene and response to methylphenidate in attention-deficit/hyperactivity disorder. Pharmacogenetics 2002; 12:497–9.
27. Cheon KA, Ryu YH, Kim JW, Cho DY. The homozygosity for 10-repeat allele at dopamine transporter gene and dopamine transporter density in Korean children with attention deficit hyperactivity disorder: relating to treatment response to methylphenidate. Eur Neuropsychopharmacol 2005; 15:95–101.
28. Stein MA, Waldman ID, Sarampote CS, et al. Dopamine transporter genotype and methylphenidate dose response in children with ADHD. Neuropsychopharmacology 2005; 30:1374–82.
29. Lott D, Kim S, Cook EH, deWitt H. Dopamine transporter genotype and amphetamine response. Neuropsychopharmacology 2005; 30:602–9.

30. Loo SK, Specter E, Stolen A, Hopfer A, Teale PD, Reite ML. Functional effects of the DAT1 polymorphism on EEG measures in ADHD. J Am Acad Child Adolesc Psychiatry 2003; 42:986–93.
31. Rohde LA, Roman T, Szobot C, Cunha RD, Hutz MH, Biederman J. Dopamine transporter gene, response to methylphenidate and cerebral blood flow in attention-deficit/hyperactivity disorder. Synapse 2003; 48:87–9.
32. Faraone SV, Doyle AE, Mick E, Biederman J. Meta-analysis of the association between the 7-repeat allele of the dopamine D(4) receptor gene and attention deficit hyperactivity disorder. Am J Psychiatry 2001; 158:1052–7.
33. Asghari V, Sanyal S, Buchwaldt S, Paterson A, Jovanovic V, Van Tol HH. Modulation of intracellular cyclic AMP levels by different human dopamine D4 receptor variants. J Neurochem 1995; 65:1157–65.
34. Van Tol HH, Wu CM, Guan HC, et al. Multiple dopamine D4 receptor variants in the human population. Nature 1992; 358:149–52.
35. Hamarman S, Fossella J, Ulger C, Brimacombe M, Dermody J. Dopamine receptor 4 (DRD4) 7-repeat allele predicts methylphenidate dose response in children with attention deficit hyperactivity disorder. J Child Adolesc Psychopharmacol 2004; 14:564–74.
36. Salee F, Newcorn JA, Allen AJ, Stein MA, McDougle C, Sethuraman S. Pharmacogenetics of atomoxetine: relevance of DRD4. Scientific Proceedings of the 51st Annual Meeting of the American Academy of Child and Adolescent Psychiatry, Washington, D.C., 2004.
37. Michelson D, Faries D, Wernicke J, et al. Atomoxetine in the treatment of children and adolescent with attention-deficit/hyperactivity disorder: a randomized, placebo-controlled, dose-response study. Pediatrics 2001; 108:E83.
38. Bobb AJ, Addington AM, Sidransky E, et al. Support for association between ADHD and two candidate genes: NET1 and DRD1. Am J Med Genet B Neuropsychiatr Genet 2005; 134:67–72.
39. Yang L, Wang Y-F, Li J, Faraone SV. Association of norepinephrine transporter gene (NET) with methylphenidate response. J Am Acad Child Adolesc Psychiatry 2004; 43:1154–8.
40. Sachse C, Brockmoller J, Bauer S, Roots I. Cytochrome P450 2D6 variants in a Caucasian population: allele frequencies and phenotypic consequences. Am J Hum Genet 1997; 60:284–95.
41. Michelson D, Read HA, Ruff D, Witcher J, Zhang S, McCracken JT. CY2D6 and clinical response to atomoxetine in children and adolescents with ADHD. J Am Acad Child Adolesc Psychiatry 2007; 46:242–51.
42. Van der Meulen EM, Bakker SC, Pauls DL, Sinnke RJ, Buitelaar J. A genome-wide quantitative trait locus analysis on methylphenidate response rate in Dutch sibpairs with attention-deficit/hyperactivity disorder. Scientific Proceedings of the 16th World Congress of the International Association for Child and Adolescent Psychiatry and Allied Professions, Berlin, Germany, 2004.
43. Spencer T, Biederman J, Wilens T, Harding M, O'Donnell D, Griffin S. Pharmacotherapy of attention deficit hyperactivity disorder across the lifespan. J Am Acad Child Adolesc Psychiatry 1996; 35:409–28.

44. Charach A, Ickowicz A, Schachar R. Stimulant treatment over five years; adherence, effectiveness, and adverse events. J Am Acad Child Adolesc Psychiatry 2004; 43:559–67.
45. McGough JJ, Biederman J, Wigal S, et al. Long-term tolerability and effectiveness of once-daily mixed amphetamine salts (Adderall XR) in children with ADHD. J Am Acad Child Adolesc Psychiatry 2005; 44:530–8.
46. Wilens T, Pelham W, Stein M, et al. ADHD treatment with once-daily OROS methylphenidate: interim 12-month results from a long-term open-label study. J Am Acad Child Adolesc Psychiatry 2003; 42:424–33.
47. Swanson JM, Kraemer HC, Hinshaw SP, et al. Clinical relevance of the primary findings of the MTA; success rates based on severity of ADHD and ODD symptoms at the end of treatment. J Am Acad Child Adolesc Psychiatry 2001; 40:168–79.
48. Rowland AS, Skipper B, Rabiner D, et al. The effectiveness of ADHD medication treatment in an epidemiologic sample. Scientific Proceedings of the 50th Annual Meeting of the American Academy of Child and Adolescent Psychiatry, Miami, FL, 2003.
49. McGough J. Attention-deficit/hyperactivity disorder pharmacogenomics. Biol Psychiatry 2005; 57:1367–73.
50. Cook EH. The early development of child pharmacogenetics. J Am Acad Child Adolesc Psychiatry 1999; 38:1478–81.
51. Goldstein DB. Pharmacogenetics in the laboratory and the clinic. N Engl J Med 2003; 348:553–6.
52. Tannock R. Attention deficit hyperactivity disorder: advances in cognitive, neurobiological, and genetic research. J Child Psychol Psychiatry 1998; 39: 65–99.
53. Greenhill LL, Halperin JM, Abikoff H. Stimulant medications. J Am Acad Child Adolesc Psychiatry 1999; 38:503–12.

34

Endophenotypes in ADHD: Rational and Progress

Russell Schachar and Jennifer Crosbie
Department of Psychiatry, Hospital for Sick Children, University of Toronto, Toronto, Ontario, Canada

Twin, family, and adoption studies provide compelling evidence that genetic risk factors contribute substantially to attention deficit hyperactivity disorder (ADHD) (1,2). Twin studies show high genetic contribution regardless of whether ADHD is defined as a category, as a continuous trait, or as an extreme of a trait ($h^2 = .64$ to .9) (3,4). Genetic linkage and association studies have proven remarkably productive in ADHD identifying a number of genetic risks for the disorder (3). Progress in ADHD was swift because scientists were forearmed with considerable knowledge about the probable role of neurotransmitter dysfunction based on the dramatic effect of stimulant medication in ameliorating behavioral and cognitive manifestations of ADHD (5,6). There have now been over 30 association reports for candidate genes including the genes for the DA transporter (DAT1), DA receptors D4 and D5, the serotonin receptors 1B and 2A, calcyon, EKN1, G(olf), and the gene for the synaptic vesicle docking fusion protein, synaptosomal-associated protein of 25 kDa (SNAP25) (3,7). Furthermore, there have been four genome wide scans on relatively small, independent samples (8–11), which are suggestive of linkage signals in the distal region of chromosome 5p.

Despite this progress, not all findings have been replicated. For example, of the many studies of DRD4, almost half have failed to replicate association or linkage (12). Moreover, the effect size of observed risks has been small. Meta-analysis of DAT1 and DRD4 linkage and association findings (12,13) indicate that the average increase in risk for ADHD associated with replicated genetic findings is approximately 1.5-fold. Similarly, a recent large joint meta-analysis of DRD5 by Lowe et al. (14) showed an overall odds ratio of 1.2. The lack of consistency in genetic findings is also evident in the largely nonoverlapping areas of linkage identified in genome scans conducted to date.

In response to the problem of nonreplication, there has been a call for application of novel strategies to facilitate gene discovery. The goal of this chapter is to detail the logic for the utility of nonclinical endophenotypes in facilitating genetic research and to propose a priori criteria by which endophenotypes should be evaluated before they are applied in molecular research. As an illustration, we summarize evidence bearing on one putative ADHD endophenotype for which considerable evidence is available—motor response inhibition—in order to illustrate the validation of an endophenotype.

SOURCES OF VARIATION IN GENETIC RESEARCH

There are various explanations for the apparent difficulty in replicating genetic association and linkage in ADHD. The first relates to the apparent complexity of the relationship between causative genes and the behavioral phenotype. ADHD is clearly not a single-gene disorder with Mendelian inheritance. One-to-one correspondence between genes and specific aspects of a disease or a syndrome as a whole is unlikely. Rather, ADHD conforms to a multifactorial polygenic threshold model of heredity. This model holds that a complex trait results from the action of a number of genes each of which exerts a small effect. These genes contribute individually or interact with other genes from the moment of conception or at any time during development and may do so in conjunction with various environmental factors. Together, these factors generate a continuous phenotypic distribution. When these contributions reach a certain threshold on this continuum, pathological manifestations occur (15) (Fig. 1). Any allelic variant or environmental risk factor can therefore be present among individuals located anywhere in the phenotypic distribution, and no single variant is either sufficient or necessary to cause individuals to cross the threshold between affected and nonaffected. If this model is correct, it is easy to see that the current categorical approach to diagnosis wastes much of the information present in the underlying distribution, and will inevitably result in nonreplicable genetic association findings. Another reason for non-replication is genetic heterogeneity: different genes might contribute to ADHD risk in different populations.

Heritability rates for ADHD vary from 50% to 90% (7,16). Therefore, a substantial component of variance is due to environmental risks (including measurement error). These environmental factors could contribute to ADHD independently or through interactions with genetic factors. A range

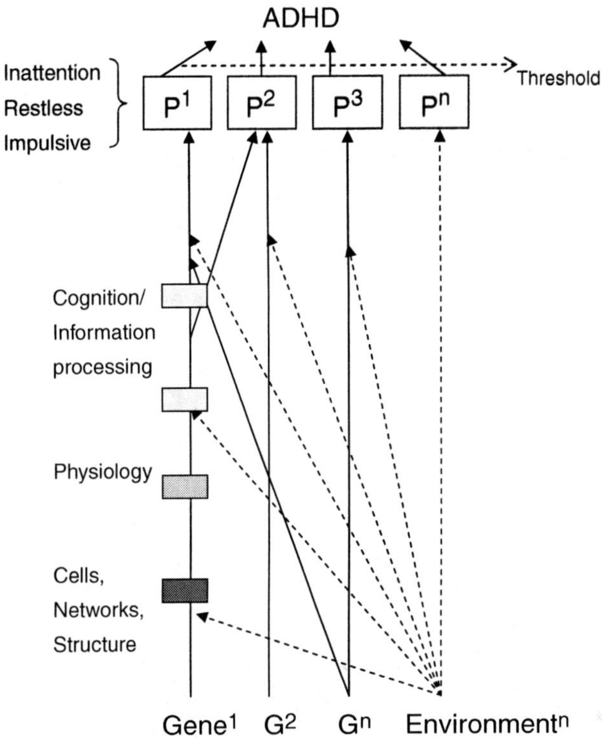

Figure 1 Locating endophenotypes with the multifactorial, polygenetic threshold model of ADHD. *Note*: Figure 1 shows various hypothetical pathways from genes (G^1,..., G^n) and environmental risks (E^1,...,E^n) to the behavioral manifestations of ADHD (Phenotype, P^1,...,P^n). The lowest level shows the effects of various genes and the highest level shows individual behavioral manifestations such as restlessness, inattentiveness, and impulsiveness. For the sake of simplicity, the figure does not include separate genetic or environmental risks for home versus school behavior, although this is a possibility. As one ascends from the level of genes toward the level of the clinical manifestations of the disorder, a greater number of genetic and environmental factors come into play and interact in the genesis of each manifestation of the behavioral outcome of ADHD. In addition, as one ascends from the level of genes to that of overt clinical manifestations, the overall effect of any single genetic or environmental risk factor becomes diluted by the contribution of other factors. A range of neurobiological processes and structures are traversed as one moves from the level of genes toward overt behavior, such as, proteins (*red bars*), cellular networks and structures (*green bars*), neurophysiology (*yellow bars*), and cognition and information processing (*blue bars*). By contrast, as one descends from the behavioral level toward the genetic level the relationship between any specific clinical manifestation and any specific genetic cause is strengthened although less of the variation in overall clinical manifestation might be explained. Putative endophenotypes such as cognitive deficits (*Caption continues on next page*)

of environmental risks are thought to contribute to ADHD including maternal smoking, perinatal insult, head injury (17–20), and psychosocial adversity (poverty, low-income housing, single-parent families, parental psychopathology and early severe deprivation; 21). Environmental factors might even be capable of generating nongenetic phenocopies of ADHD. The converse is also possible: environmental protective factors could yield cases in which genetic risks are present but disorder is absent. The genetic and nongenetic factors which contribute to ADHD could differ across populations and families, making replication difficult.

The prevailing diagnostic approach is based on clusters of symptoms, clinical characteristics, and natural history (22). The resulting ADHD diagnosis may be clinically informative although it may not describe homogenous and genetically relevant subtypes. It is not yet possible to distinguish subtypes of ADHD that arise from different combinations of genetic and/or nongenetic factors. For example, ADHD occurs following traumatic brain injury in approximately 20% of injured children (19). No research to date has identified specific markers of these two ADHD variants.

Phenotypic variation across genetic studies could also derive from disparities among informants, variation in the way ADHD subtypes are handled, or the inclusion of comorbid conditions. There is only modest agreement between parents and teachers in their report of ADHD symptoms (~.4) and different informants identify different children as disordered (23). Twin studies indicate that both parent and teacher ratings of ADHD behaviors are highly heritable (24–27). Yet, there is evidence that parents and teachers may be identifying genetically unique traits (25,28,29). ADHD cases vary considerably in the nature of their behavioral manifestations—some have a predominance of inattentive symptoms, some a predominance of hyperactive and impulsive symptoms and some exhibit both of these clusters to approximately equal extents. It is not yet known whether genetic and environmental factors operate in the same way across these subtypes (4,30,31). There may be distinct sets of genes involved at various levels of ADHD severity and with various subtypes, or, subtypes and severity could reflect variable manifestations of a common set of genes (pleiotrophism) as is seen in conditions such as Marfan's syndrome (32). Another source of

---

(*blue bars*) are genetically informative because they are closer to the expression of a smaller set of underlying genes. The model represents the complexity of the possible relationships, one gene (G^1) may contribute to multiple subphenotypes (P^1, P^2), or any single subphenotype (P^1) may be influenced by multiple genes (such as, $G^1 \times G^3$; $G^1 + G^2$, G^1 or G^2). Moreover, in the case of ADHD a range of more complex models are likely, involving multiple genes and environment factors (such as, $G^2 \times G^1 + E^2$ results in P^3) that may be interacting or functioning in an additive way.

genetic heterogeneity could arise from the various "subtypes" that are delineated by the presence of a comorbid disorder. Comorbidity with conduct, learning, and emotional disorders is very common in ADHD (33). ADHD and conduct disorder (CD) and ADHD and reading disorder share common and unique genetic influences (34,35). Treating ADHD as a quantitative trait does eliminate the issue of the arbitrary threshold that is imposed on the diagnosis of ADHD, however it does not mitigate other sources of error such as those introduced by the presence of comorbidity.

THE POTENTIAL OF ENDOPHENOTYPES

Genetic risks in complex medical and psychiatric diseases may be more clearly and reliably expressed in nonclinical endophenotypes (from the Greek *endo* meaning within and *phainen* meaning to show) than they are in clinical phenotypes as presently defined (36–39). Endophenotypes are manifestations of gene action that are in the same genetic pathway linking genes to complex clinical manifestations of disorder, but are closer to the mechanism of action of the genes involved in the disorder (36–39). The closer one gets to the immediate effects of genes and the farther one is from the clinical phenotype, the fewer the number of genetic and nongenetic factors that are likely to affect the trait. The interplay among genetic and environmental risk factors and phenotypic variation is illustrated in Figure 1.

A valid endophenotype should be more strongly associated with specific susceptibility genes than other complex clinical endpoints even if it is not associated with all of the alleles that confer risk for the broader ADHD phenotype. Linkage and association could be stronger in a subgroup of individuals who show a particular endophenotype. Even if endophenotypes are themselves multifactorial and multigenic, as is likely to be the case, they could nevertheless be useful in genetic research if they are influenced by a smaller set of genetic and environmental factors than the clinical manifestations of the disorder (39). Accordingly, endophenotypes could increase the power of genetic linkage and association analyses by identifying individuals with particular genetic susceptibilities across samples, subtypes, situations, levels of severity, and presence of comorbidity.

Endophenotypes could be used to identify individuals at genetic risk even in the absence of overt disorder (spectrum phenotypes) (40). Some individuals with the disease genotype might not express the disease phenotype per se but rather might exhibit subclinical or alternative phenotypes because of incomplete genetic penetrance, pleiotropy, or the absence of necessary interacting genetic or environmental risks. This pattern is thought to be at work in other psychiatric disorders such as schizophrenia where nonschizophrenic monozygotic twins may not exhibit schizophrenia per se but manifest schizoid personality disorder. Both twins have an equal tendency to transmit the disorder to their offspring indicating that the schizoid personality is a marker of similar genetic risk (41,42). In the case of autism, unaffected siblings tend to exhibit language learning disorders more often than expected (43). We do not yet know the phenotypic spectrum of ADHD: there might be a range of behavioral and nonbehavioral (including endophenotypic) expressions of the various genotypes (pleiotropy). In addition to identifying spectrum phenotypes, endophenotypes could delineate subgroups with increased etiological homogeneity (affected individuals with the endophenotype). Finally, endophenotypes could be used as a quantitative trait with a wide range of scores in place of a binary diagnosis as is typical employed in research into the genetics of psychiatric disease. The net effect of a valid endophenotype could be an increase in statistical power to detect linkage or association.

There is considerable optimism that valid and useful endophenotypes can be identified because a good deal is known about the pathophysiology of ADHD. A wide range of potential endophenotypes are currently proposed and many twin and genetic studies include a panel of putative endophenotypes (what we call "candidate" endophenotypes to mirror the concept of a candidate gene). However, few if any of these candidate endophenotypes have been tested to see if they meet a priori criteria for a valid endophenotype. Ultimately the validity of a candidate endophenotype will be evident in its ability to increase the power to detect functional genetic variants in ADHD. But, given the limitations and expense of clinical research, it is not possible to include in any particular study every measure that has a purported relationship to ADHD. Moreover, poorly chosen measures could yield associations that prove to be false positives or false negatives. Next, we review the criteria by which a candidate endophenotype should be evaluated before inclusion in genetic research (36–39) (Table 1).

CRITERIA FOR GENETIC ENDOPHENOTYPES

Sensitivity and Specificity

An endophenotype should be common in affected individuals (i.e., sensitive), relatively if not completely unique to the disorder (i.e., specific),

Table 1 Criteria for Genetic Endophenotypes

Sensitivity and specificity
Heritability, genetic sensitivity, and genetic specificity
Familial aggregation
Presence in unaffected family members
State-independence
Biological plausibility
Sound psychometric properties
Feasibility

and relatively uncommon among unaffected individuals in the general population (44). However, there is an important limitation to this criterion that it concerns only phenotypic sensitivity and specificity. Phenotypic sensitivity to ADHD may not be high for a candidate endophenotype if some apparently unaffected individuals are carriers of risk genes with reduced penetrance. Given the high prevalence of ADHD in the general population it is likely that common allelic variants are involved in ADHD. Therefore, we can expect that many unaffected individuals will carry susceptibility genes without manifesting the ADHD phenotype at a diagnostic level. ADHD may also share some genetic risks with other psychiatric disorders. Genetic risks that are shared among disorders could contribute to the elevated rate of comorbidity that is evident in ADHD (45,46). It is easy to see how this could be the case for ADHD and reading disorder, for example, where both disorders could share common genes affecting cognitive processes such as temporal processing, working memory, or inhibitory control. In ADHD, these cognitive deficits could result in behavioral manifestations (e.g., inattention), whereas in reading disability the deficit could result in impaired phonological decoding. In such cases, the specificity of an endophenotype would not be high although it might still increase power for detecting genetic risks for each disorder. Although nonspecific genetic risks for child psychopathology may be quite common, the ideal starting point for ADHD genetics should be the identification of endophenotypes that are both genetically sensitive and specific to ADHD.

Heritability, Genetic Sensitivity, and Genetic Specificity

Endophenotypes should be heritable, meaning that the endophenotypic variation in the population should be partly caused by genetic variation between individuals. Typically, when endophenotypes are discussed, it is said that "...the endophenotype must be as heritable as or more heritable than the behavioral phenotype" (31). This criterion for the validity of an endophenotype is only partially correct. It is not likely that any endophenotype can be more heritable than ADHD (approximate $h^2 \approx 80\%$) (7,16). However, putative endophenotypes do have to be heritable otherwise they would not be useful for genetic studies. What is crucial is that the genetic structure of the putative endophenotype be simpler than the clinical "exophenotype" that it is meant to dissect. If an endophenotype is sensitive and specific to a disorder, has even moderate heritability ($\approx 50\%$), and is genetically simpler (i.e., affected by fewer loci), it could lead to significant increases in power to detect disease alleles for the associated disorder.

To determine whether an endophenotype is valid and useful for increasing power in molecular genetic research, a decisive criterion would be that the phenotypic covariance between the ADHD phenotype and the putative endophenotype at least partly be due to shared genes. Multivariate quantitative genetic modeling (i.e., simultaneously analyzing two or more traits) can be used with twin data to estimate the degree of genetic correlation between traits (47). The genetic correlation measures the extent to which two phenotypes are influenced by the same genetic factors regardless of their respective heritability (48). The higher the genetic correlation between a candidate endophenotype and a disorder, the more likely it is that identifying polymorphisms for the former will amount to finding disease alleles for the latter. If ADHD is a genetically heterogeneous disorder as is likely, then endophenotypes that have high genetic correlation with some subsets of ADHD symptoms or dimensions but not others may be useful in the genetic "dissection" of ADHD.

Finally, multivariate genetic modeling between a genetically sensitive ADHD endophenotype and disorders that are comorbid with ADHD (e.g., reading and CDs) can allow us to assess the "genetic specificity" of the endophenotype to ADHD. For example, a genetically specific endophenotype to ADHD would be one that shows strong genetic correlation with ADHD, but only weak or no genetic correlation with reading and/or other disorders.

Familial Aggregation

A candidate endophenotype should be evident in relatives of affected individuals. Full siblings, for example, share 50% of their genes on average. If the endophenotype is influenced by shared genetic factors, then the deficit should be found in at least some relatives of affected probands. Of course, the fact that a trait is familial does not ensure that it is heritable because shared environmental influences can generate familial similarity. Twin or adoption designs are required to assess heritability.

Presence in Unaffected Family Members

A corollary of familial aggregation is that an endophenotype should be present even in the unaffected relatives of affected probands. If the severity of overt clinical symptoms and the extent of the endophenotype are independent it would demonstrate that the endophenotype has the capacity to detect asymptomatic genetic carriers or those with incomplete penetrance of the disease-causing genotype (49). One would also predict covariance for the endophenotype among relatives. That is, the relatives of ADHD individuals with a particular endophenotype should be more likely to manifest the endophenotype than relatives of ADHD individuals who do not manifest the endophenotype, whether they are affected or not.

State-Independence

A valid endophenotype will not vary with disease progression or treatment and will not vary with measurement technique. If such an endophenotype marks genetic risk despite fluctuations in overt manifestations of the disease, then one would expect that individuals of all ages would exhibit the genetic marker pre- and postonset of the disease. In addition, individuals who once manifested the endophenotype would continue to do so even if they had "outgrown" the overt disorder due to treatment or to altered environmental circumstances (unless these also affect the endophenotype) or if the original disorder had morphed into another disorder (heterotypic continuity).

Biological Plausibility

Biological plausibility, i.e., a functional relation between a putative endophenotype and the disorder, is a vital feature of a putative endophenotype. A good deal is known about the biological basis of ADHD from which to generate predictions about the nature of a potential endophenotype. Imaging and pharmacological studies indicate that structural or functional abnormalities in cortical–subcortical pathways supporting executive function are central to the disorder. Individuals with a diagnosis of ADHD have smaller prefrontal cortical volumes than controls particularly in the right inferior prefrontal cortex, corpus callosum, caudate, and cerebellum (50–52) and there is a relationship of prefrontal morphology and the clinical characteristics of ADHD (53,54). Functional imaging studies in ADHD show less activation compared to controls in frontal and cingulate regions (55,56) and there is a correlation between activation and clinical characteristics in ADHD (52,57). Subcortical structures are also implicated. Most studies show smaller caudate and globus pallidus volumes in ADHD (55,58,59) and there is a demonstrated link between volume and asymmetry of caudate nucleus and performance on executive function tasks in ADHD (60,61). Functional neuroimaging studies report differences in the amount of activation in the caudate, putamen, and globus pallidus during performance of executive function tasks (62). Dopamine transporters are particularly common in subcortical structures that are otherwise implicated in ADHD and in executive function. As a result, genes in the dopamine system have been targeted with success in molecular research. Therefore, a logical choice for an endophenotype would be any neuropsychological process, neurochemical, or structural abnormality that is affected by variation in these neurotransmitters, that responds to stimulant administration or that activates brain regions presumed to be abnormal in ADHD.

Sound Psychometric Properties

Candidate endophenotypes should be reliable if they reflect enduring traits. Standardized measures would be particularly helpful especially if the endophenotype varies with age or sex in a systematic way as is likely to be the case for cognitive processes. Furthermore, it would be advantageous for statistical analyses for the putative endophenotype to be quantitative rather than categorical.

Feasibility

The biology of ADHD reviewed above suggests that structural brain abnormalities might be fruitful candidate endophenotypes. Durston et al. (105) investigated the validity of markers of brain structure in ADHD by comparing individuals with a confirmed diagnosis of ADHD and their unaffected siblings. They found reduced prefrontal gray matter and left occipital gray and white matter in both children with ADHD and their unaffected siblings. Despite the promise of this research, it seems highly unlikely that structural imaging can be incorporated easily and economically in most genetic designs. Candidate endophenotypes should be easy to measure and noninvasive in order to facilitate research in affected children, their relatives, and the general population.

EXECUTIVE FUNCTIONS AS CANDIDATE ENDOPHENOTYPES

There is a strong case to be made for the importance of executive function deficits in ADHD. Executive functions refers to those neuropsychological processes that are necessary to organize, integrate, and influence perceptions, emotions, and responses across time in order to meet the needs and goals of the organism (63,64). Executive function comes into play when one is required to prepare, withhold, inhibit, or switch responses, to monitor one's performance for errors, to manage delay, and to maintain and manipulate information held temporarily in memory. Executive functions are important to behavioral self-regulation, academic achievement, and development of cognitive skills (65,66). Various aspects of executive function are involved in overlapping and sequential ways in the performance of most tasks (67). Yet, each component appears to be somewhat distinct judging from their unique developmental trajectories (68–71), the limited intercorrelations that are observed among functions (72) and their dependence on partially segregated, although functionally inter-related, frontal-subcortical circuits (64,69,73).

Deficits in executive functions are readily apparent and reproducible in ADHD (74) and several theories posit that these deficits are central to the disorder (66,75,76). Executive functions depend on the same neural circuits and transmitters that are implicated in ADHD (77) and improve with administration of methylphenidate (78–80). The few twin studies published suggest that some executive function measures are heritable (81,82).

Various executive functions distinguish ADHD from controls (83) and could serve as potentially valid endophenotypes. While few have been evaluated formally as candidate endophenotypes, there is considerable evidence pertaining to the validity of a proposed executive function endophenotype in motor response inhibition. We now review this literature from the perspective of the validity criteria proposed above.

INHIBITORY CONTROL AS A CANDIDATE ENDOPHENOTYPE FOR ADHD

Motor response inhibition is a crucial executive function that comes into play when one tries to withhold or interrupt an ongoing or planned response. The stop signal task a commonly laboratory paradigm used to study this type of inhibition. In the paradigm, participants perform two concurrent tasks—a primary or go task and a secondary or stopping task. The primary or go task involves a choice response: e.g., if an X appears, a right-hand response is made; if a Y appears, a left-hand response is made. The secondary task involves a stop signal on a subset of go trials. When the stop signal appears, the participant instructed to stop their response on that trial. In the stop signal task (Fig. 2), the stop signal is typically a tone which follows the presentation of the go signal. The delay between presentation of the go and the stop signals is dynamically adjusted. If a participant stops successfully on a given trial, the delay is increased for the next trial making it more difficult to stop. If the participant fails to stop, the delay is decreased making it easier to stop on the next stopped trial. As dynamic tracking proceeds, it converges on the delay at which the participant is able to stop 50% of the time. With knowledge of the latency of the go response and of the delay between go and stop signals at which the two processes are tied, one can estimate the latency of the unobserved stopping process known as stop signal reaction time (SSRT; 84). Longer SSRT indicates poorer inhibitory control.

Sensitivity and Specificity

Deficient inhibitory control, manifest in significantly longer SSRT, is a replicated deficit in ADHD (76,85–88). Willcutt et al. (83) reviewed a number of cognitive tasks and found that differences between ADHD and normal control groups in SSRT was a consistent finding; 22 of 27 studies in which ADHD and control groups were compared yielded a significant group difference ($p < .05$) with a weighted mean effect size of 0.61. The task has been shown to have an effect size of .74, sensitivity of .80, and specificity of .67 (86). Moreover, differences between ADHD and normal controls is not a function of associated CD, anxiety, or learning disability, and is independent of age or intelligence (83,86). Leblanc et al. (106) studied motor response inhibition in a group of children who suffered traumatic brain injury while controlling for preinjury history of ADHD. Inhibition was impaired by head injury whether it was associated with secondary ADHD or

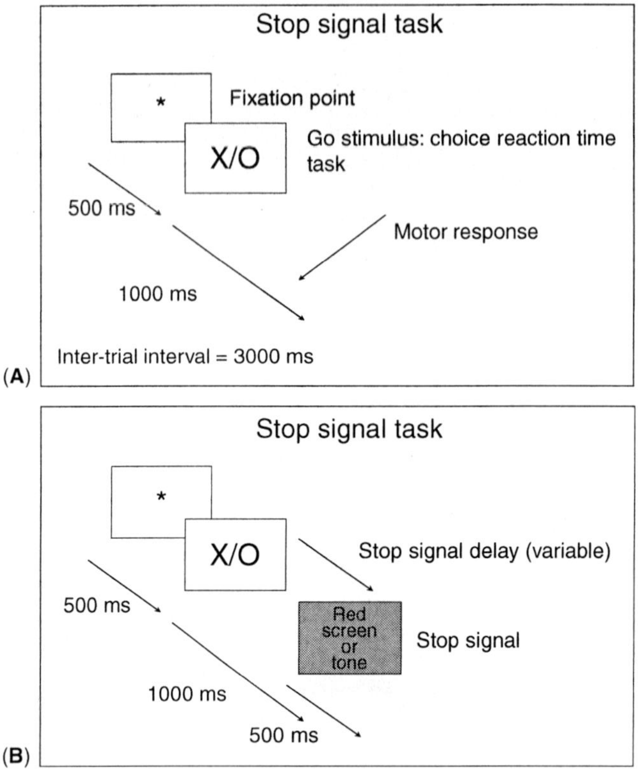

Figure 2 Stop signal task. The stop signal task involves two component tasks. In the go task (**A**), participants must respond as quickly and as accurately as they can to either an "X" or an "O" presented on a computer screen. In the stop task (**B**), a stop signal (e.g., tone), instructs the participant to cancel their response on that particular trial.

not. Moreover, deficit in inhibitory control discriminated between primary and acquired ADHD. More importantly, initial inhibition deficits normalized within 2 years postinjury.

Heritability, Genetic Sensitivity, and Genetic Specificity

Although there is preliminary evidence that various executive functions in normal control individuals are heritable (89), the heritability of motor response inhibition in the stop task or of other candidate ADHD endophenotypes has not been investigated extensively. Kuntsi and Stevenson (90) obtained evidence for genetic influence for several indices of performance on the stop signal task but did not report heritability for the primary index of inhibitory control (SSRT). Groot et al. (91) studied heritability of performance in a go no-go task but found that it was not possible to distinguish between genetic (A), shared environmental (C), and unique environmental (E) effects, thus leaving unanswered the question of heritability. There is, however, evidence for the heritability of the neural substrate of inhibition and those brain regions implicated in ADHD. Pennington et al. (92) reported heritability of .56–.97 for subcortical and cortical volumes, left and right neocortex, and total cerebral volume (93). Furthermore, Durston et al. (105) found reduced prefrontal gray matter, left occipital gray, and white matter in both ADHD and their unaffected siblings.

Familial Aggregation

Crosbie and Schachar (107) found that deficient inhibition in ADHD children delineated a particularly familial subgroup of ADHD. They observed that ADHD children with poor inhibition were four times more likely than those with good inhibition to have a first-degree family member affected with ADHD regardless of comorbidity with CD or reading disability (RD), symptom severity, or level of impairment. By contrast, good and poor inhibition groups did not differ in history of neurobiological risk, psychosocial adversity, symptom severity, or intelligence.

Presence in Un-Affected Family Members

Further evidence of the familial nature of inhibitory control deficit was reported by Schachar et al. (108). They compared five groups of participants. Groups one and two were rigorously diagnosed ADHD participants and their ADHD siblings. Groups three and four were ADHD participants and their unaffected siblings. The fifth group consisted of normally developing participants. The probands and their affected siblings both showed significant inhibition deficit compared to normal controls. Unaffected siblings of ADHD probands showed an intermediate deficit in inhibition that was not attributable to the severity of their ADHD symptoms, or by the extent of exposure to neurobiological risks or psychosocial adversity. Moreover, ADHD participants in Groups 1 and 3 with inhibition deficit were more likely than those without to have a sibling in Groups 2 or 4 with inhibition deficit. Slaats Willemse et al. (109) also observed clustering in ADHD siblings of response inhibition as measured in the go no-go task as well as performance on measures of attentional control and fine visuomotor skills. These studies indicate that unaffected siblings of affected ADHD probands show deficits in executive function.

State-Independence

Deficient inhibition has been detected in ADHD individuals at every age indicating that it is a trait that does not disappear despite the usual diminution over time in overt ADHD behaviors. Deficient inhibition has been detected in children, adolescents, and adults with an ADHD diagnosis although the effect was weaker in ADHD adults (94,95). We tested a group of nonmedicated ADHD children repeatedly over the course of a day using the stop task and measured their behavior at the same time. Not surprisingly, we found that the children became progressively more restless, less cooperative and less attentive as the day wore on. Nevertheless, performance on the stop task was stable, indicating that inhibition can be measured independent of concurrent behavior (96). In addition, inhibitory control improves along with behavior when stimulant medication is administered (97).

Biological Plausibility

Aron and Poldrack (110) conducted a meta-analysis of all functional MRI studies of motor response inhibition that have used either the go no-go or stop signal tasks. These studies indicate that the right inferior prefrontal cortex is critical to response inhibition. fMRI evidence converges nicely with lesion-deficit studies which show that the amount of damage to the right inferior prefrontal cortex is significantly correlated with SSRT in patients with unilateral frontal damage (98). The striatum is also involved in inhibition (99) as would be expected from current theories of motor control (100,101). The striatum is a critical relay station in the corticostriatal motor loop involved in controlling ongoing movement both in human and primates and is strongly influenced by dopaminergic and glutamaturgic neurotransmission. Human electrophysiological studies confirm the role of the dorsolateral prefrontal cortex in inhibitory control (102).

Sound Psychometric Properties

Soreni et al. (96) studied 14 nonmedicated children once a week in the morning for three consecutive weeks using the stop task to measure response inhibition. Interclass correlations showed high reliability and stability of this measure.

Feasibility

The stop signal task could be easily administered to individuals of ages 7 to 80 years (103). The function relating age to SSRT is basically "U" shaped: inhibitory control improves through childhood and adolescent and peaks in early adulthood, following which there is a slow increase into old age even though inhibitory control is well preserved even in old age. The results of the Williams study (103) serve as basic norms.

PUTTING ENDOPHENOTYPES TO WORK IN GENETIC RESEARCH

Only a few studies have applied inhibitory control or other endophenotypes in the search for genetic risks in ADHD. Crosbie et al. (in preparation) investigated the relationship of three candidate genes in ADHD: the dopamine transporter (DAT1), dopamine receptor D4 (DRD4), and synaptosomal-associated protein of 25 kDa (SNAP25) and two candidate endophenotypes inhibitory control (measured with the stop task) and working memory (measured with digit span). The 4-repeat allele of the 48 bp repeat located in the third exon of DRD4 was associated with better inhibitory control and SNAP25 was associated with poor inhibition. No relationship was found between inhibitory control and DAT1. Langley et al. (111) observed that children with the 7-repeat allele had shorter mean reaction times for incorrect responses on the stop signal task (116.6 vs. 134.1 msec) than children without the allele, but did not report the relationship risk alleles and inhibitory control. Children with the allele also displayed higher activity levels. The children with and without the allele did not differ significantly in number of ADHD symptoms when the symptoms were split into the areas of inattention and hyperactivity/impulsivity.

CONCLUSIONS

The primary goals of this chapter were to describe the ways in which endophenotypes might advance research into the genetic basis of ADHD, to lay out criteria for validation of an endophenotype prior to its use in molecular genetic research, and to illustrate, using the example of motor response inhibition, the progress that has been made in validating and applying endophenotypes in the search for genetic susceptibility to ADHD. The commonly mentioned criteria of familial aggregation and presence in nonaffected family members are merely corollaries of the truly indispensable criterion of heritability. The criteria of phenotypic sensitivity and specificity are not enough, because genetic sensitivity and specificity are truly what matter for the genetic usefulness of an endophenotype. Finally, the other commonly recognized criterion of biological plausibility was discussed, arguing that it is a desirable although not a necessary characteristic of a valid endophenotype.

Motor response inhibition meets many of the proposed criteria for a valid endophenotype and has already proved useful for refining the search for genetic risks in ADHD. Inhibition has a well-established neurological basis which overlaps considerably with the proposed biology of ADHD. Deficient response inhibition measured in the stop signal task is a replicated and fairly specific deficit in ADHD. Inhibitory deficit is a marker for a particularly familial form of ADHD and the deficit is found in siblings of affected individuals whether they have ADHD or not. Inhibition is a reliable and stable trait that is found in affected individuals of all ages. The measure is easily administered and is feasible for use in general population studies. However, there are notable areas for further research. Twin studies are needed to determine whether putative endophenotypes such as inhibition are heritable and genetically correlated with aspects of the clinical phenotype, and not with other disorders.

No claim is made that deficient motor response inhibition is the sole or the most important potential marker of genetic risk for ADHD. There most certainly are other cognitive deficits in ADHD such as in delay management, error detection, and working memory. These cognitive deficits may divide ADHD into etiologically meaningful subtypes. Sonuga Barke (112) has proposed a dual pathway model of ADHD in which some cases arise from dysfunctions that affect mesocortical pathways and motor inhibition and other cases arise from genetic influences on mesolimbic pathways that affect motivation, reward, and capacity to tolerate delay. Support for this hypothesis derives from a study showing that both deficient inhibition and delay aversion, a putative marker of mesolimbic pathway dysfunction, were both present in a group of ADHD cases, but that these deficits were found in different individuals to a considerable extent. Together, delay aversion and deficient inhibition accounted for the majority of ADHD cases (104). Similarly, Schachar et al. (108) measured performance monitoring, another proposed marker of mesolimbic pathway function, in a group of ADHD children. They found abnormality in both inhibition and performance monitoring and a nonsignificant correlation between the two. Given the proposed polygenic influence on ADHD it is likely that various genetically informative executive function deficits will be identified. If multiple, etiologically distinct deficits are evident in ADHD then it may not be correct to aggregate performance measures in an attempt to increase statistical power, as has occasionally been proposed (74). On the other hand, if clusters of cognitive deficits can be found, then aggregated measures may increase power over that achieved with a single measure.

Endophenotypes will not be the panacea that will overcome all problems in genetic research into complex disorders. Not every gene involved in ADHD may be expressed in a cognitive deficit and not every deficit in ADHD may serve as an indicator of an underlying genetic mechanism. Some performance deficits in ADHD could be manifestations of the disorder itself while others may reflect environmental influences rather than being steps along a pathway from genes to phenotype. Variation in executive control might be attributable to a subset of ADHD genes and still have a considerable amount of genetic heterogeneity. Some cognitive deficits may be highly influenced by environmental factors. Nevertheless, executive function deficits could be useful markers of genetic risk in ADHD given the importance of these processes in ADHD, their association with the proposed biological basis of ADHD, and the ease with which these markers could be exploited in clinical and general population samples. There will still be a need to test putative endophenotypes of different kinds such as functional deficits derived from neuroimaging studies, variation in life course, presence of comorbidity, or treatment response.

REFERENCES

1. Biederman J, Faraone SV, Keenan K, et al. Further evidence for family-genetic risk factors in attention deficit hyperactivity disorder. Patterns of comorbidity in probands and relatives psychiatrically and pediatrically referred samples. Arch Gen Psychiatry 1992; 49:728–38.
2. Sprich S, Biederman J, Crawford MH, Mundy E, Faraone SV. Adoptive and biological families of children and adolescents with ADHD. J Am Acad Child Adolesc Psychiatry 2000; 39:1432–7.
3. Khan SA, Faraone SV. The genetics of ADHD: a literature review of 2005. Curr Psychiatry Rep 2006; 8:393–7.
4. Levy F, Hay DA, McStephen M, Wood C, Waldman I. Attention-deficit hyperactivity disorder: a category or a continuum? Genetic analysis of a large-scale twin study. J Am Acad Child Adolesc Psychiatry 1997; 36:737–44.
5. Douglas VI, Barr RG, O'Neill ME, Britton BG. Short term effects of methylphenidate on the cognitive, learning and academic performance of children with attention deficit disorder in the laboratory and the classroom. J Child Psychol Psychiatry 1986; 27:191–211.
6. Spencer T, Biederman J, Wilens T, Harding M, O'Donnell D, Griffin S. Pharmacotherapy of attention-deficit hyperactivity disorder across the life cycle [see comments]. J Am Acad Child Adolesc Psychiatry 1996; 35: 409–32.
7. Faraone SV, Perlis RH, Doyle AE, et al. Molecular genetics of attention-deficit/hyperactivity disorder. Biol Psychiatry 2005; 57:1313–23.
8. Arcos-Burgos M, Castellanos FX, Pineda D, et al. Attention-deficit/hyperactivity disorder in a population isolate: linkage to loci at 4q13.2, 5q33.3, 11q22, and 17p11. Am J Hum Genet 2004; 75:998–1014.
9. Bakker SC, van der Meulen EM, Buitelaar JK, et al. A whole-genome scan in 164 Dutch sib pairs with attention-deficit/hyperactivity disorder: suggestive evidence for linkage on chromosomes 7p and 15q. Am J Hum Genet 2003; 72: 1251–60.
10. Hebebrand J, Dempfle A, Saar K, et al. A genome-wide scan for attention-deficit/hyperactivity disorder in 155 German sib-pairs. Mol Psychiatry 2006; 11:196–205.
11. Smalley SL, Kustanovich V, Minassian SL, et al. Genetic linkage of attention-deficit/hyperactivity disorder on chromosome 16p13, in a region implicated in autism. Am J Hum Genet 2002; 71:959–63.
12. Faraone SV, Doyle AE, Mick E, Biederman J. Meta-analysis of the association between the 7-repeat allele of the dopamine D(4) receptor gene and attention deficit hyperactivity disorder. Am J Psychiatry 2001; 158: 1052–7.
13. Maher BS, Marazita ML, Ferrell RE, Vanyukov MM. Dopamine system genes and attention deficit hyperactivity disorder: a meta-analysis. Psychiatry Genet 2002; 12:207–15.
14. Lowe N, Kirley A, Hawi Z, et al. Joint analysis of the DRD5 marker concludes association with attention-deficit/hyperactivity disorder confined to the predominantly inattentive and combined subtypes. Am J Hum Genet 2004; 74:348–56.

15. Lander ES, Schork NJ. Genetic dissection of complex traits [erratum appears in Science 1994 Oct 21; 266(5184):353]. Science 1994; 265:2037–48.
16. Waldman ID, Gizer IR. The genetics of attention deficit hyperactivity disorder. Clin Psychol Rev 2006; 26:396–432.
17. Aronson M, Hagberg B, Gillberg C. Attention deficits and autistic spectrum problems in children exposed to alcohol during gestation: a follow-up study. Develop Med Child Neurol 1997; 39583–7.
18. Ernst M, Moolchan ET, Robinson ML. Behavioral and neural consequences of prenatal exposure to nicotine. J Am Acad Child Adolesc Psychiatry 2001; 40:630–41.
19. Max JE, Lansing AE, Koele SL, et al. Attention deficit hyperactivity disorder in children and adolescents following traumatic brain injury. Dev Neuropsychol 2004; 25:159–77.
20. Milberger S, Biederman J, Faraone SV, Jones J. Further evidence of an association between maternal smoking during pregnancy and attention deficit hyperactivity disorder: findings from a high-risk sample of siblings. J Clin Child Psychol 1998; 27:352–8.
21. Roy P, Rutter M, Pickles A. Institutional care: associations between overactivity and lack of selectivity in social relationships. J Child Psychol Psychiatry 2004; 45:866–73.
22. American Psychiatric Association. Diagnostic and Statistical Manual of Mental Disorders. 4th ed. (DSM-IV). Washington, D.C.: American Psychiatric Association, 1994.
23. Mitsis EM, McKay KE, Schulz KP, Newcorn JH, Halperin JM. Parent-teacher concordance for DSM-IV attention-deficit/hyperactivity disorder in a clinic-referred sample. J Am Acad Child Adolesc Psychiatry 2000; 39: 308–13.
24. Eaves LJ, Silberg JL, Meyer JM, et al. Genetics and developmental psychopathology: 2. The main effects of genes and environment on behavioral problems in the Virginia Twin Study of Adolescent Behavioral Development. J Child Psychol Psychiatry 1997; 38:965–80.
25. Martin N, Scourfield J, McGuffin P. Observer effects and heritability of childhood attention-deficit hyperactivity disorder symptoms. Br J Psychiatry 2002; 180:260–5.
26. Sherman DK, Iacono WG, McGue MK. Attention-deficit hyperactivity disorder dimensions: a twin study of inattention and impulsivity-hyperactivity. J Am Acad Child Adolesc Psychiatry 1997; 36:745–53.
27. Sherman DK, McGue MK, Iacono WG. Twin concordance for attention deficit hyperactivity disorder: a comparison of teachers' and mothers' reports. Am J Psychiatry 1997; 154:532–5.
28. Nadder TS, Silberg JL, Rutter M, Maes HH, Eaves LJ. Comparison of multiple measures of ADHD symptomatology: a multivariate genetic analysis. J Child Psychol Psychiatry 2001; 42:475–86.
29. Szatmari P, Offord DR, Siegel LS, Finlayson MA, Tuff L. The clinical significance of neurocognitive impairments among children with psychiatric disorders: diagnosis and situational specificity. J Child Psychol Psychiatry 1990; 31:287–99.

30. Levy F, McStephen M, Hay DA. The diagnostic genetics of ADHD symptoms and subtypes. In: Levy F, Hay D, eds. Attention Genes and ADHD. Philadelphia, PA: Brunner-Routledge, 2001:35–58.
31. Stevenson J, Asherson P, Hay D, et al. Characterizing the ADHD phenotype for genetic studies. Dev Sci 2005; 8:115–21.
32. Pyeritz RE. The Marfan syndrome. Annu Rev Med 2000; 51:481–510.
33. Jensen PS, Martin D, Cantwell DP. Comorbidity in ADHD: implications for research, practice, and DSM-V. J Am Acad Child Adolesc Psychiatry 1997; 36:1065–79.
34. Nadder TS, Rutter M, Silberg JL, Maes HH, Eaves LJ. Genetic effects on the variation and covariation of attention deficit-hyperactivity disorder (ADHD) and oppositional-defiant disorder/conduct disorder (ODD/CD) symptomatologies across informant and occasion of measurement. Psychol Med 2002; 32: 39–53.
35. Willcutt EG, Pennington BF, DeFries JC. Twin study of the etiology of comorbidity between reading disability and attention-deficit/hyperactivity disorder. Am J Med Genet 2000; 96:293–301.
36. Almasy L, Blangero J. Endophenotypes as quantitative risk factors for psychiatric disease: rationale and study design. Am J Med Genet 2001; 105:42–4.
37. Gottesman II, Gould TD. The endophenotype concept in psychiatry: etymology and strategic intentions. Am J Psychiatry 2003; 160:636–45.
38. Rutter M. The interplay of nature, nurture, and developmental influences: the challenge ahead for mental health. Arch Gen Psychiatry 2002; 59:996–1000.
39. Tsuang MT, Faraone SV, Lyons MJ. Identification of the phenotype in psychiatric genetics. Eur Arch Psychiatry Clin Neurosci 1993; 243:131–42.
40. Cannon TD, Gasperoni TL, van Erp TG, Rosso IM. Quantitative neural indicators of liability to schizophrenia: implications for molecular genetic studies. Am J Med Genet 2001; 105:16–9.
41. Fischer M. Psychoses in the offspring of schizophrenic monozygotic twins and their normal co-twins. Br J Psychiatry 1971; 118:43–52.
42. Gottesman II, Bertelsen A. Confirming unexpressed genotypes for schizophrenia. Risks in the offspring of Fischer's Danish identical and fraternal discordant twins. Arch Gen Psychiatry 1989; 46:867–2.
43. Szatmari P, MacLean JE, Jones MB, et al. The familial aggregation of the lesser variant in biological and nonbiological relatives of PDD probands: a family history study. J Child Psychol Psychiatry 2000; 41:579–86.
44. Biederman J, Faraone SV, Mick E, et al. High risk for attention deficit hyperactivity disorder among children of parents with childhood onset of the disorder: a pilot study. Am J Psychiatry 1995; 152:431–5.
45. Caron C, Rutter M. Comorbidity in child psychopathology: concepts, issues and research strategies. J Child Psychol Psychiatry 1991; 32:1063–80.
46. Pennington BF. From single to multiple deficit models of developmental disorders. Cognition 2006; 101:385–413.
47. Plomin R, DeFries JC. Multivariate behavioral genetic analysis of twin data on scholastic abilities. Behav Genet 1979; 9:505–17.
48. Neale MC, Cardon LR. Methodology for Genetic Studies in Twins and Families. Dordrecht: Kluwer Academic Publishers, 1992.

49. Cornblatt BA, Malhotra AK. Impaired attention as an endophenotype for molecular genetic studies of schizophrenia. Am J Med Genet 2001; 105:11–5.
50. Castellanos FX, Lee PP, Sharp W, et al. Developmental trajectories of brain volume abnormalities in children and adolescents with attention-deficit/hyperactivity disorder. JAMA 2002; 288:1740–8.
51. Sowell ER, Thompson PM, Welcome SE, Henkenius AL, Toga AW, Peterson BS. Cortical abnormalities in children and adolescents with attention-deficit hyperactivity disorder. Lancet 2003; 362:1699–707.
52. Yeo RA, Hill DE, Campbell RA, et al. Proton magnetic resonance spectroscopy investigation of the right frontal lobe in children with attention-deficit/hyperactivity disorder. J Am Acad Child Adolesc Psychiatry 2003; 42:303–10.
53. Casey BJ, Tottenham N, Fossella J. Clinical, imaging, lesion, and genetic approaches toward a model of cognitive control. Dev Psychobiol 2002; 40: 237–54.
54. Filipek PA, Semrud-Clikeman M, Steingard RJ, Renshaw PF, Kennedy DN, Biederman J. Volumetric MRI analysis comparing subjects having attention-deficit hyperactivity disorder with normal controls. Neurology 1997; 48: 589–601.
55. Rubia K. The dynamic approach to neurodevelopmental psychiatric disorders: use of fMRI combined with neuropsychology to elucidate the dynamics of psychiatric disorders, exemplified in ADHD and schizophrenia. Behav Brain Res 2002; 130:47–56.
56. Schulz KP, Fan J, Tang CY, et al. Response inhibition in adolescents diagnosed with attention deficit hyperactivity disorder during childhood: an event-related FMRI study. Am J Psychiatry 2004; 161:1650–7.
57. Teicher MH, Anderson CM, Polcari A, Glod CA, Maas LC, Renshaw PF. Functional deficits in basal ganglia of children with attention-deficit/hyperactivity disorder shown with functional magnetic resonance imaging relaxometry. Nat Med 2000; 6:470–3.
58. Bush G, Frazier JA, Rauch SL, et al. Anterior cingulate cortex dysfunction in attention-deficit/hyperactivity disorder revealed by fMRI and the Counting Stroop. Biol Psychiatry 1999; 45:1542–52.
59. Valera EM, Faraone SV, Biederman J, Poldrack RA, Seidman LJ. Functional neuroanatomy of working memory in adults with attention-deficit/hyperactivity disorder. Biol Psychiatry 2005; 57:439–47.
60. Casey BJ, Castellanos FX, Giedd JN, et al. Implication of right frontostriatal circuitry in response inhibition and attention-deficit/hyperactivity disorder. J Am Acad Child Adolesc Psychiatry 1997; 36:374–83.
61. Semrud-Clikeman M, Steingard RJ, Filipek P, Biederman J, Bekken K, Renshaw PF. Using MRI to examine brain-behavior relationships in males with attention deficit disorder with hyperactivity. J Am Acad Child Adolesc Psychiatry 2000; 39:477–84.
62. Durston S. A review of the biological bases of ADHD: what have we learned from imaging studies? Ment Retard Dev Disabil Res Rev 2003; 9:184–95.
63. Miller EK, Cohen JD. An integrative theory of prefrontal cortex function. Annu Rev Neurosci 2001; 24:167–202.

64. Stuss DT, Alexander MP. Executive functions and the frontal lobes: a conceptual view. Psychol Res 2000; 63:289–98.
65. Barkley RA. ADHD and The nature of Self-control. New York: The Guilford Press, 1997.
66. Barkley RA. Attention-deficit/hyperactivity disorder, self-regulation, and time: toward a more comprehensive theory. J Dev Behav Pediatrics 1997; 18:271–9.
67. Mesulam MM. From sensation to cognition. Brain 1998; 121:1013–52.
68. Baddeley A. The episodic buffer: a new component of working memory? Trends Cogn Sci 2000; 4:417–23.
69. Levy R, Goldman-Rakic PS. Segregation of working memory functions within the dorsolateral prefrontal cortex. Exp Brain Res 2000; 133:23–32.
70. Owen AM. The role of the lateral frontal cortex in mnemonic processing: the contribution of functional neuroimaging. Exp Brain Res 2000; 133:33–43.
71. Petrides M, Alivisatos B, Frey S. Differential activation of the human orbital, mid-ventrolateral, and mid-dorsolateral prefrontal cortex during the processing of visual stimuli. Proc Natl Acad Sci U S A 2002; 99:5649–54.
72. Miyake A, Friedman NP, Emerson MJ, Witzki AH, Howerter A, Wager TD. The unity and diversity of executive functions and their contributions to complex "Frontal Lobe" tasks: a latent variable analysis. Cogn Psychol 2000; 41:49–100.
73. Posner MI, Rothbart MK. Attention, self-regulation and consciousness. Philos Trans R Soc Lond B Biol Sci 1998; 353:1915–27.
74. Doyle AE, Faraone SV, Seidman LJ, et al. Are endophenotypes based on measures of executive functions useful for molecular genetic studies of ADHD? J Child Psychol Psychiatry 2005; 46:774–803.
75. Pennington BF, Ozonoff S. Executive functions and developmental psychopathology. J Child Psychol Psychiatry 1996; 37:51–87.
76. Schachar R, Mota VL, Logan GD, Tannock R, Klim P. Confirmation of an inhibitory control deficit in attention-deficit/hyperactivity disorder [In Process Citation]. J Abnorm Child Psychol 2000; 28:227–35.
77. Castellanos FX, Giedd JN, Marsh WL, et al. Quantitative brain magnetic resonance imaging in attention-deficit hyperactivity disorder. Arch Gen Psychiatry 1996; 53:607–16.
78. Arnsten AF, Steere JC, Hunt RD. The contribution of alpha 2-noradrenergic mechanisms of prefrontal cortical cognitive function. Potential significance for attention-deficit hyperactivity disorder. Arch Gen Psychiatry 1996; 53:448–55.
79. Solanto MV. Neuropsychopharmacological mechanisms of stimulant drug action in attention-deficit hyperactivity disorder: a review and integration. Behav Brain Res 1998; 94:127–52.
80. Vaidya CJ, Austin G, Kirkorian G, et al. Selective effects of methylphenidate in attention deficit hyperactivity disorder: a functional magnetic resonance study. Proc Natl Acad Sci U S A 1998; 95:14494–9.
81. Ando J, Ono Y, Wright MJ. Genetic structure of spatial and verbal working memory. Behav Genet 2001; 31:615–24.
82. Stins JF, de Sonneville LM, Groot AS, Polderman TC, van Baal CG, Boomsma DI. Heritability of selective attention and working memory in preschoolers. Behav Genet 2005; 35:407–16.

83. Willcutt EG, Doyle AE, Nigg JT, Faraone SV, Pennington BF. Validity of the executive function theory of attention-deficit/hyperactivity disorder: a meta-analytic review. Biol Psychiatry 2005; 57:1336–46.
84. Logan GD, Schachar RJ, Tannock RT. Impulsivity and inhibitory control. Psychol Sci 1997; 8:60–4.
85. Oosterlaan J, Logan GD, Sergeant JA. Response inhibition in AD/HD, CD, comorbid AD/HD + CD, anxious, and control children: a meta-analysis of studies with the stop task. J Child Psychol Psychiatry 1998; 39:411–25.
86. Schachar R, Logan GD. Impulsivity and inhibitory control in normal development and childhood psychopathology. Dev Psychol 1990; 26:710–20.
87. Schachar R, Tannock R. Test of four hypotheses for the comorbidity of attention-deficit hyperactivity disorder and conduct disorder. J Am Acad Child Adolesc Psychiatry 1995; 34:639–48.
88. Schachar RJ, Tannock R, Logan G. Inhibitory control, impulsiveness, and attention deficit hyperactivity disorder. Clin Psychol Rev 1993; 13:721–39.
89. Fan J, Wu Y, Fossella JA, Posner MI. Assessing the heritability of attentional networks. BMC Neurosci 2001; 2:14.
90. Kuntsi J, Stevenson J. Psychological mechanisms in hyperactivity. II. The role of genetic factors. J Child Psychol Psychiatry 2001; 42:211–9.
91. Groot AS, de Sonneville LM, Stins JF, Boomsma DI. Familial influences on sustained attention and inhibition in preschoolers. J Child Psychol Psychiatry 2004; 45:306–14.
92. Pennington BF, Filipek PA, Lefly D, et al. A twin MRI study of size variations in human brain. J Cogn Neurosci 2000; 12:223–32.
93. Carmelli D, Swan GE, DeCarli C, Reed T. Quantitative genetic modeling of regional brain volumes and cognitive performance in older male twins. Biol Psychol 2002; 61:139–55.
94. Lijffijt M, Kenemans JL, Verbaten MN, van Engeland H. A meta-analytic review of stopping performance in attention-deficit/hyperactivity disorder: deficient inhibitory motor control? J Abnorm Psychol 2005; 114:216–22.
95. Murphy P. Inhibitory control in adults with attention-deficit/hyperactivity disorder. J Atten Disord 2002; 6:1–4.
96. Soreni N, Crosbie J, Ickowicz A, Schachar R. Across the day stability of sustained attention and inhibitory control in ADHD children. Manuscript submitted for publication. Journal of Attention Disorders 2007.
97. Tannock R, Schachar RJ, Carr RP, Chajczyk D, Logan GD. Effects of methylphenidate on inhibitory control in hyperactive children. J Abnorm Child Psychol 1989; 17:473–91.
98. Aron AR, Fletcher PC, Bullmore ET, Sahakian BJ, Robbins TW. Stop-signal inhibition disrupted by damage to right inferior frontal gyrus in humans. Nat Neurosci 2003; 6:115–6.
99. Liddle PF, Kiehl KA, Smith AM. Event-related fMRI study of response inhibition. Hum Brain Mapp 2001; 12:100–9.
100. Band GP, Van Boxtel GJ. Inhibitory motor control in stop paradigms: review and reinterpretation of neural mechanisms. Acta Psychol (Amst) 1999; 101: 179–211.

101. Vink M, Kahn RS, Raemaekers M, van den Heuvel M, Boersma M, Ramsey NF. Function of striatum beyond inhibition and execution of motor responses. Hum Brain Mapp 2005; 25:336–44.
102. van Boxtel GJ, van der Molen MW, Jennings JR, Brunia CH. A psychophysiological analysis of inhibitory motor control in the stop-signal paradigm. Biol Psychol 2001; 58:229–62.
103. Williams BR, Ponesse JS, Schachar RJ, Logan GD, Tannock R. Development of inhibitory control across the life span. Dev Psychol 1999; 35:205–13.
104. Solanto MV, Abikoff H, Sonuga-Barke E, et al. The ecological validity of delay aversion and response inhibition as measures of impulsivity in AD/HD: a supplement to the NIMH multimodal treatment study of AD/HD. J Abnorm Child Psychol 2001; 29:215–28.
105. Durston S, Hulshoff Pol HE, Schnack HG, Buitelaar JK, Steenhuis MP, Minderaa RB, et al. Magnetic resonance imaging of boys with attention-deficit/hyperactivity disorder and their unaffected siblings. J Am Acad Child Adolesc Psychiatry 2004; 43(3):332–40.
106. Leblanc N, Chen S, Swank PR, Levin H, Schachar R. Impairment and recovery in inhibitory control after traumatic brain injury in children: effect of age at injury, injury severity and lesion location. Brain Cogn 2006; 60(2): 208–9.
107. Crosbie J, Schachar R. Deficient inhibition as a marker for familial ADHD. Am J Psychiatry 2001; 158(11):1884–90.
108. Schachar RJ, Crosbie J, Barr CL, Ornstein TJ, Kennedy J, Malone M, et al. Inhibition of motor responses in siblings concordant and discordant for attention deficit hyperactivity disorder. Am J Psychiatry 2005; 162(6):1076–82.
109. Slaats-Willemse D, Swaab-Barneveld H, de Sonneville L, van der Meulen E, Buitelaar J. Deficient response inhibition as a cognitive endophenotype of ADHD. J Am Acad Child Adolesc Psychiatry 2003; 42(10):1242–48.
110. Aron AR, Poldrack RA. The cognitive neuroscience of response inhibition: relevance for genetic research in attention-deficit/hyperactivity disorder. Biol Psychiatry 2005; 57(11):1285–92.
111. Langley K, Marshall L, Van Den Bree M, Thomas H, Owen M, O'Donovan M, et al. Association of the dopamine D(4) receptor gene 7-repeat Allele with neuropsycological test performance of children with ADHD. Am J Psychiatry 2004; 161(1):133–8.
112. Sonuga-Barke EJ, Dalen L, Daley D, Remington B. Are planning, working memory, and inhibition associated with individual differences in preschool ADHD symptoms? Dev Neuropsychol 2002; 21(3):255–72.

35

Can Attention Itself Be Trained? Attention Training for Children At-Risk for ADHD

Leanne Tamm

Center for Advanced ADHD Research, Treatment, and Education, University of Texas Southwestern Medical Center, Dallas, Texas, U.S.A.

Bruce D. McCandliss

Sackler Institute for Development Psychology, Weill Medical College of Cornell University, New York, New York, U.S.A.

Angela Liang and Tim L. Wigal

Child Development Center, University of California Irvine, Irvine, California, U.S.A.

Michael I. Posner

Department of Psychology, University of Oregon, Eugene, Oregon, U.S.A.

James M. Swanson

Child Development Center, University of California Irvine, Irvine, California, U.S.A.

WHAT IS ATTENTION TRAINING?

Attention training (ATT) is based on the concept that efficiency increases after repetitive practice of specific cognitive operations of attention (1) because practice produces adaptations in the underlying neuroanatomical networks linked to these processes (2). This concept has origins in the field of cognitive rehabilitation where attention process training (APT), using tasks such as listening for descending number sequences, shifting set, and visual cancellation, has been used to activate and train sustained, alternating, and divided attention (3). It should be noted that the term "ATT" has also been used to refer to different approaches, including (1) neurofeedback or biofeedback, (2) electronic equipment designed to give the child feedback when he/she is off task, and (3) cognitive training techniques, which involve training the child to self-talk to keep themselves on task and paying attention. We do not review these approaches in this chapter. Instead, we specifically refer to ATT methodologies as those using adaptive tasks specific to attentional functions thought to have certain corresponding neural bases which are changed through repetition and practice.

Several randomized controlled trials have been conducted to investigate the efficacy of ATT in different populations, including traumatic brain injury and stroke. The majority of these studies report positive findings and demonstrate transfer of improvements on untrained assays of attention components such as sustained attention and executive function (4–10).

One criticism that has been levied against ATT methodologies is that they have not been based on a theoretical model or framework of attention (7). Some ATT approaches have focused on training sustained attention, while others focus on alternating or divided attention or executive conflict, making it difficult to compare results. Posner and colleagues have suggested a framework by which to understand attention based on neuroanatomical and neuroimaging evidence (1). This model suggests that attention includes three major functions: alerting, orienting, and executive control, associated with specified neuroanatomical networks (i.e., different networks of interconnected brain areas). The alerting network is involved in establishing a vigilant state and maintaining readiness to react. Imaging studies show that the alerting network depends largely on frontal and parietal areas of the right hemisphere (11,12). Orienting involves selectively focusing on one or two items out of many candidate inputs. The orienting network utilizes superior and inferior parts of the parietal lobe in conjunction with frontal and subcortical structures related to eye movements (13). The executive control network has been related to the control of goal-directed behavior, target detection, error detection, conflict resolution, and inhibition of automatic responses. The executive control network involves frontal areas including the anterior cingulate and lateral prefrontal cortex (14). Each of these neuroanatomical networks appears to undergo intense postnatal development (15). Individuals with attention deficit hyperactivity disorder (ADHD) tend to show specific deficits in these functions, especially in alerting and executive control (16).

Efforts to develop an assessment measure of these three functions has resulted in the attention network test (ANT) with versions for adults (17), school-aged children (18), and preschool children [CHOC-UCI Initiative for the Development of Attention and Readiness (CUIDAR), described later in the chapter]. The ANT task is a combination of a cued reaction time and flanker task (17). Studies suggest that performance on the ANT task follows a roughly normal distribution (19), and that performance is stable within normal adult subjects across a wide age range with no gender differences.

It has also been shown that practice or previous experience has little impact on the attentional measures although overall reaction time is somewhat reduced (19), making it a good candidate as an outcome measure for ATT of alerting, orienting, and executive control.

Posner (20) proposed testing the utility of the idea that implementing ATT early in development may actually enhance attention and executive control networks. Neuropsychological studies suggest extensive development of attention and executive control functions between the ages of 3 and 5, which correlate with developments in brain structure and function. Although the neurological basis of the effect of ATT is not yet understood, evoked potential measures and fMRI evidence suggest that ATT is impacting brain function (7,21). Implementing ATT with preschool-aged children may have a long term impact on the functional development of these systems. Further, implementing ATT with children at risk for the development of attention and behavior problems may prevent or arrest impairments of attention. Evidence suggests that computerized gamelike tasks can be utilized to assess and/or train attentional functions in preschool-aged children (22). Thus, researchers have adapted ATT materials to be developmentally appropriate for both typically developing and "at-risk" preschoolers.

APPLICATIONS OF ATT FOR ADHD POPULATIONS

Since ADHD is by its very nature a disorder of attention, ATT has been considered as a possible nonpharmacological alternative to treatment with stimulant medication. There are few studies investigating the utility of ATT in the ADHD population, however. Williams (23) utilized adult-based ATT materials with a group of six ADHD children. Forty hours of ATT yielded significant improvements in pre- and post-measures of attention. In a somewhat larger study ($n = 33$) by the same researcher, latency-aged children (8 to 12 years of age) diagnosed with ADHD were tested before and after an 18-week period, during which children were divided into a no-treatment control (NTC) group and an treatment group that received 36 sessions of ATT using materials augmented with problem-solving activities developed for adults. Significant treatment group effects were reported for measures of both sustained and executive attention. A cancellation task that involved discriminating between several potential targets showed a 32% improvement for the ATT group versus an 8% increase for the NTC group. An auditory discrimination target counting task showed a 56% ATT improvement versus an 18% improvement for the NTC group. These results represent an average treatment group and pre- and post-assessment effect size of 1.01. Despite the lack of age-appropriate materials, their findings suggest that ATT shows promise as form of treatment for children diagnosed with ADHD.

Thomson and colleagues (24) recognized the need to adapt attention assessment and training materials to the specific needs of children in an age-appropriate fashion. Kerns, et al. (2) used child-appropriate adaptations of the adult APT materials (3) and conducted a randomized active treatment control study of the effects of training sustained and executive attention skills in ADHD children (7 to 11 years of age; $n = 14$). Half the subjects were assigned to APT for 16, 30-min sessions per week over 8 weeks, and half were assigned to a video game control (VGC) group that was assigned to play age-appropriate video games with social praise from the experimenters for an equivalent amount of time. On a measure of sustained attention (Underlining Boxes test) the APT group improved by 32% whereas the VGC group improved only 6%, and on a measure of effortful processing (a Math Efficiency measure based on the number of age-appropriate problems completed within a fixed time), the APT group showed a 55% improvement compared to 20% for the VGC group. At the level of generalization, the APT group showed a greater reduction in teacher ratings of ADHD symptoms than the VGC group, but this difference was only marginally significant ($p < .066$). At the cognitive level, this study demonstrated significant treatment-specific benefits of APT in tasks related to sustained attention and executive attention measures.

Klingberg et al. (25) developed a version of ATT with a central focus on nonverbal working memory skills. Their study evaluated the impact of 25, 30-min sessions of ATT on a group of children with ADHD ($n = 14$, 11 ± 2.5 years of age). The treatment was delivered by computer in an adaptive fashion (i.e., each trial was dynamically adjusted to each child's ability to preserve high success and an element of challenge). In a randomized controlled study in which the assessment team was blind to assignment to "high" dose (experimental) or "low" dose (control) groups, the experimental group ($n = 7$) produced significantly greater gains on cognitive measures of sustained and executive attention reflecting performance on visual-spatial working memory, digit span, and Stroop tasks. Also, the treatment effects were significant for a measure of restlessness: the number of head movements was reduced by 74% in the experimental group, yet increased by 8% in the control group (an effect size of 1.75), which is comparable to the 62% reduction in head movement typically reported following 0.4 mg/kg methylphenidate in a similar paradigm and population (26). However, treatment effects on reaction time latency or variability did not reach statistical significance. An imaging study showed that the working memory treatment was effective in improving activation of brain areas related to working memory (21).

Shalev et al. (27) conducted a study of a version of ATT designed to adaptively challenge children in tasks that required sustained attention, selective attention, spatial orienting, resolving conflict, and dual task management. The study included children diagnosed with ADHD from

6 to 13 years of age randomly assigned to 16 sessions of ATT using the progressive attentional training (PAT) system ($n = 24$) versus a VGC ($n = 17$). Performance on an effortful, timed, passage copying task demonstrated a 48.7% improvement for the ATT group in the number of words copied, whereas the VGC group demonstrated a nonsignificant increase of 1.8%. Most strikingly, parental rating scores for the ATT group were reduced for ratings of inattention (by 23%) and hyperactivity (by 19%), but no significant reduction was found for the VGC group on these pre- and postmeasures assessed by raters blind to treatment condition.

Taken together, these studies provide significant support for the notion that adaptive training of executive function skills and sustained attention skills may positively impact the developing attention skills of elementary school-aged children with ADHD, and such increases may, under some circumstances, generalize to ecologically valid assays of real-world effortful task performance and expression of ADHD symptoms.

ATT FOR PRESCHOOL CHILDREN

Posner and colleagues have recently completed a three-year project funded by the McDonnell Foundation to investigate the impact of ATT on typically developing preschool children (28,29). ATT activities were adapted from a nonhuman primate study by Rumbaugh and Washburn (30) that demonstrated significant gains in attentional abilities of primates following adaptive (i.e., progressive increases in the amount of challenge on sustained attention and other attention skills) computer-based activities. Adapting these procedures for use with preschool children involved creating animated animal characters, and gamelike motivational schemes for a battery of interactive exercises. For example, one activity that required planning and maintaining information over a delay period was reconceptualized as a game of tag between a duck and a cat character, in which the child controlled the cat character, and the duck character would present challenges such as disappearing into a pond in a way that required the child to remember the duck's path, and anticipate and plan for the duck's return. Difficulty was adapted by manipulating the duration of the delay and the relative speed of the two characters in the "tag" game.

To evaluate the impact of these activities on typically developing preschoolers, Rueda and colleagues (18) conducted a randomized controlled trial with two groups of children aged 4- to 5-years old. The study contrasted the impact of 5 days of ATT ($n = 24$) with a randomly assigned control group ($n = 24$) that watched videos with an interactive component. Following training, children in the ATT group showed more adultlike performance in the conflict network of the ANT task than the control children and this performance was also reflected in an event-related potentials component associated with the ability to resolve conflict. In addition, the ATT group showed a significantly greater pre- and post-change in a preschool analog of the Raven's Progressive Matrices Test, the Kaufman Brief Intelligence Test (K-BIT) Nonverbal IQ score (31), when compared to controls.

This preliminary research demonstrates that computer-based ATT activities developed for adult- and school-aged children can be adapted for use with preschool children. It also provides support for the hypothesis that such training can influence relevant behavior, generalize beyond the training tasks, and influence the underlying attentional network. Thus, it is plausible that ATT might be utilized as a possible intervention for preschoolers with attention problems.

Dowsett and Livesey demonstrated that some forms of ATT might be effectively adapted for preschool children at risk for attention difficulties (32). They studied 47 children (age 3 to 5) that had significant difficulties inhibiting responses during an age-appropriate go/nogo task. Children receiving three sessions of executive function training (dimensional card sort task, change task) demonstrated significant improvements on the go/nogo task, in contrast to both a no-intervention control group and a practice control group that received no training but three sessions of practice on the same go/nogo task.

ATT AND THE CUIDAR PROGRAM

New developments from the cognitive neurosciences about brain plasticity (33) set the stage for a collaboration of investigators at University of California, Irvine (UCI) and the Sackler Institute to investigate ATT, which challenged the consensus views (34). The traditional view has been that ADHD symptoms are due to fixed biological differences (e.g., a dopamine deficit) and that effective treatments (e.g., pharmacological intervention with stimulant medication or even behavioral interventions with token systems) offer "symptomatic relief" but have no carryover benefits and thus must be used chronically.

A new hypothesis purports that ADHD symptoms may be due to inefficient neural networks that could be strengthened during early development by specific experiences delivered by adaptive training (35). A fortunate collaboration between clinicians and scientists at the UCI, Child Development Center, and the Children's Hospital of Orange County (CHOC) provided an opportunity to test the cognitive neuroscience vision of ATT in preschool children at risk for ADHD. In 2000, California Proposition 10 imposed a statewide tax on tobacco products, with the proceeds specifically designated to fund service delivery programs to enhance school readiness. In 2001, a group of clinicians from UCI and CHOC proposed a service delivery program for preschool children at risk for ADHD, which was labeled the CHOC-UCI Initiative for the Development of Attention and Readiness (CUIDAR), funded by the Children and Families Commission of Orange County.

Parent Groups

CUIDAR is based on application of an early intervention and prevention model for preschoolers with behavior problems suggesting risk for later diagnosis of ADHD. The primary intervention is a once-a-week, 10-session community parent education (COPE) program, which is supplemented by concurrent social skills/child care for the preschool children. After completion of the COPE program, an optional medical clinic evaluation of ADHD is provided. Thus, CUIDAR provides service via a psychosocial intervention (COPE) before diagnosis and consideration of pharmacological intervention. Over the past three years, this approach has been used with over 1500 families, and has been well-regarded by participating families, pediatricians, and schools. The program has been especially well received by the Spanish-speaking Latino/Hispanic population, a group that underutilizes behavioral health services. A discussion of issues related to designing and implementing the CUIDAR model is provided by Tamm et al. (36). Preliminary information from the start-up experience (rather than a controlled clinical trial), show that parents report overwhelming satisfaction with the program, significant gains in parenting skills, and a reduction in child behavior problems.

Parent education was selected as the main method of intervention because it has a long history of demonstrated efficacy in reducing child behavior problems (37–42). This psychosocial intervention is also more acceptable to parents and professionals than pharmacological intervention, in part due to the weaker evidence base for the efficacy of medication at this age, and the potential of greater side effects of medication in young children (38,40,42). While many different approaches to teaching parenting skills have been shown to be effective, most approaches teach a similar curriculum based on behavior modification and social learning principles.

In the COPE model (43,44) parenting skills are taught in a unique, interactive approach to a group of 20–25 parents. The large group is subdivided by the COPE facilitator into small discussion groups of 4–5 parents, and these groups are systematically led through the COPE curriculum that focuses on teaching the following parenting strategies: (1) praise and attending, (2) rewards, (3) planned ignoring, (4) transitional warnings, (5) when-then statements, (6) planning ahead, (7) point systems, (8) time out, (9) time out from reinforcement—loss of privileges, and (10) problem solving. A primary feature of each COPE session is watching a videotaped vignette of a parenting error related to a topic of the curriculum, followed by a discussion within the small groups to identify the error and to offer suggestions for more appropriate parent–child interaction in that context. The COPE facilitator uses the group-generated solutions (1) to model appropriate parent behavior, (2) to demonstrate situations in which the strategies could be applied, (3) to practice in role-playing exercises, and (4) to propose homework for home implementation of the strategy before the next session.

Child Groups

The CUIDAR program provides a social skills intervention for children while their parents participate in the evening COPE parenting groups. The child groups follow a specific structure with a focus on prosocial behaviors. Components of the group structure include: (1) settling activity (story/coloring), (2) circle time (games/songs), (3) introduction of a social skill (using puppets), (4) role play of social skill (also using puppets), (5) activity time, (6) snack time, (7) movie. Throughout, a reward-based point system is used to promote positive behavior. The social skills covered in the 10-week program include following the rules of the "red sign" (observing a "red sign" for silence or required hand-raising to speak), listening and participating, ignoring, sharing, saying nice things, "calm body," and helping others. Debriefing with an experienced COPE facilitator occurs after each group to facilitate communication between the childcare/social skills providers and group leaders, and to allow problem solving for managing more difficult children.

ATT in CUIDAR

CUIDAR delivers services annually to about 700 families with preschool children at risk for ADHD (see www.CUIDAR.net). This provided an infrastructure to work directly with the children in these child care groups (while their parents attend the traditional COPE parent training groups) and created an opportunity to develop materials for ATT. Our goal was to develop and refine ATT materials to make the "games" appropriate for at-risk preschool children, and eventually to test the hypothesis that neural networks of attention (i.e., alerting and executive control as defined by Posner) can be strengthened by targeted adaptive training, as proposed by McCandliss for an intervention for children with reading disorders (35). The Sackler Institute and the Orange County Proposition 10 Commission provided start-up funding to adapt the materials initially developed for ATT in normal toddlers (28) for use with the preschool children at risk for ADHD, and a grant from the National Institute of Child Health and Development (NICHD) provided funds to conduct a pilot project with the CUIDAR families. Subsequent NIH applications have not been well received, perhaps due to the perception that this approach to implement and evaluate a program to prevent or "cure" ADHD is too radical.

The CUIDAR team focused on modifying the ANT task to be appropriate for preschoolers, since their performance was at approximately chance levels on the school-aged ANT (18). A preschool-appropriate ANT version was developed that assesses alerting, orienting, and executive control, and that has good test–retest reliability. This allows the ANT to be employed as a "probe" task of functioning levels of the attentional network components.

As part of an integrated development plan to create a more direct link between targeted cognitive skills and ATT modules, our team designed new training tasks to impact alerting and executive control. We created prototype versions of computer applications to reinforce and challenge preschoolers' ability to sustain attention and resolve conflict.

Alerting

The alerting activity involves a simple goal of attempting to wait and remain in a ready-to-respond state for an extended period of time, in order to rapidly respond to an infrequent and very brief event. In adapting this paradigm for children we created a "fly-catching" character, "HippityHop, the frog." Children are instructed to help "HippityHop" by pressing the space bar to catch as many flies as fast as they can from a jar, but they must also follow two rules: (1) the button can only be pressed when the flies exit the jar, (2) the child must wait for the fly despite an auditory cue (buzzing) on some trials. Children are told that in some trials they will hear a buzz before the fly exits the jar but they are still to withhold their response until after the fly exits the jar. The game is adaptive in that the "catch" time changes to maintain a success rate of 50% for the uncued (nonbuzzing) flies. It also slowly lengthens the wait time as children successfully catch the flies at a higher rate.

Executive Control

Similar adaptations and programming were used to produce a conflict resolution task based on the dimensional change control task (DCCT) paradigm (45). The DCCT paradigm was used to design a preschooler's game, using a character called Monster Zoo Keeper whose task it is to feed the monsters. On each trial the child is given an object and must decide which of two monsters should eat it, a truck-eating monster that likes red things, or a flower-eating monster that likes blue things. The rules whether the monsters are hungry for colors or hungry for shapes vary (i.e., during the day, the monsters are hungry for colors, and during the evening for shapes). Adaptive algorithms adjust the frequency of the rule change and the number of items that pose a direct conflict between the stated rule and recently reinforced, but currently inappropriate, decision responses.

We performed a pilot study to investigate the feasibility of implementing a randomized clinical trial with children of parents participating in the

CUIDAR COPE groups, as well as to test the feasibility of using the initial modules we developed for our version of ATT and a control task. We screened commercial video games from the Children's Software Review database (www.childrenssoftware.com), which reviews over 2500 video games, and chose Atari's "Tonka Firefighter" as an appropriate VGC example for comparison to ATT (e.g., "Hippity Hop" frog game and monster zoo game). In the Tonka Firefighter game, children play the role of a firefighter and help save the day by choosing and controlling a vehicle such as a fire truck, chopper, pump truck, or fire dozer. Children chose from a variety of activities such as saving stranded kittens, putting out blazing fires, cleaning up parks, and creating a fireworks show. Children were randomly assigned to an ATT group ($n = 14$, 5 sessions with the Alerting task) or a VGC group ($n = 13$, 5 sessions with the Tonka Firefighter game). The preschool version of the ANT task was administered pre and post.

The outcome of our initial feasibility study confirmed our experience and those of others of the benefits of ATT over VCG, and demonstrated that our ATT intervention in preschool children results in improvements after just 5 sessions that are about the same magnitude as those reported in the literature on elementary school-aged children with ADHD. The results of our initial pilot study will be presented in a later publication by our group. We utilized our experience with the feasibility study to modify and refine the prototypes of the alerting and executive control tasks. For example, additional "skins" and related "cover-stories" were developed so that the key task elements and paradigm are preserved, but the surface level of the task modified to be interesting for a child performing the task several times.

We are now conducting a randomized clinical trial to investigate the specificity of the alerting and executive control tasks. Preschool children in the CUIDAR childcare groups have been randomly assigned to an alerting training (AT) group ($n = 9$) or an executive control (EC) training group ($n = 8$). Each group is receiving 6 ATT sessions with the alerting task or the executive control task, respectively. The preschool ANT task and the KBIT administered pre and post will serve as primary outcome measures, and we anticipate that the ANT alerting scores will be improved for the AT group and the ANT executive control scores will be improved for the EC group. We are also exploring whether these tasks can be adapted upwards to be age appropriate for a school-aged population (ages 7 to 12), and utilized as a treatment for ADHD.

CAN ATTENTION BE TRAINED?

Although far from conclusive, it does appear that attention can be trained. Further, it appears that ATT can be adapted successfully for preschoolers, and has promising evidence as an intervention for children at-risk for or diagnosed with ADHD. Future studies should examine the specificity of ATT tasks, utilize imaging techniques to explore the impact of ATT on brain function, and investigate whether attentional gains are generalizable to other settings.

REFERENCES

1. Posner MI, Raichle ME. Images of Mind. New York: Scientific American Books, 1994.
2. Kerns KA, Eso K, Thompson J. Investigation of a direct intervention for improving attention in young children with ADHD. Dev Neuropsychol 1999; 16:273–95.
3. Sohlberg MM, Mateer CA. Introduction to Cognitive Rehabilitation: Theory and Practice. New York: Guilford, 1989.
4. Ethier M, Braun CMJ, Baribeau JMC. Computer-dispensed cognitive-perceptual training of closed head injury patients after spontaneous recovery. Study 1: speeded tasks. Can J Rehabil 1989; 2:223–33.
5. Finlayson MAJ, Alfano DP, Sullivan JF. A neuropsychological approach to cognitive remediation: microcomputer applications. Can Psychol 1987; 28:180–90.
6. Gray JM, Robertson IH. Remediation of attentional difficulties following brain injury: three experimental single case studies. Brain Inj 1989; 3:163–70.
7. Mateer CA, Mapou R. Understanding, evaluating, and managing attention disorders following traumatic brain injury. J Head Trauma Rehabil 1996; 11:1–16.
8. Penkman L. Remediation of attention deficits in children: a focus on childhood cancer, traumatic brain injury and attention deficit disorder. Pediatr Rehabil 2004; 7:111–23.
9. Sohlberg MM, Mateer CA. Effectiveness of an attention-training program. J Clin Exp Neuropsychol 1987; 9:117–30.
10. Thompson JB, Kerns KA. Cognitive rehabilitation of the child with mild traumatic brain injury. In: Press OU, ed. Neuropsychological Management of Mild Traumatic Brain Injury. New York: Oxford University Press, 1995.
11. Coull JT, Frith CD, Frackowiak RS, Grasby PM. A fronto-parietal network for rapid visual information processing: a PET study of sustained attention and working memory. Neuropsychologia 1996; 34:1085–95.
12. Posner MI, Petersen SE. The attention system of the human brain. Annu Rev Neurosci 1990; 13:25–42.
13. Corbetta M, Kincade JM, Ollinger JM, McAvoy MP, Shulman GL. Voluntary orienting is dissociated from target detection in human posterior parietal cortex. Nat Neurosci 2000; 3:292–7.
14. Bush G, Luu P, Posner MI. Cognitive and emotional influences in anterior cingulate cortex. Trends Cogn Sci 2000; 4:215–22.
15. Ruff H, Rothbart MK. Attention in Early Development: Themes and Variations. New York: Oxford University Press, 1996.
16. Swanson JM, Posner MI, Cantwell D, et al. Attention-deficit/hyperactivity disorder: symptom domains, cognitive processes & neural networks. In: Parasuraman R, ed. The Attentive Brain. Boston: MIT Press, 1998:445–60.

17. Fan J, McCandliss BD, Sommer T, Raz A, Posner MI. Testing the efficiency and independence of attentional networks. J Cogn Neurosci 2002; 14:340–7.
18. Rueda MR, Fan J, McCandliss BD, et al. Development of attentional networks in childhood. Neuropsychologia 2004; 42:1029–40.
19. Fan J, Yanhong W, Fossella JA, Posner MI. Assessing the heritability of attentional networks. BMC Neurosci 2001; 2:14.
20. Posner MI. Issues in psychology: domain specificity of skills and knowledge. Unpublished manuscript, 2002.
21. Olesen PJ, Westerberg H, Klingberg T. Increased prefrontal and parietal activity after training of working memory. Nat Neurosci 2004; 7:75–9.
22. Berger A, Jones L, Rothbart MK, Posner MI. Computerized games to study the development of attention in childhood. Behav Res Meth Instrum Comput 2000; 32:297–303.
23. Williams DJ. A process-specific training program in the treatment of attention deficits in children. Seattle: University of Washington, 1989.
24. Thomson JB, Seidenstrang L, Kerns KA, Sohlberg MM, Mateer CA. Pay Attention! Puyallup, WA: Association for Neuropyschological Research and Development, 1984.
25. Klingberg T, Forssberg H, Westerberg H. Training of working memory in children with ADHD. J Clin Exp Neuropsychol 2002; 24:781–91.
26. Teicher MH, Anderson CM, Polcari A, Glod CA, Maas LC, Renshaw PF. Functional deficits in basal ganglia of children with attention deficit/hyperactivity disorder shown with functional magnetic resonance imaging relaxometry. Nat Med 2000; 6:470–3.
27. Shalev L, Tsal Y, Mevorach C. Computerized progressive attentional training (CPAT) program: effective direct intervention for children with ADHD. Paper presented at the Journal of Cognitive Neuroscience, San Francisco, 2004.
28. Posner MI. Development of attentional networks. Paper presented at the 10th Annual George Miller Presidential Lectureship of the Annual Meeting of the Cognitive Neuroscience Society, San Francisco, CA, 2004.
29. Rueda MR, Rothbart MK, McCandliss BD, Saccamanno L, Posner MI. Training, maturation and genetic influences on the development of executive attention. Proceedings of National Academy of Sciences 2005; 102:14931–6.
30. Rumbausgh DM, Washburn DA. Attention and memory in relation to learning: a comparative adaptation perspective. In: Krasnegor Grlna, ed. Attention, Memory and Executive Function. Baltimore, MD: Brookes, 1995:199–219.
31. Kaufman AS, Kaufman NL. Kaufman Brief IntelligenceTest—Manual. Circle Pines: American Guidance Service, 1990.
32. Dowsett SM, Livesey DJ. The development of inhibitory control in preschool children: effects of "executive skills" training. Dev Psychobiol 2000; 36:161–74.
33. Posner MI. Developing brains: the works of the Sackler Institute. Clin Neurosci Res 2001; 1:258–66.
34. Swanson JM, Sergeant JA, Taylor E, Sonuga-Barke EJ, Jensen PS, Cantwell DP. Attention-deficit hyperactivity disorder and hyperkinetic disorder. Lancet 1998; 351:429–33.
35. McCandliss BD, Noble KG. The development of reading impairment: a cognitive neuroscience model. Ment Retard Dev Disabil Res Rev 2003; 9:196–204.

36. Tamm L, Swanson JM, Lerner MA, et al. Intervention for preschoolers at risk for attention-deficit/hyperactivity disorder (ADHD): Service Before Diagnosis. Clinical Neuroscience Research 2005; 5:247–53.
37. Barkley RA. Defiant Children: A Clinician's Manual for Parent Training. London: Guilford Press, 1987.
38. Endo GT, Sloane HN, Hawkes TW, Jenson TW. Reducing child whining through self-instructional parent training materials. Child Fam Behav Ther 1991; 13:41–58.
39. Forehand R, McMahon RJ. Helping the Noncompliant Child: A Clinician's Guide to Parent Training. New York: Guilford, 1981.
40. Forehand R, Rogers T, McMahon RJ, Wells KC, Griest DL. Teaching parents to modify child behavior problems: an examination of some follow-up data. J Pediatr Psychol 1981; 6:313–22.
41. Patterson G. Beyond technology: the next stage in developing an empirical base for parent training. In: L'Abate L, ed. Handbook of Family Psychology and Therapy. Homewood, IL: Dorsey Press, 1985:1344–79.
42. Webster-Stratton C. Modification of mother's behaviors and attitudes through videotape modeling group discussion. Behav Ther 1981; 12:634–42.
43. Cunningham CE. Large group, community based, parenting courses. In: Barkley RA, ed. Attention Deficit Hyperactivity: A handbook for Diagnosis and Treatment. New York: Guilford Press, 1998.
44. Cunningham CE, Bremner R, Boyle M. Large group community-based parenting programs for families of preschoolers at risk for disruptive behavior disorders: utilization, cost effectiveness, and outcome. J Child Psychol Psychiatry 1995; 36:1141–59.
45. Zelazo PD, Frye D, Rapus T. An age-related dissociation between knowing rules and using them. Cogn Develop 1996; 11:37–63.

Index